D0884718

Salivary Glands
in
Health and Disease

Salivary Glands in Health and Disease

D. K. MASON

BDS, MD, FDS(Ed. & Glasg.), FRCS(Glasg.), MRCPath

Professor, Department of Oral Medicine and Pathology, Glasgow Dental Hospital and School, University of Glasgow, Glasgow.

D. M. CHISHOLM

BDS, PhD

Lecturer, Department of Oral Medicine and Pathology, Glasgow Dental Hospital and School, University of Glasgow, Glasgow.

1975

W. B. Saunders Company Ltd   London · Philadelphia · Toronto

W. B. Saunders Company Ltd: 12 Dyott Street
London WC1A 1DB

West Washington Square
Philadelphia, Pa. 19105

833 Oxford Street
Toronto, Ontario M8Z 5T9

Library of Congress Cataloging in Publication Data
Mason, D   K
  Salivary glands in health and disease.
  1. Salivary glands—Diseases. 2. Salivary glands.
I. Chisholm, D. M., joint author. II. Title.
DNLM: 1. Salivary glands—Physiology. 2. Salivary gland diseases. W1230 M398s
RC815.5.M37   616.3'1   75-1402
ISBN 0-7216-6135-1

© 1975 by W. B. Saunders Company Ltd. All rights reserved. This book is protected by
copyright. No part of it may be reproduced, stored in a retrieval system, or transmitted in
any form or by any means, electronic, mechanical, photocopying, recording, or otherwise,
without written permission from the publisher.

Printed at The Lavenham Press Ltd, Lavenham, Suffolk, England.

Preface

Knowledge of the function of salivary glands and their secretions in health and disease has accumulated slowly. Some famous anatomists, physiologists and surgeons in earlier times have made major contributions to salivary gland research. Dental surgeons and, more recently, gastro-enterologists, psychologists, endocrinologists, rheumatologists, general physicians have all been interested in aspects of salivary function in various disease processes, as have general and plastic surgeons. As a result, there has been a very considerable literature on those subjects spread over many different scientific journals. In the same period some new methods of investigating salivary gland function in man have emerged and some older and well-tried techniques have been refined.

This book has two main objectives: firstly, to present an up-to-date review of salivary glands and their secretions in health and disease; secondly, to detail and evaluate different methods which have been described for the investigation of salivary gland disease, thus facilitating their use by clinicians and other investigators.

Glasgow, 1974

D. K. MASON
D. M. CHISHOLM

Acknowledgements

We have much pleasure in acknowledging the help we have received from many of our colleagues, in particular Dr H. W. Noble (Chapter 1), Dr J. A. Beeley (Chapter 3), Mr T. W. MacFarlane (Chapter 3 and Chapter 20), Mr T. Gibson (Chapter 14) and Dr W. N. Mason (Chapter 17), who all have made major contributions. We would also like to thank colleagues in other disciplines with whom we have worked closely over the years; Dr R. McG Harden, University of Dundee, and Dr W. D. Alexander and Professor W. W. Buchanan, University of Glasgow. For clinical and radiographic data we are grateful to Mr I. A. McGregor (Figures 14.3 to 14.5), Mr K. W. Stephen (Table 8.5) and Dr G. L. Schall (Figures 18.2 and 18.3). Our thanks are due also to the authors, editors and publishers of the following journals and books for permission to reproduce their copyright material:

Acta Radiologica—Table 10.4, Figures 10.21, 10.23; *Archives of Oral Biology*—Figure 16.1; *British Dental Journal*—Figures 10.5, 10.10, 10.15, 15.1, 18.1, 19.3; *British Journal of Oral Surgery*—Figures 5.3, 5.4, 5.7; *British Medical Journal*—Figure 12.5; *Cancer*—Figures 2.9, 2.11, 9.10, Table 9.3; *Clinical Science*—Table 10.6; *Journal of Clinical Pathology*—Figure 19.2; *Journal of Dental Research*—Figures 16.2, 16.4, 16.5; *Journal of Oral Medicine*—Figures 8.1, 16.7; *Journal of Oral Pathology*—Figures 13.1, 13.2, 13.3; *Journal of Physiology*—Table 3.9; *Modern Problems in Pediatrics*—Figures 8.3, 8.4; *Oral Surgery, Oral Medicine, Oral Pathology*—Tables 8.2, 8.3, 17.2, 17.3, 17.4; *Quarterly Journal of Medicine*—Tables 10.1, 10.7, Figure 10.6; *Radiology*—Figures 4.10, 17.6, 17.9, 17.16, 17.18; *Surgery, Gynaecology and Obstetrics with International Abstracts of Surgery*—Figure 14.2; World Health Organisation—Table 9.4.

We wish to acknowledge our gratitude to Mr John Davis, Department of Medical Illustration, Glasgow Dental Hospital and School, for the preparation of photographs and Mr Gabriel Donald and his staff, Department of Medical Illustration, Glasgow Western Infirmary, for all the line drawings and diagrams.

It gives us great pleasure to thank Mrs C. Bell who typed the manuscript and gave unfailing help and assistance.

Finally, we would like to express our thanks to Mr David Inglis and the staff of W. B. Saunders Company Ltd. for their help, encouragement and assistance.

Contents

Preface

Acknowledgements

PART I

Salivary Glands and their Secretions

CHAPTER 1

Embryology, Applied Anatomy and Innervation

The development of the salivary glands is the same irrespective of location or size. The glandular primordia stem from proliferating buds of oral epithelial cells (Figures 1.1 to 1.3). These cells continue to divide and the epithelial bud invades the underlying mesenchyme. The first salivary gland to develop is the parotid gland, about the 4th week of intra-uterine life, followed by the submandibular (6th week), sublingual (8th week) and the minor salivary glands about the 12th week. A detailed investigation of the manner of development of the submandibular and sublingual glands in the human embryo was contributed by Thoma (1919). After budding, the distal portions branch and form the ducts which end as bulbous terminals—the acini. It has been shown that the process of branching is induced by the mesenchyme surrounding the epithelium (Grobstein, 1953). At first, these buds are solid structures, but later, the ductal areas begin to hollow out; this does not occur until about the 6th month in utero. The secretory cells do not assume function during fetal development. The early development of the parotid gland around the facial nerve has been described by Gasser (1970).

Although the anlage of the parotid is the first to appear, the submandibular and sublingual are the first to become arranged into solid and encapsulated organs. Condensation of the mesenchyme surrounding the developing parotid occurs late in embryonic life and as a consequence, small lymph nodes, some containing salivary tissue, may become enclosed within the gland. It is of interest that salivary tissue has been found in lymph nodes outside the capsule of the parotid (Godwin, 1952). Salivary tissue, however, has not been noted in lymph nodes in the region of the developing submandibular and sublingual glands (Thompson and Bryant, 1950). Sebaceous gland elements are occasionally found within the parotid gland and are thought to originate from intercalated and striated ducts that end blindly (Meza-Chavez, 1949). Heterotropic elements, such as lymphoid tissue and sebaceous glands, may become the sites of neoplastic transformation. The proliferative behaviour of differentiating cells in the developing rat parotid gland (Redman and Sreebny, 1970) and rat submandibular and sublingual glands (Leblond, 1964) support the view that the division of cells in advanced stages of differentiation may be important in the growth of salivary glands. Increased total DNA content of gland, together with presence of mitotic figures in well-differentiated acinar cells (Redman and Sreebny, 1970), has provided strong evidence that the rat parotid acinar cells may be categorised as an expanding population as defined by Leblond (1964). Acinar epithelium is not an end product of differentiation and its replacement or regeneration may arise from pre-existing acini and also from proliferative activity of cells of duct origin (Evans and Cruickshank, 1970).

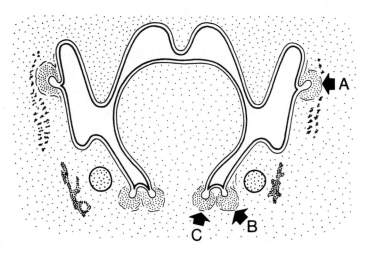

Figure 1.1. Coronal section of human embryo at seven weeks approximately. Nasal cavities are still not separate from oral cavity. Buds of epithelium (arrowed) show sites of origin of (A) parotid, (B) sublingual and (C) submandibular major salivary glands.

The origin of the myoepithelial cell in salivary glands remains unknown. Applying immunohistochemical techniques to post-natal development of rat submandibular glands, Line and Archer (1972) concluded that myoepithelial cells were not derived from acini. They suggest that the terminal tubule epithelial cell may serve as a stem cell for both myoepithelium and acini. The possibility of an undifferentiated precursor from a source external to the basement membrane migrating at an early stage to a position among tubule cells cannot be excluded (Line and Archer, 1972).

APPLIED ANATOMY

Major salivary glands
The three major salivary glands are paired and situated bilaterally. They are the parotid, submandibular and sublingual glands. The relation between the size of the parotid gland on the right and left sides is very close (Ericson, 1970).

(a)

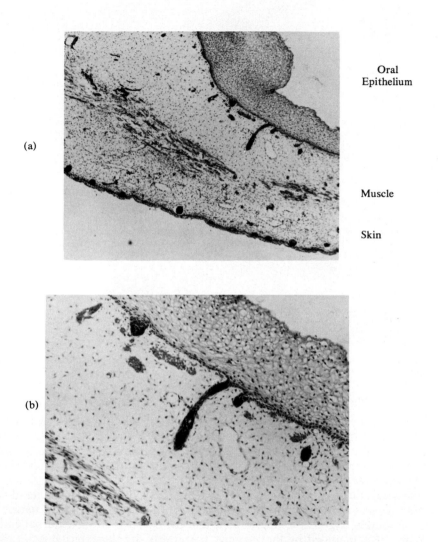

Oral
Epithelium

Muscle

Skin

(b)

Figure 1.2. Early development of human labial salivary glands (60 mm C.R.) a. full thickness section through lower lip. Note budding and proliferation of primitive oral epithelium. Skin appendages are developing in relation to primitive dermis (× 20). b. Budding of oral epithelium (× 60).

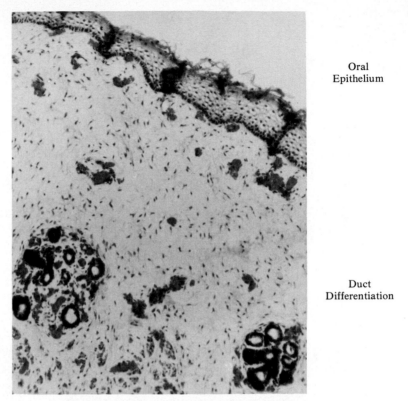

Oral
Epithelium

Duct
Differentiation

Figure 1.3. Development of labial salivary glands (135 mm C.R.) Hollowing out of epithelial buds to form early duct structures (× 60).

Parotid gland

The parotid is the largest of the salivary glands; it lies beneath the skin and extends deeply posterior to the ascending ramus (Figures 1.4 and 1.5). It is surrounded by fascia of varying thickness, which is thickest laterally and inferiorly over the gland. Deep extensions of this fascia divide the gland into smaller compartments or lobules.

The parotid gland weighs from 14 to 28 g and the outline of the gland is irregular and partially shaped by its confines of adjacent structures, namely the mandible, zygoma, temporal bone and the cartilage of the external ear. Above, it is bounded by the zygoma; posteriorly, by the external auditory meatus, mastoid process and sterno-mastoid muscle. Inferiorly, it extends down to the lower border of the mandible; anteriorly, the superficial portion extends for varying distances over the masseter muscle and the ascending ramus of the mandible. Deeply; it extends into the pterygomandibular space lying on the posterior belly of the digastric muscle, branches of the carotid artery, jugular vein, pharynx and styloid process just above it. Many authors feel that the parotid is a bi-lobed structure (e.g. McCormack, Cauldwell and Anson, 1945), but this is of little importance to the surgeon as dissection of

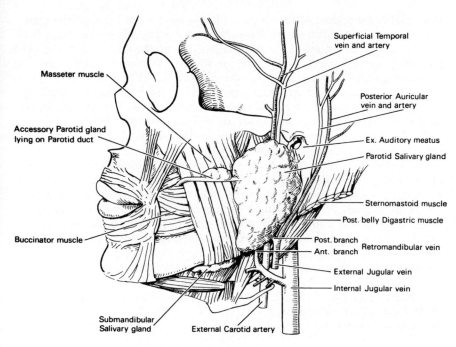

Figure 1.4. Lateral view of relations of parotid gland.

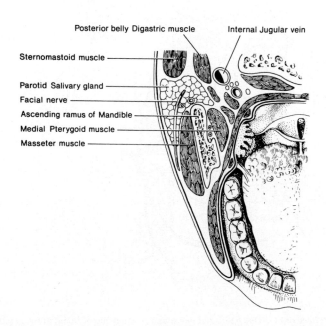

Figure 1.5. Horizontal cross section of parotid gland at level of occlusal surfaces of lower teeth.

the facial nerve seldom follows a path of easy separation through the gland.

The accessory parotid gland is somewhat dissociated from the main body and lies along the principal excretory duct, that is, the duct of Stensen. The parotid duct is located at the level of the ear lobe and travels over the masseter muscle. On reaching the anterior border of this muscle, it bends medially to invade the bucco-pharyngeal fascia, the buccinator muscle and the buccal mucosa. It terminates as a papillary orifice in the buccal epithelium at the level of the upper second molar tooth. In the adult, the parotid is a pure serous gland. However, in the early post-embryonic period, some mucous cells are often found to be present.

The facial nerve is associated with the parotid gland for an important part of its course during which it divides into its main terminal branches. Immediately after it emerges from the stylo-mastoid foramen at the base of the skull it gives off three small branches, the posterior auricular, the posterior digastric and the stylo-hyoid nerves. It then enters the parotid gland passing superficial to the external carotid artery and the posterior facial vein. At this stage the nerve usually divides into two main divisions, the temporofacial and the cervicofacial; these in turn subdivide into at least five main branches: temporal, zygomatic, buccal, mandibular and cervical as shown in Figure 1.6. The various patterns of branching have been described by McCormack, Cauldwell and Anson (1945) and will be considered further under surgical treatment of salivary gland disease (Chapter 14).

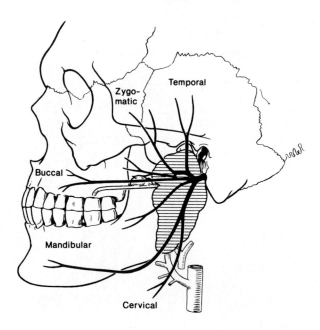

Figure 1.6. Pattern of branching of facial nerve and relationship of facial nerve to parotid gland and duct.

Blood supply. The external carotid artery appears from under cover of the digastric and stylo-hyoid muscles, ascends through the deepest part of the gland and under shelter of the posterior border of the vertical ramus of the mandible to the neck where it divides into the maxillary and superficial temporal artery. Branches from the external carotid artery supply the gland. Venous return is to the retromandibular vein.

Lymph drainage. Beneath the parotid fascia lymph glands lie on the surface and within the substance of the gland. Other lymph glands of the pre-auricular group lie superficial to the parotid fascia just beneath the skin (Figures 1.7a, b). Lymph drains to intra- and extra-glandular nodes and thence via the external carotid artery to the jugulo-digastric and other glands of the antero-superior group of deep cervical lymph glands.

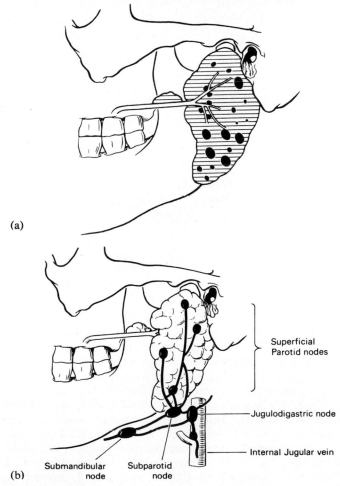

(a)

(b)

Superficial Parotid nodes

Jugulodigastric node

Internal Jugular vein

Submandibular node

Subparotid node

Figure 1.7. a. Distribution of lymph nodes within parotid salivary gland. **b.** Lymphatic drainage of parotid salivary gland.

9

Submandibular gland

This is the second largest of the major salivary glands. It is about half as large as the parotid and weighs 10 to 15 g. These glands are located in the floor of the oral cavity (Figures 1.8 and 1.9) and are contained, for the most part, in the submandibular triangle, extending anteriorly to the belly of the digastric muscle and posteriorly to the stylo-mandibular ligament. The name of the submandibular gland is derived from its location and close association with the mandible, and it is a mixed gland. The secretory units may be mixed or exclusively serous, the latter predominating. However, some sections may demonstrate acini, which appear to be composed entirely of muco-serous elements. Serous crescents are often observed surrounding the mucous cells.

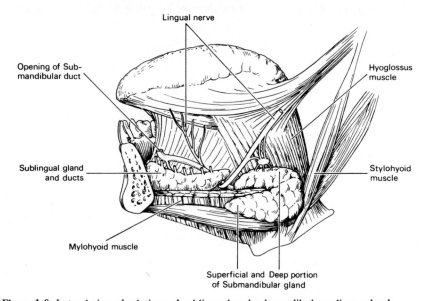

Figure 1.8. Lateral view of relations of sublingual and submandibular salivary glands.

The principal excretory duct is the duct of Wharton which emerges from the medial surface of the gland, and proceeds forwards and upwards towards the floor of the mouth. The duct lies at first on the hyo-glossus muscle under cover of the mylo-hyoid, from which it is separated by the deep part of the gland, with the lingual nerve above it and the hypoglossal nerve below. It next passes on to the genio-glossus, where the sublingual gland separates it from the mylo-hyoid, and the lingual nerve twists round it, crossing it superficially from above downwards at the anterior border of the hyo-glossus, and then passing upwards deep to it (Figure 1.6). When compared with the main excretory duct of the parotid, two conspicuous differences are noted. The first is a diminution in calibre with a corresponding decrease in wall thickness. Since the submandibular gland is substantially smaller than the parotid, the difference in the diameter of the lumen is not striking. The second difference involves the presence of isolated smooth muscle strands

10

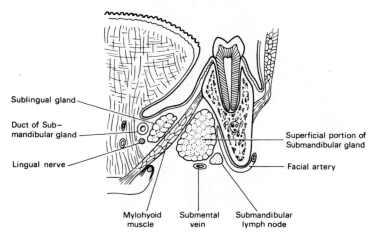

Figure 1.9. Coronal section of sublingual and submandibular salivary glands at the level of the 1st molar tooth.

around the duct. The exit of the submandibular or Wharton's duct is marked by a minute orifice on the crest of the sublingual papilla (sublingual caruncle) which is located lateral to the lingual frenulum in the sublingual sulcus. This elevation may be observed easily by rolling the tongue back in the mouth.

Blood supply. The blood supply to the submandibular gland is principally via branches of the facial and the lingual arteries and its veins drain into the common facial vein.

Lymph drainage. Lymph passes to the submandibular lymph nodes which lie on the surface of the submandibular salivary gland and thence mainly to the postero-inferior (jugulo-omo-hyoid) and also to the antero-superior (jugulo-digastric) groups of deep cervical glands (Figure 1.10).

Sublingual gland

The sublingual gland is the smallest of the major salivary glands and usually weighs less than 2 g. This gland is a flattened almond-shaped organ measuring a little over 1 inch in length and situated in the middle region of the sublingual sulcus. The superior surface is bordered by the sublingual mucosa and the inferior surface rests on the mylo-hyoid muscle. The capsule surrounding the gland is not so well defined as in the other major glands. The acini are composed of both serous and mucous elements but the latter predominate. Unique features which characterise the sublingual gland include the scarcity of pure serous acini and the presence of sero-mucous cells. The duct system has also certain peculiar features, as described below. The principal excretory duct is known as Bartholin's duct. This may fuse with the submandibular duct, in which case a common orifice on the

11

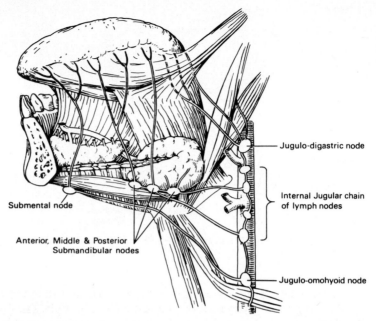

Jugulo-digastric node

Internal Jugular chain of lymph nodes

Submental node

Anterior, Middle & Posterior Submandibular nodes

Jugulo-omohyoid node

Figure 1.10. Lymphatic drainage of sublingual and submandibular salivary glands.

sublingual papilla is shared. More commonly, the principal duct remains independent and, with other smaller ducts, is provided with external orifices, in close proximity to that of the submandibular duct on the sublingual caruncle and along the crest of the sublingual fold on the floor of the oral cavity. The minor ducts are known as the ducts of Rivinus.

Blood supply. This is supplied by the lingual artery and by branches of the submental artery which pursue the mylo-hyoid muscle to reach the gland. The venous return is by corresponding veins. It is innervated via a similar pathway to the submandibular gland.

Lymph drainage. Lymph drainage is to the submental and submandibular lymph glands and thereafter to the superior and inferior deep cervical glands.

Minor salivary glands

The minor salivary glands are located beneath the epithelium in almost every part of the oral cavity, except in the gingivae and the anterior regions of the hard palate. In certain areas, i.e. sublingual, labial, buccal, palatal, lingual and labial, there are concentrations of these glands. Apart from the dorsal lingual glands which are entirely serous (von Ebner's glands), all these minor glands are mucous or predominantly mucous, with few serous acini.

12

Salivary ducts

With few exceptions, there are three types of duct present in all salivary glands. These vary in their distribution and in their histological appearance (Chapter 2). Intercalated ducts lined by cuboidal epithelium convey the secretion from the alveoli to the wider striated ducts which are lined by more columnar cells containing many mitochondria, accounting for the striated appearance. Lastly, the saliva passes through excretory ducts which are lined by clear cuboidal epithelium until near the duct orifice when the epithelium becomes of stratified squamous type. The striated ducts, which are intra-lobular, are thought to be the most active in modifying the composition of saliva. Much evidence supports the view that these ducts have an important role in the formation of saliva, as the cells are histologically much more complex than mere conducting cells need be. Certain areas of these ducts have been shown to have specific purposes (Cohen, Logothetopoulos and Myant, 1955; Burgen and Seeman, 1958; McGee, Mason and Duguid 1967; Ferguson and Stephen, 1972) and some animals have been found to have a duct segment specialising in water and electrolyte metabolism which, structurally, is similar to the convoluted tubules of the kidney (Junqueira, 1964).

INNERVATION

The control of oral glandular secretions, both salivary and mucous glands, is regulated by the autonomic nervous system.

Secretion is subject to reflex stimulation, which may be of a physical or psychic nature. Both peripheral stimuli, transmitted via the afferent nerve pathways from the oral cavity and psychic stimuli from other sensory centres such as taste, smell and sight converge on the salivary nuclei in the medulla oblongata.

The efferent pathway is via the parasympathetic and sympathetic parts of the autonomic nervous system.

Parotid

Secreto-motor fibres arise from cell bodies in the otic ganglion and reach the parotid gland by 'hitch-hiking' along the auriculo temporal nerve. The pre-ganglionic fibres arise from cell bodies in the inferior salivatory nucleus in the medulla and travel by way of the glossopharyngeal nerve, its tympanic branch, the tympanic plexus and the lesser superfacial petrosal nerve to the otic ganglion. The sympathetic fibres reach the gland from the superior cervical ganglion by way of the plexus on the external carotid and middle meningeal arteries. The gland itself receives sensory fibres from the auriculo temporal nerve, but the parotid fascia receives its sensory innervation from the great auricular nerve (Figure 1.11).

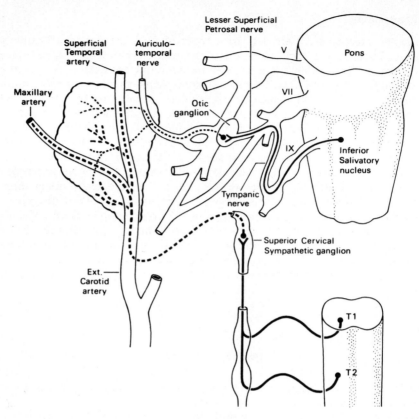

Figure 1.11. Parotid gland—autonomic nerve supply.

Submandibular and sublingual

Secreto-motor fibres to the submandibular and sublingual glands have their cell bodies in the submandibular ganglion or in small ganglionic masses on the surface of the gland itself. The pre-ganglionic fibres pass from cell bodies in the superior salivatory nucleus in the pons by way of the nervus intermedius and travel with the facial nerve as far as the stylo-mastoid canal. They leave the facial nerve in the chorda tympani (in company with taste fibres to the anterior two-thirds of the tongue) and passing across the lateral wall of the middle ear leave the skull through the petro-tympanic fissure. The chorda tympani passing downwards joins the lingual nerve from behind. Sympathetic innervation reach the glands from the superior cervical ganglion by way of vascular nerve plexuses around the facial artery (Figure 1.12).

Although the parasympathetic produces the main secreto-motor effect, some salivary flow is caused by stimulation of the sympathetic. Whether the latter is a secreto-motor or purely motor function has been disputed, but recently Hodgson and Speirs (1974) and Garret and Harrop (1974) have demonstrated that sympathetic nerves are involved in the reflex secretion of

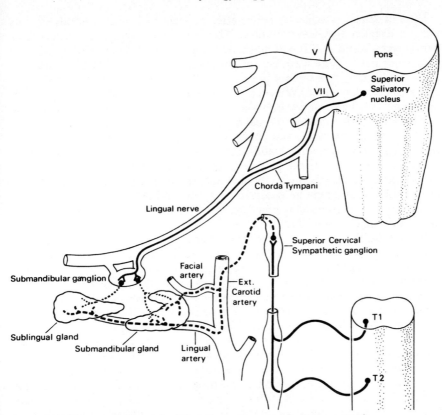

Figure 1.12. Submandibular and sublingual glands —autonomic nerve supply.

amylase from parotid acinar cells in the rat. Speirs, Hodgson and Bennett (1974) have provided some evidence that the sympathetic innervation may play a part in amylase secretion by human parotid gland acini.

Control of salivary secretion is a more complex matter than was previously assumed. As Emmelin (1972) has described and demonstrated mainly in animal experiments, there are various ways in which the amount and composition of the saliva poured into the mouth can be varied at the neuroeffector level. Nerves affect the different types of acinar cell and vary the rate of flow of primary saliva. Nerves may affect the duct cells which the saliva passes as it is secreted. Sympathetic and parasympathetic nerves influence the glandular cells differently, and on the sympathetic side a and β receptors may control different processes. Nerves acting to constrict or dilate the blood vessels may also affect the secretory activity by altering the blood supply and its distribution to the gland and by way of the myoepithelial cells the nerves may vary the time of contact and exchange between saliva and the different parts of the duct system. In addition, hormones and locally released biologically active agents other than chemical transmitters may act on blood vessels, gland cells and myoepithelium and thus play a role when saliva is formed.

15

Ultrastructural studies of neuro-effector sites in salivary glands of cats were undertaken by Garrett (1966, 1972). In the earlier study no intra-acinar nerves were found and it was suggested that neuro-effector sites within the glands occurred where a vesicle containing axon in an interstitial Schwann-axon bundle had a free surface in relatively close approximation to an effector cell. However, Creed and Wilson (1969) and Shackleford and Wilborn (1970) have reported the presence of axons within the acinar basement membrane and between acinar cells in the cat submandibular gland. In his later study Garrett (1972) observed axons beneath the basement membrane of acinar cells in cat submandibular gland and also showed intra-acinar axons to be easily demonstrated in rat parotid gland. With regard to vascular inner-vation, many axons, the majority of which are adrenergic though some may be non-adrenergic, may be detected close (around 2000 Å) to outer smooth muscle cells of the muscular blood vessels and endothelial cells of capillaries in cat and rat (Garrett, 1972).

In human material no axons were detected beneath the parenchymal basement membrane of parotid or submandibular glands in reports by Ferner and Gansler (1961), Garrett (1967) and Norberg, Hökfelt and Eneroth (1969). Axons at this site, however, have been observed in human submandibular gland (Tandler, 1965) and labial glands (Tandler and Ross, 1969). Garrett (1972) has concluded that two types of neuro-effector sites are present in salivary glands: those relatively close, (about 1000 Å) to a parenchymal cell; and those beneath parenchymal basement membrane separated from the effector cell by less than 200 Å. This latter type of innervation is more common with parasympathetic axons. Garrett (1972) stressed that there is no uniform pattern of innervation for salivary glands and that variation occurs in different species, within the same species and even in cells within the same gland. It is clear that these varying patterns must be borne in mind when interpreting experimental data.

REFERENCES

Burgen, A. S. V. & Seeman, P. (1958) The role of the salivary duct system in the formation of saliva. *Canadian Journal of Biochemistry and Physiology,* **37,** 359.

Cohen, B., Logothetopoulos, J. H. & Myant, N. B. (1955) Autoradiographic localisation of iodine-131 in the salivary glands of the hamster. *Nature (London),* **176,** 1268.

Creed, K. E. & Wilson, J. A. F. (1969) The latency of response of secretory acinar cells to nerve stimulation in the submandibular gland of the cat. *Australian Journal of Experimental Biology and Medical Science,* **47,** 135.

Emmelin, N. (1972) Control of salivary glands. In *Oral Physiology* (Eds) Emmelin, N. & Zotterman, Y. pp.1-14. Oxford: Pergamon Press.

Ericson, S. (1970) The normal variation of the parotid size. *Acta Oto-laryngologica,* **70,** 294.

Evans, R. W. & Cruickshank, A. H. (1970) *Epithelial Tumours of the Salivary Glands.* Philadelphia: W. B. Saunders Company.

Ferguson, M. M. & Stephen, K. W. (1972) Sex differences in the autoradiographic pattern of ^{125}Iodide uptake in mouse submandibular salivary gland. *Archives of Oral Biology,* **17,** 1117.

Ferner, H. & Gansler, H. (1961) Electronen-mikroskopische Untersuchungen an der Glandula submandibularis and parotis des Menschen. *Zeitschrift für Zellforschung und mikro-skopische Anatomie,* **55,** 148.

Garrett, J. R. (1966) The innervation of salivary glands. II. The ultrastructure of nerves in normal glands of the cat. *Journal of the Royal Microscopical Society*, **85,** 149.

Garrett, J. R. (1967) The innervation of normal human submandibular and parotid salivary glands. Demonstrated by cholinesterase histochemistry, catecholamine fluorescence and electron microscopy. *Archives of Oral Biology*, **12,** 417.

Garrett, J. R. (1972) Neuro-effector sites in salivary glands. In *Oral Physiology* (Eds) Emmelin, N. & Zotterman, Y. p. 83. Oxford & New York: Pergamon Press.

Garrett, J. R. & Harrop, T. J. (1974) Effects of preganglionic sympathectomy on morphological changes in parotid glands of rats on eating. *Journal of Dental Research*. In press.

Gasser, R. F. (1970) The early development of the parotid gland around the facial nerve at its branches in man. *Anatomical Record*, **167,** 63.

Godwin, J. T. (1952) Benign lymphoepithelial lesion of the parotid gland. *Cancer*, **5,** 700.

Grobstein, C. (1953) Analysis in vitro of the early organisation of the rudiment of the mouse submandibular gland. *Journal of Morphology*, **93,** 19.

Hodgson, C. & Speirs, R. L. (1974) Neural control of amylase secretion from the rat parotid gland. *Journal of Dental Research*. In press.

Junqueira, L. C. U. (1964) Studies on the physiology of rat and mouse salivary glands. III. On the function of the striated ducts of the mammalian salivary glands. In *Salivary Glands and their Secretions, International Series of Monographs on Oral Biology* (eds) Sreebny, L. M. & Meyer, J. p. 123. Oxford: Pergamon Press.

Leblond, C. P. (1964) Classification of the cell populations on the basis of their proliferative behaviour. *National Cancer Institute Monographs*, **14,** 119.

Line, S. E. & Archer, F. L. (1972) The post-natal development of myoepithelial cells in the rat submandibular gland: An immunohistochemical study. *Virchows Archiv; Abteilunga: Pathologische Anatomie (Berlin)*, **10,** 253.

Meza-Chavez, L. (1949) Sebaceous glands in normal and neoplastic parotid glands. Possible significance of sebaceous glands in respect to the origin of tumors of the salivary glands. *American Journal of Pathology*, **25,** 627.

McCormack, L. J., Cauldwell, E. W. & Anson, B. J. (1945) The surgical anatomy of the facial nerve. *Surgery, Gynecology and Obstetrics*, **80,** 620.

McGee, J. O'D., Mason, D. K. & Duguid, W. P. (1967) The site of iodide concentration in hamster salivary glands as demonstrated by autoradiography. *Archives of Oral Biology*, **12,** 1189.

Norberg, K.-A., Hökfelt, T. & Eneroth, C.-M. (1969) The autonomic innervation of human submandibular and parotid glands. *Journal of Neuro-Visceral Relations*, **31,** 280.

Redman, R. S. & Sreebny, L. M. (1970) Proliferative behaviour of differentiating cells in the developing rat parotid gland. *Journal of Cell Biology*, **46,** 81.

Shackleford, J. M. & Wilborn, W. H. (1970) Ultrastructural aspects of cat submandibular glands. *Journal of Morphology*, **131,** 253.

Speirs, R. L., Hodgson, C. & Bennett, H. (1974) The effects of selective denervation on the amylase levels in reflexly produced rat parotid saliva. *Journal of Dental Research*. In press.

Tandler, B. (1965) Ultrastructure of the human submaxillary gland. III. Myoepithelium. *Zeitschrift für Zellforschung und mikroskopische Anatomie*, **65,** 852.

Tandler, B. & Ross, L. L. (1969) Observations of nerve terminals in human labial salivary glands. *Journal of Cell Biology*, **42,** 339.

Thoma, K. H. (1919) A contribution to the knowledge of the development of the submaxillary and sublingual salivary glands in human embryos. *Journal of Dental Research*, **1,** 95.

Thompson, A. S. & Bryant, H. C. (1950) Histogenesis of papillary cystadenoma lymphomatosum (Warthin's tumor) of the parotid gland. *American Journal of Pathology*, **26,** 807.

CHAPTER 2

Histology and Histochemistry

In this chapter an account is presented of the histology and histochemistry of the salivary glands. In addition a brief description is given of the morphological changes observed during secretory cell activity. It should be noted that our knowledge concerning these aspects of the salivary glands has been gained from the study of animals, especially rodents, and is not always applicable to humans.

HISTOLOGY

Comprehensive reviews concerning salivary gland histology have been given by Zimmerman (1927), Stormont (1932), Burgen and Emmelin (1961) and Leeson (1967). Accounts have been given of the fine structure of human glands (Tandler, 1962, 1963, 1965; Kurtz, 1964; Tandler et al, 1969, 1970) and rodent (Scott and Pease, 1964; Tamarin and Sreebny, 1965; Hand, 1970a). The salivary glands are composed of secretory end-pieces, a system of intra-lobular ducts and excretory or extra-lobular ducts (Figure 2.1). The secretory unit or lobule is made up of the secretory end-piece and the intra-lobular ducts. The cells of the secretory end-piece are pyramidal in shape and are arranged around a central lumen. Each lobule is separated by neurovascular structures and intra-lobular connective tissue, although this is sparse. Intercellular canaliculi (secretory capillaries) are present and continuous with the lumen at the interface between acinar cells. The acinar cells rest upon a basement membrane and myoepithelial cells are interposed between the basement membrane and the acinar cells. Acinar cells, either mucous or serous or an admixture of the two (seromucous) and myoepithelial cells are the cell types of the secretory end-piece. Morphologically, salivary glands may be classified as being mucous, serous or mixed according to the relative proportions of different acinar cell types. The lumen enclosed by mucous acinar cells is larger than that bounded by serous cells. In mixed glands, serous cells tend to be confined to the distal portion of the secretory end-piece and are often referred to as the 'crescents of Gianuzzi'. These serous cells communicate with the lumen via secretory capillaries. The intra-lobular duct system comprises intercalated and striated duct cells,

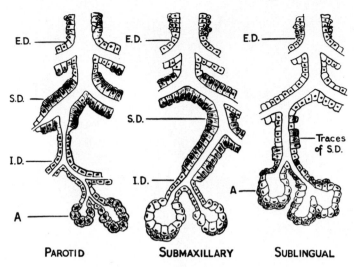

Figure 2.1. Diagrammatic representation of the human salivary gland duct system (after Jenkins, 1966). Acini (A), intercalated ducts (I.C.), striated ducts (S.D.) and excretory ducts (E.D.) are shown.

which lead to the extra-lobular duct system, the excretory ducts, which in turn open into the oral cavity.

In giving an account of the main histological features of these cells, it is important to realise that the morphological characteristics depend upon the functional state of the cell when examined. Furthermore, gradual transitional change may be observed at various locations throughout the duct system.

Acinar cells

Acinar cells may be classified according to the relative amounts of neutral and acidic polysaccharides (Shackleford and Klapper, 1962), so that the following cell types may be distinguished—mucous cells, having much acidic carbohydrate, serous cells containing largely neutral carbohydrate, and 'seromucous' cells with considerable amounts of both. Serous cells produce a 'watery' secretion, whilst the secretion of mucous cells is viscous and rich in muco-polysaccharide (Munger, 1964).

Mucous cells

Mucous cells are relatively large, pyramidal-shaped cells that rest on a basement membrane and stain a pale blue colour with routine haematoxylin and eosin. The nucleus, which stains darkly, is angular in shape and located towards the basal portion of the cell (Figure 2.2a, b). Ultrastructurally, the mucous cell is characterised by the presence of abundant endoplasmic reticulum and secretory droplets. Other fine structural constituents include

19

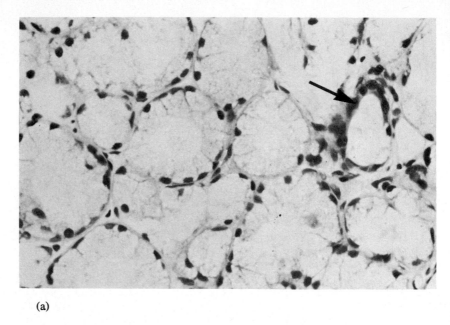

(a)

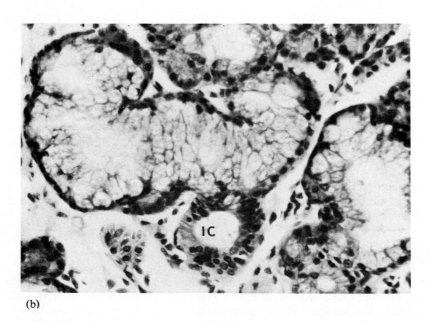

(b)

Figure 2.2a. Mucous acini with pale cytoplasm, pyramidal shape and basally located nuclei. Intercalated duct cell is present (arrowed). Labial salivary glands ($\times$ 30). b. Mucous acini from labial salivary glands. Intercalated duct is present (IC) ($\times$ 50).

the Golgi apparatus, mitochondria, lipid droplets and desmosomal attachments (Figure 2.3). The interphase between cells is fairly smooth with few interdigitations.

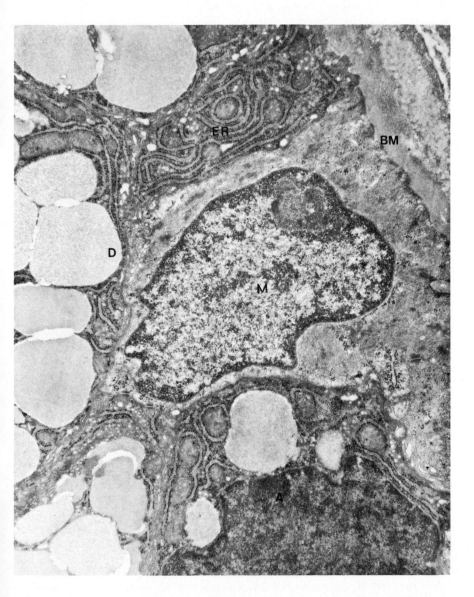

Figure 2.3. Fine structural features of myoepithelial cell (M) and acinar cell (A). Endoplasmic reticulum (ER) and acinar secretory droplets (D) are shown. The basement membrane is indicated (BM) ($\times$ 7050).

Serous cells

Serous cells are roughly pyramidal in shape. The nucleus is located in the basal third of the cells and the cytoplasm stains intensely with haematoxylin and eosin giving the cell a characteristic darkly basophilic colour (Figure 2.4 and 2.5). The cell rests upon a basement membrane, 500 Å thick, and is associated with an elaborate system of intercellular canaliculi or secretory capillaries. Ultrastructurally, abundant endoplasmic reticulum, the Golgi apparatus, mitochondria, desmosomal attachments and secretory droplets are observed. Microvilli are encountered at the luminal border and intercellular space. Helical filaments have been noted within dilated intracristal spaces of rat salivary gland mitochondria (Hand, 1970b) and may represent DNA or DNA protein.

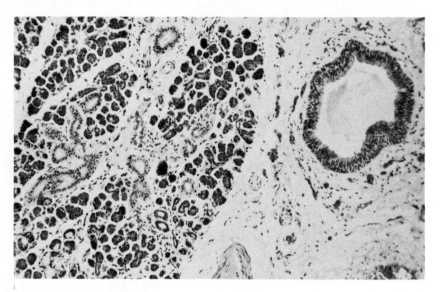

Figure 2.4. Submandibular gland showing predominately serous acinar cells. An excretory duct with double-layered epithelial lining lies in the stroma on the right (× 25).

Duct cells

Intercalated duct cells

Intercalated duct cells are low cuboidal cells (Figure 2.2a) the cytoplasm of which stains faintly with conventional staining techniques. The cell rests upon a basement membrane and the nucleus is centrally placed. They are relatively sparsely distributed in sublingual and labial glands. Ultrastructurally, the cell is characterised by the paucity of cytoplasmic organelles. However, endoplasmic reticulum and membrane-bound secretory granules are usually observed and the Golgi apparatus tends to be prominent. The luminal surface shows a few stubby microvilli.

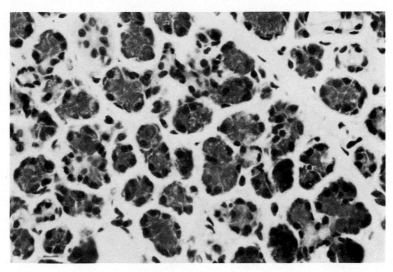

Figure 2.5. Serous acini staining darkly with haematoxylin and eosin: submandibular salivary gland (× 40).

Striated duct cells

Striated duct cells are low columnar cells which rest on a basement membrane and stain a bright eosinophilic colour with haematoxylin and eosin. The nuclei of the cells tend to be centrally placed (Figure 2.6 and 2.7). The fine structural features of the striated duct cells reflects their secretory function. Infolding of both the basal and lateral plasma membranes, 400 to 650 Å in width and projecting into adjacent cells, is marked whilst the luminal surface exhibits numerous short, stubby microvilli (Figure 2.8). Basal striations are uncommon in labial striated cells (Tandler et al, 1969). Mitochondria are arranged in a characteristic fashion within the cell, being distributed in parallel rows in the basal portion. Desmosomal attachments, lipid inclusions and membrane-bound secretion granules are other ultrastructural features (Figure 2.9). The endoplasmic reticulum and Golgi are not well developed. Chains of vesicles are noted in relation to the elaborately folded basal membranes, which greatly increase membrane surface area and may be equated with the free and fast transport of water and ions.

Excretory duct cells

The histological features of the cells which comprise the excretory duct system vary with location (Figures 2.4 and 2.10). Excretory duct cells within the oral epithelium are of the stratified squamous type whilst within the connective tissue stroma of the lamina propria they may be pseudo-stratified or simply tall columnar. A double-layered structure for the excretory duct is characteristic (Figure 2.4). The fine structure of the excretory duct of the rat

23

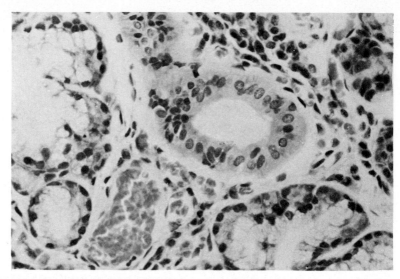

Figure 2.6. Striated duct within human labial salivary glands. Occasional inflammatory cells, mucous acini and blood vessel are present (× 40).

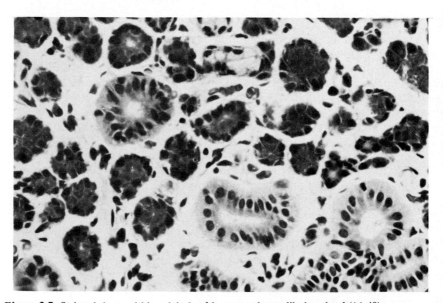

Figure 2.7. Striated ducts within a lobule of human submandibular gland (× 40).

and cat have been studied by Shackleford and Schneyer (1971) and Shackleford and Wilborn (1970). Three principal cell types are recognised—light, dark and basal cells. Light cells, which are the most numerous, are characterised by basal infolding and bulbous distal portions and are not unlike striated cells. Dark cells are basophilic and have highly developed

24

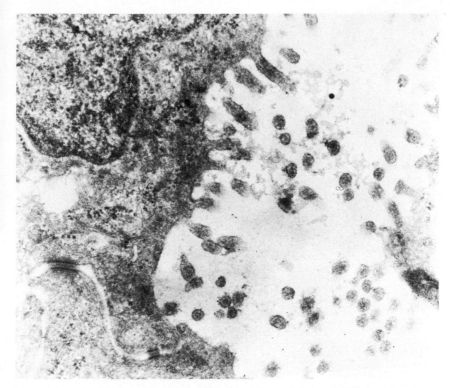

Figure 2.8. Electronmicrograph showing luminal surface of duct cell. Stubby microvilli are present ($\times$ 42 250).

microvilli, whilst basal cells are characterised by the presence of hemi-desmosomes. It is of interest that micropuncture and perfusion studies (Young et al, 1967) strongly suggest a secretory function for this portion of the duct system, such that isotonic perfusion fluid is converted to an hypotonic end product.

Myoepithelial cells

Myoepithelial cells are interposed between the base of the acinar and intercalated duct cells and the basement membrane. They have close functional and morphological similarity to smooth muscle cells. At a light-microscopic level, however, they present a problem of identification. The following observations are relevant to the matter of recognition of myoepi-thelial cells. In the past, judgement as to the identification of myoepithelial cells has been made largely on staining characteristics of cells under the light microscope, special histochemical stains being employed (Zimmermann, 1898; Silver, 1954; Travill and Hill, 1963; Shear, 1964, 1966; Garrett and Harrison, 1970). However, Garrett and Harrison (1970) have used alkaline phosphatase and adenosine triphosphatase histochemical reactions and

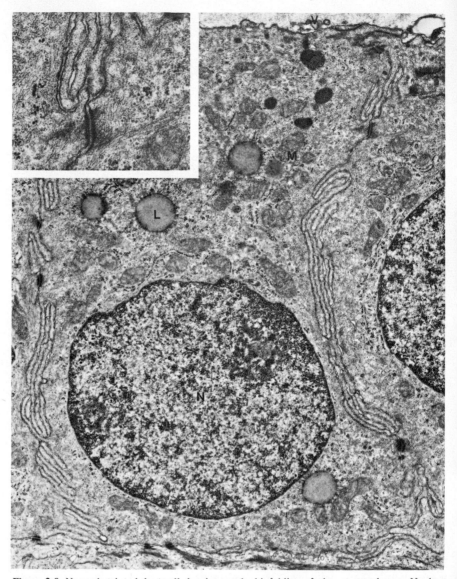

Figure 2.9. Normal striated duct cell showing marked infolding of plasma membrane. Nucleus (N), mitochondria (M), lipid droplets (L) and microvilli (V) are indicated ($\times$ 7050). Inset shows desmosmal attachment ($\times$ 26 320).

shown that neither technique can be regarded as a universal marker for salivary myoepithelial cells. With regard to the origin of the myoepithelial cell some workers have described the presence of cells with characteristics of both epithelial and myoepithelial cells, regarding them as transitional forms in the differentiation of secretory epithelial cells to myoepithelium (Goldstein, 1961; Tandler, 1965; Hamperl, 1970). It is to be noted that myoepithelial

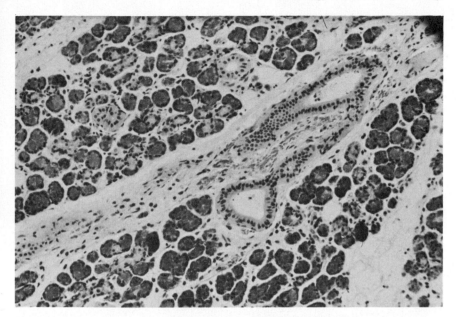

Figure 2.10. Normal light-microscopic appearance of human submandibular salivary glands. Serous acini and intra- and extra-lobular ducts are shown. Connective tissue divides the glands into lobules ($\times$ 168).

cells and smooth muscle cells have close morphological and functional similarities and share a closely related or identical protein which shows immunological cross-reactivity with actomyosin (Archer and Kao, 1968). The contractile function of myoepithelium has been demonstrated by Emmelin, Garrett and Ohlin (1968). A recent study employing fluorescein-labelled antibody against human uterine actomyosin as an immunohistochemical marker for myoepithelial cells during the early stages of rat submandibular gland development failed to determine the exact origin of the myoepithelial cell (Line and Archer, 1972). A mesodermal origin is unlikely since desmosomal connections between myoepithelial and contiguous cells are observed. Such connections are not a feature of cells of mesenchymal derivation (Fawcett, 1966). However, the ultrastructural features of the myoepithelial cell are characteristic. The cells are stellate in shape with elongated, tapering processes. The nucleus is elongated and centrally placed, whilst desmosomal attachments bind the myoepithelial cell to the secretory cells. The cytoplasm contains numerous myofilaments measuring approximately 50 Å in diameter and which are distributed in parallel in the long axis of the cell (Figure 2.11). These myofilaments frequently aggregate to form electron-dense structures similar to the dark bodies observed in smooth muscle cells (Rhoden, 1962). Attachment devices anchor the myofilaments to the plasma membrane. Mitochondria are not abundant but appear to be evenly distributed throughout the cell. Glycogen particles appear to be numerous whilst the endoplasmic reticulum consists of only a few cisternae. Non-filamentous and filamentous portions of the cytoplasm are recognised,

27

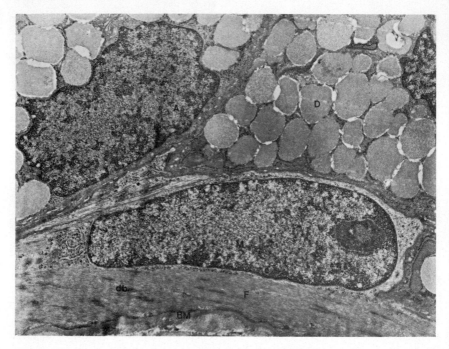

Figure 2.11. Fine structural features of myoepithelial cell (M) and acinar cells (A). Myofilament (F) with dense bodies (db) and basement membrane (BM) are indicated, as are acinar secretory droplets (D). ($\times$ 7425.)

filaments tending to be present towards the basement membrane (Tandler et al, 1970). 'Clear cells' have been described (Tandler, 1965) as accompanying myoepithelial cells and may represent a precursor cell. Pinocytotic vesicles and solitary cilia have been described (Tandler et al, 1970), whilst Tamarin (1966) has estimated myoepithelium to comprise nine per cent of total intra-lobular parenchyma volume for rat submandibular gland. Freeze-etched replicas have been employed to confirm the location of myoepithelial cells (Leeson and Leeson, 1971).

Oncocytes

Oncocytes may be defined by morphological criteria as large epithelial cells with characteristic granular and deeply eosinophilic cytoplasm. They are observed with increasing frequency with increasing age of the individual (Chapter 13). No specific function for oncocytes has been demonstrated and it is probable that they represent effete or degenerating cells. However, characteristically they stain heavily with oxidative enzymes. The fine structural characteristics include the presence of large numbers of enlarged mitochondria. The oncocyte of the salivary gland appears to exist in three recognisable ultrastructural forms (Hübner, Paullussen and Kleinsasser,

28

1967; Tandler, Hugger and Erlandson, 1970). The most common is the large, polyhedral epithelial oncocyte, the variants being the 'condensed' oncocyte and the 'myoepithelial' oncocyte.

Sex dimorphism in rodent salivary glands

Lacassagne (1940) first described a sex difference in the mouse submandibular salivary gland. In mice, before puberty, the cells of the intra-lobular ducts are cuboidal in shape with a clear cytoplasm and centrally located nuclei. In the adult male mouse there is a preponderance of intra-lobular ducts over acini and in the proximal portion of these ducts the cells are tall columnar containing numerous granules (Figure 2.12) and basally placed nuclei. In the adult female, however, these cells or granular tubules are low columnar, contain fewer granules and are present in approximately equal proportion to acinar cells. In the adult rat submandibular gland tubule diameter is greater in males than females. Experimental study has demonstrated that the secretory function of the granular tubules is under hormonal control (Raynaud, 1960).

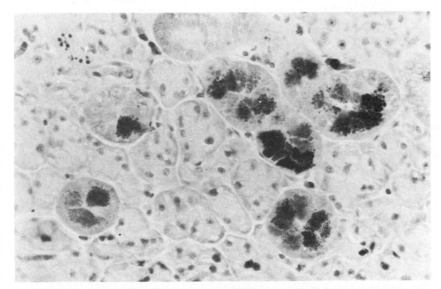

Figure 2.12. Adult male submandibular gland. Granular tubules. Aniline acid fuchsin—picric acid ($\times$ 159).

HISTOCHEMISTRY

Comparative histochemical studies dealing with salivary glands have shown marked species variation with regard to morphological and histochemical features (Arvy, 1962; Shackleford and Klapper, 1962) Quintarelli, 1963;

Spicer and Duvenci, 1964; Leppi et al, 1967). A single type of histo-chemically defined glycoprotein, for example, may be synthesised in a particular gland of certain species, whereas others elaborate admixtures of mucins. The effect of age, sex and hormonal state may be responsible for the wide histochemical and histological changes observed in the sub-mandibular gland of rodents. The critical importance of the age factor may be attributed to the prolonged post-natal development of the rodent sub-mandibular gland. In the rat (Jacoby and Leeson, 1959) and the hamster (Devi and Jacoby, 1966) the acinar cells complete their differentiation well in advance of the granular cells which are not completely differentiated until the animal reaches full maturity.

Accounts of the histochemistry in human salivary glands have been given by Quintarelli (1961), Munger (1964), Leppi and Spicer (1966) and Eversole (1972a, b).

Carbohydrates

In the acinar cells of all mammalian species examined, the presence of amylase-resistant PAS-positive material can be demonstrated. In general, a higher concentration of this material is present in mucous than in serous cells. The relative amounts of neutral and acidic carbohydrates, as deter-mined by the alcian blue, colloidal iron and Periodic Acid Schiff reactions, varies considerably within the secretory unit of different mammalian species (Shackleford and Klapper, 1962). Biochemical characterisation of salivary mucous secretions has shown sialic acid (neuraminic acid) to be one of the more consistently found carbohydrates. With the use of the enzyme neur-aminidase (Spicer and Warren, 1960) and by mild acid hydrolysis (Quintarelli 1961) it has been established that sialic acid is responsible for most of the alcian blue and colloidal iron positive staining of salivary gland tissue sections. This acidic carbohydrate is probably present in considerable quantities in mucous-secreting glands. Johnson, Johnson and Helwig (1962) have shown that some salivary glands elaborate sialomucin or sulfomucin, whereas other glands produce an admixture of the two.

Amylase-resistant PAS-positive material is present in the intra-lobular ducts especially in the apical cytoplasm. Glycogen, demonstrated by a positive PAS reaction not resistant to amylase digestion, is present in the cytoplasm of duct cells (Hill and Bourne, 1954). Histochemical evaluation of mucin elaborated by human minor sublingual and submandibular glands shows the existence of a heterogeneous population of muco-substances (Eversole, 1972a, b). Mucous acinar cells synthesise neutral, carboxy- and sialomucins whilst seromucous and demilunar cells elaborate sialomucins. Sub-mandibular serous cells synthesise a zymogen-like neutral glycan. Differences in staining characteristics may be observed in the same minor glands obtained from different subjects and may reflect different stages in secretory cycles or those factors (Chapter 3) which alter salivary composition. In rat sublingual gland, using PA-silver methanamine and colloidal thorium, Enomoto and Scott (1971) have shown at an ultrastructural level that mucous acinar cell granules, but not demilunar cell granules, comprise muco-substances containing vicinol glycols and polyanions.

A classification of mucins has been advanced by Spicer, Leppi and Stoward (1965). Basically, Type I represents neutral muco-substances; Type II, carboxylated; and Types III and IV, sulphated mucins.

Phosphatases

Alkaline phosphatase is generally localised in myoepithelium although varying quantities have been reported in the other main epithelial cells. The presence of adenosine triphosphatase in myoepithelial cells has been demonstrated by Shear (1964). However, in a recent study Garrett and Harrison (1970) employed alkaline phosphatase and adenosine triphosphatase histochemical reactions and showed that neither technique could be regarded as a universal marker for salivary myoepithelial cells. Indeed, inconsistencies in activity were observed within the myoepithelium of individual glands, species variation was marked and even the appropriate technique could not be relied upon to demonstrate all the myoepithelial cells present in a tissue section.

There is considerable variability in the localisation of acid phosphatase in salivary glands. The enzyme activity appears to be confined to the cytoplasm of serous acinar and duct cells (Chauncey and Quintarelli, 1961).

Esterases

Cholinesterase is concentrated mainly in the nerve fibres which are found principally in relation to the main ducts of the salivary glands. The enzyme is present in rat parotid acinar and duct cells and granular cells of the submandibular gland.

Dehydrogenases

In rodents, marked succinic dehydrogenase activity has been demonstrated in the duct cells of the major salivary glands whilst moderate activity has been found in acinar cells. The distribution of the enzyme accords well with that of mitochondria (Duwey, 1958).

It is clear that little uniformity exists with regard to the enzyme content of salivary cells as revealed by histochemical techniques. This is true especially for acinar cells. However, the presence of protease, esterase, alkaline phosphatase and succinic dehydrogenase in duct cells appears less variable and provides strong evidence for an important role which these cells make to the final secretory product.

MORPHOLOGICAL CHANGES DURING SECRETION

The ultrastructural basis of the secretory process in exocrine cells has been defined by Palade (1959, 1961). Fine structural changes during secretion in rodent parotid acinar and striated cells was described initially by Parks (1962).

In acinar cells, prior to secretory activity, the cells are characterised by an extensive and highly organised rough-surfaced endoplasmic reticulum (RER), whilst the Golgi apparatus is prominent, consisting of stacks of flattened cisternae and numerous small vesicles. At this stage the nucleus is centrally placed and secretory droplets are almost completely absent. As secretory activity progresses, the endoplasmic reticulum involutes and the Golgi cisternae become distended and form vacuoles. Eventually, the apical cytoplasm becomes filled with secretory droplets and the nucleus is displaced basally. The mode of discharge of secretory granules from mucous cells may be by a merocrine process (Trier and Rubin, 1965), although there is evidence that apocrine secretion may take place in human labial mucous cells (Tandler et al, 1969), rat sublingual mucous cells (Kim, Nasjleti and Han, 1972) and goblet cells (Neutra and Leblond, 1966a, b).

The formation of secretory granules, the role of the Golgi apparatus in synthesis and transport of carbohydrates and protein and modes of discharge of the secretory product have been extensively studied in exocrine glands using techniques such as auto-radiography and electronhistochemistry.

The Golgi apparatus plays a key role in the elaboration of mucus. The stacked cisternae of the Golgi apparatus appear to be the site of carbohydrate synthesis (Neutra and Leblond, 1967a, b). The presence of nucleoside diphosphatase activity may reflect the role of the Golgi apparatus in the addition of carbohydrates to the secretory proteins (Hand, 1971). The synthesis and transport of secretory proteins in salivary acinar cells is similar to that mechanism demonstrated in pancreatic exocrine cells (Neutra and Leblond, 1966a, b; Jamieson and Palade, 1967a, b). Protein for transport is synthesised by ribosomes on the endoplasmic reticulum (ER), transferred to the cisternae of the ER and is then transported to the condensing vacuole via the ER cisternae, transitional elements and the peripheral vesicles of the Golgi apparatus. The Golgi lamellae do not appear to be involved in protein transport but rather add a second component to the condensing vacuole.

Acid phosphatase activity has been shown in the condensing vacuoles of the Golgi apparatus and may be a mechanism for lysosomal regulation of the secretory process (Hand, 1971). Lysosomes may be involved in the removal or degradation of excessive membraneous material which may form in secretory cells. Herzog and Miller (1970) have suggested the existence of an increasing entry-exit concentration gradient for peroxidase in the stacked cisternae of the Golgi apparatus, peroxidase being one of the enzymes secreted by salivary glands. Auto-radiographic evidence indicates that concentration of secretory product occurs in the distal cisternae and associated vacuoles of the Golgi stacks. The rate of intracellular processing and storage of secretory proteins may be slower and more prolonged in rabbit parotid acinar cells than in exocrine pancreatic cells (Castle, Jamieson and Palade, 1972).

Unusual crystal-like structures have been observed in secretory granules and, although considered to be glycoprotein in nature, their function remains unknown (Luzzatto, Procicchiani and Rosati, 1968). The mechanism by which secretory substances discharge in mucous and serous cells of pancreas and salivary glands has been the subject of many investigations (Palade, 1961; Amsterdam, Ohad and Schramm, 1969; Tandler et al, 1969; Hand, 1970a; Kim, Nasjleti and Han, 1972). In serous cells, the secretory granules discharge their content by establishing a continuity between membranes of the granule and the apical cell surface. Secretory granules in secretory cells are bound by membranes that show a trilaminar structure (Tamarin and Sreebny, 1965; Yohro, 1970; Martinez-Hernandez, Nakane and Pierce, 1972).

For mucous acinar cells, secretory granules are discharged through gaps in the apical cell surface, whilst in serous acinar cells a continuity between granule membrane and cell membrane is established. Thus, the essential difference lies in the behaviour of the membranes. Amsterdam, Ohad and Schramm (1969) have shown that in rat serous cells the granule membrane, once connected with the lumen, acts as a lumen membrane, resulting in an enlargement of the lumen space. Following discharge, reduction in lumen size is achieved by withdrawal of the lumen membrane in the form of small, smooth vesicles. Following the initial membrane fusion, the granule membrane is capable of fusing subsequently with additional deeper located granules. This sequential fusion is probably controlled by cyclic AMP. The subsequent fate of the granule membrane has been investigated by Amsterdam et al (1971) and they conclude that the membrane is not re-utilised and that the protein of the membrane is degraded after secretion. Membranolytic agents or lysosomes may play a role in this process (Martinez-Hernandez, Nakane and Pierce, 1972). Amsterdam et al (1971) further suggest that the protein of membrane is synthesised de novo concomitantly with the exportable protein in the RER. The fusion of mucous granules before and during secretion appear to protect the cell cytoplasm from exposure to the luminal extra-cellular space. However, on occasion the entire cell content may be extruded into the lumen (Tandler et al, 1969).

REFERENCES

Amsterdam, A., Ohad, I. & Schramm, M. (1969) Dynamic changes in the ultrastructure of the acinar cell of the rat parotid gland during the secretory cycle. *Journal of Cell Biology*, **41**, 753.

Amsterdam, A., Schramm, M., Ohad, I., Solomon, Y. & Selinger, Z. (1971) Concomitant synthesis of membrane protein and exportable protein of the secretory granule in rat parotid gland. *Journal of Cell Biology*, **50**, 187.

Archer, F. L. & Kao, V. C. Y. (1968) Immunohistochemical identification of actomyosin in myoepithelium of human tissues. *Laboratory Investigation*, **18**, 669.

Arvy, L. (1962) Les enzymes des glandes salivaires. In *Handbuch der Histochemie, Vol. 7*. Stuttgart: Springer.

Burgen, A. S. V. & Emmelin, N. G. (1961) *Physiology of the Salivary Glands*. London: Arnold.

Castle, J. D., Jamieson, J. D. & Palade, G. E. (1972) Radioautographic analysis of the secretory process in the parotid acinar cell of the rabbit. *Journal of Cell Biology*, **53**, 290.

Chauncey, H. H. & Quintarelli, G. (1961) Localization of acid-phosphatase, non-specific esterases and β-D-galactosidase in parotid and submaxillary glands of domestic and laboratory animals. *American Journal of Anatomy*, **108**, 263.

Devi, N. S. & Jacoby, F. (1966) The submaxillary gland of the golden hamster and its post-natal development. *Journal of Anatomy*, **100**, 269.

Duwey, M. M. (1958) A histochemical and biochemical study of the parotid gland in normal and hypophysectomized rats. *American Journal of Anatomy,* **102,** 243.

Emmelin, N., Garrett, J. R. & Ohlin, P. (1968) Neural control of salivary myoepithelial cells. *Journal of Physiology,* **196,** 381.

Enomoto, S. & Scott, B. L. (1971) Intracellular distribution of mucosubstances in the major sublingual gland of the rat. *Anatomical Record,* **169,** 71.

Eversole, L. R. (1972a) The mucoprotein histochemistry of human mucous acinar cell containing salivary glands: submandibular and sublingual glands. *Archives of Oral Biology,* **17,** 43.

Eversole, L. R. (1972b) The histochemistry of mucosubstances in human minor salivary glands. *Archives of Oral Biology,* **17,** 1225.

Fawcett, D. W. (1966) *An Atlas of Fine Structure.* Philadelphia: W. B. Saunders Company.

Garrett, J. R. & Harrison, J. D. (1970) Alkaline-phosphatase and adenosine-triphosphatase histochemical reactions in the salivary glands of cat, dog and man with special reference to the myoepithelial cells. *Histochemie,* **24,** 214.

Goldstein, D. J. (1961) On the origin and morphology of myoepithelial cells of apocrine sweat glands. *Journal of Investigative Dermatology,* **37,** 301.

Hamperl, H. (1970) The myothelia (myoepithelial cells). Normal state, regressive changes, hyperplasia; tumors. *Current Topics in Pathology,* **53,** 161.

Hand, A. R. (1970a) The fine structures of Von Ebner's gland of rat. *Journal of Cell Biology,* **44,** 340.

Hand, A. R. (1970b) Intracristal helices in salivary gland mitochondria. *Anatomical Record,* **168,** 565.

Hand, A. R. (1971) Morphology and cytochemistry of the Golgi apparatus of rat salivary gland acinar cells. *American Journal of Anatomy,* **130,** 141.

Herzog, V. & Miller, F. (1970) Die Lokalisation Endogener Peroxydase in der Glandula Parotis der Ratte. *Zeitschrift für Zellforschung und mikroskopische Anatomie,* **107,** 403.

Hill, C. R. & Bourne, G. H. (1954) The histochemistry and cytology of the salivary gland duct cells. *Acta Anatomica,* **20,** 116.

Hübner, G., Paulussen, F. & Kleinsasser, O. (1967) The fine structure and genesis of oncocytes. *Virchows Archiv für pathologische Anatomie und Physiologie und für klinische Medizin,* **343,** 34.

Jacoby, F. & Leeson, C. R. (1959) The post-natal development of the rat submaxillary gland. *Journal of Anatomy,* **93,** 102.

Jamieson, J. D. & Palade, G. E. (1967a) Intracellular transport of secretory proteins in the pancreatic exocrine cell. I. Role of the peripheral elements of the Golgi apparatus. *Journal of Cell Biology,* **34,** 577.

Jamieson, J. D. & Palade, G. E. (1967b) Intracellular transport of secretory proteins in the pancreatic exocrine cell. II. Transport to condensing vacuoles and zymogen granules. *Journal of Cell Biology,* **34,** 597.

Johnston, W. C., Johnson, G. B. & Helwig, E. B. (1962) Effect of varying the pH on reactions for acid mucopolysaccharides. *Journal of Histochemistry and Cytochemistry,* **10,** 684.

Kim, S. K., Nasjleti, C. E. & Han, S. S. (1972) The secretion processes in mucous and serous secretory cells of the rat sublingual gland. *Journal of Ultrastructure Research,* **38,** 371.

Kurtz, S. M. (1964) The salivary glands. In *Electron Microscopic Anatomy* (ed.) Kurtz, S. M. New York: Academic Press.

Lacassagne, A. (1940) Dimorphisme sexuel de la glande sous-maxillaire chez la souris. *Comptes Rendus des Séances de la Société de Biologie et de ses Filiales,* **133,** 180.

Leeson, C. R. (1967) Structure of salivary glands. In *Handbook of Physiology; Alimentary Canal. II.* (Ed.) Code, C. F. Washington, D.C.: American Physiological Society.

Leeson, T. S. & Leeson, C. R. (1971) Myoepithelial cells of the exorbital lacrimal and parotid glands of the rat in frozen-etched replicas. *American Journal of Anatomy,* **132,** 133.

Leppi, T. J. & Spicer, S. S. (1966) The histochemistry of mucins in certain primate salivary glands. *American Journal of Anatomy,* **118,** 833.

Leppi, T. J., Spicer, S. S., Henson, J. C. & Fioravanti, J. (1967) Correlated histochemical staining and $S^{35}O_4$ labelling of salivary gland mucosubstances. *Journal of Histochemistry and Cytochemistry,* **15,** 745.

Line, S. E. & Archer, F. L. (1972) The post-natal development of myoepithelial cells in the rat submandibular gland. An immunohistochemical study. *Virchows Archiv Abteilung B. Zell Pathologie,* **10,** 253.

Luzzatto, A. C., Procicchiani, G. & Rosati, G. (1968) Rat submaxillary gland: An electron microscopic study of the secretory granules of the acinus. *Journal of Ultrastructure Research,* **22,** 185.

Martinez-Hernandez, A., Nakane, P. K. & Pierce, G. B. (1972) The secretory granules of the acinar cells of the mouse submaxillary gland. *American Journal of Anatomy,* **133,** 259.

Munger, B. L. (1964) Histochemical studies on seromucous and mucous-secreting cells of human salivary glands. *American Journal of Anatomy,* **115,** 411.

Neutra, M. & Leblond, C. P. (1966a) Synthesis of the carbohydrate of mucin in the Golgi complex as shown by electron microscope radioautography of goblet cells from rats injected with glucose—H^3. *Journal of Cell Biology,* **30,** 119.

Neutra, M. & Leblond, C. P. (1966b) Radioautographic comparison of the uptake of galactose H^3 and glucose-H^3 in the Golgi region of various cells secreting glycoproteins of mucopolysaccharides. *Journal of Cell Biology,* **30,** 137.

Palade, G. E. (1959) Functional changes in the structure of cell components. In *Subcellular Particles* (Ed.) Hayashi, T. New York: Ronald Press Co.

Palade, G. E. (1961) The secretory process of the pancreatic exocrine cell. In *Electronmicroscopy in Anatomy* (eds) Boyd, J. D., Johnson, F. R. & Lever, J. D. Baltimore: Williams and Wilkins Co.

Parks, H. F. (1962) Morphological study of the extrusion of secretory materials by the parotid glands of mouse and rat. *Journal of Ultrastructure Research,* **6,** 449.

Quintarelli, G. (1961) Histochemical studies on human mucous-secreting salivary glands. *Acta Histochemica,* **12,** 1.

Quintarelli, G. (1963) Histochemical identification of salivary mucins. *Annals of the New York Academy of Sciences,* **106,** 339.

Raynaud, J. (1960) Controle hormonal de la glande sous-maxillaire de la souris. *Bulletin de Biologique France et Belgique,* **94,** 400.

Rhodin, J. A. G. (1962) Fine structure of vascular walls in mammals with special reference to smooth muscle components. *Physiology Review,* **42,** 48.

Scott, B. L. & Pease, D. C. (1964) Electron microscopy of induced changes in the salivary gland of the rat. In *Salivary Glands and Their Secretions* (Eds) Sreebny, L. M. & Meyer, J. New York: Macmillan.

Shackleford, J. M. & Klapper, C. E. (1962) Structure and carbohydrate histochemistry of mammalian salivary glands. *American Journal of Anatomy,* **111,** 25.

Shackleford, J. M. & Wilborn, W. H. (1970) Ultrastructural aspects of cat submandibular glands. *Journal of Morphology,* **131,** 253.

Shackleford, J. M. & Schneyer, L. H. (1971) Ultrastructural aspects of the main excretory duct of rat submandibular gland. *Anatomical Record,* **169.** 679.

Shear, M. (1964) Histochemical localisation of alkaline phosphatase and adenosine triphosphatase in the myoepithelial cells of rat salivary glands. *Nature (London),* **203,** 770.

Shear, M. (1966) The structure and function of myoepithelial cells in salivary glands. *Archives of Oral Biology,* **11,** 769.

Silver, I. A. (1954) Myoepithelial cells in the mammary and parotid glands. *Journal of Physiology (London),* **125,** 8.

Spicer, S. S. & Duvenci, J. (1964) Histochemical characteristics of mucopolysaccharides in salivary and exorbital lacrimal gland. *Anatomical Record,* **149,** 333.

Spicer, S. S. & Warren, L. (1960) The histochemistry of sialic acid containing mucoproteins. *Journal of Histochemistry and Cytochemistry,* **8,** 135.

Spicer, S. S., Leppi, T. J. & Stoward, P. J. (1965) Suggestions for a histochemical terminology of carbohydrate-rich tissue components. *Journal of Histochemistry and Cytochemistry,* **13,** 599.

Stormont, D. L. (1932) The salivary glands. In *Special Cytology* (Ed.) Cowdry, E. V. New York: Hoeber.

Tamarin, A. (1966) Myoepithelium of the rat submaxillary gland. *Journal of Ultrastructure Research,* **16,** 320.

Tamarin, A. & Sreebny, L. M. (1965) The rat submaxillary salivary gland. A correlative study by light and electron microscopy. *Journal of Morphology,* **117,** 295.

Tandler, B. (1962) Ultrastructure of the human submaxillary gland. I. Architecture and histological relationships of the secretory cells. *American Journal of Anatomy,* **111,** 287.

Tandler, B. (1963) Ultrastructure of the human submaxillary gland. II. The base of the striated duct cells. *Journal of Ultrastructure Research,* **9,** 65.

Tandler, B. (1965) Ultrastructure of the human submaxillary gland. III. Myoepithelium. *Zeitschrift für Zellforschung,* **68,** 852.

Tandler, B., Denning, C. R., Mandel, I. D. & Kutscher, A. H. (1969) Ultrastructure of human labial salivary glands. I. Acinar secretory cells. *Journal of Morphology,* **127,** 383.

Tandler, B., Denning, C. R., Mandel, I. D. & Kutscher, A. H. (1970) Ultrastructure of human labial salivary glands. III. Myoepithelium and ducts. *Journal of Morphology,* **130,** 227.

Tandler, B., Hugger, R. V. P. & Erlandson, R. A. (1970) Ultrastructure of oncocytoma of the parotid gland. *Laboratory Investigation,* **23,** 567.

Travill, A. A. & Hill, M. F. (1963) Histochemical demonstration of myoepithelial cell activity. *Quarterly Journal of Experimental Physiology and Cognate Medical Sciences,* **48,** 423.

Trier, J. S. & Rubin, C. E. (1965) Electron microscopy of the small intestine: A review. *Gastroenterology,* **49,** 574.

Yohro, T. (1970) Development of the secretory units of mouse submandibular gland. *Zeitschrift für Zellforschung,* **110,** 173.

Young, J. A., Frömter, E., Schögel, E. & Hamann, K. F. (1967) Micropuncture and perfusion studies of fluid and electrolyte transport in the rat submaxillary gland. In *Secretory Mechanisms of Salivary Glands,* (Eds) Schneyer, L. H. & Schneyer, C. A. New York: Academic Press.

Zimmermann, K. W. (1898) Beiträge zur Kenntniss einiger Drüsen and Epithelien. *Archiv für mikroskopische Anatomie,* **52,** 552.

Zimmermann, K. W. (1927) Die Speicheldrüsen der Mundhöhle und die Bauchspeicheldrüse. In *Handbuch der Mikroskopischen Anatomie,* (Ed.) Von Möllendorff, P. Berlin: Springer.

CHAPTER 3

Saliva

GENERAL REVIEW AND PHYSICAL PROPERTIES

The salivary glands of man consist of three pairs of large glands (parotid, submandibular, sublingual) and the smaller glands (labial, lingual, palatal, buccal). All secrete into the oral cavity and contribute to the mixed saliva which has many important functions. Saliva keeps the mouth moist, facilitates speech and lubricates food for chewing and swallowing. As it renders food substances soluble, saliva aids in the full appreciation of taste sensation. Human saliva contains the a-amylase ptyalin which, when mixed with food by chewing, begins the digestion of starch. Its action continues as the food passes down into the body of the stomach. Saliva is also secreted in response to noxious substances and dilutes them and helps to cleanse the mouth. Its bicarbonate and protein content contribute to the buffering power of saliva, which is important in restoring the physiological pH of the oral cavity.

The rate of secretion of individual salivary glands ranges from barely perceptible during sleep (Schneyer et al, 1956) to as high as 4 ml/min on maximal stimulation. Although several standard textbooks state that the total daily salivary volume is 1 to 1.5 litres, the experimental evidence for these figures is lacking. The measured daily volume of saliva in two patients with oesophageal fistulae has been recorded as about 500 ml (McKeown and Dunstone, 1959); Jenkins (1966a) has suggested c. 620 ml as being a more realistic estimate, based partly on data of Becks and Wainwright (1943). As there is considerable variation in flow rates between individuals, especially under 'resting' conditions (Becks and Wainwright, 1943; Kerr, 1961), there will also be a large range for the normal daily mixed saliva volume.

The specific gravity of saliva varies between 1.000 and 1.010 and increases with increasing rate of flow (Kerr, 1961). The osmotic pressure is between one-half and three-quarters that of blood (Wilsmore, 1937). The viscosity of saliva depends upon the contribution of the three main glands to the saliva formed. The relative viscosities of the three main glandular secretions after citric acid stimulation were found by Schneyer (1955) to be: parotid, 1.5; submandibular, 3.4; sublingual, 13.4 centipoises. Thus the viscosity is directly proportional to the percentage of mucous-secreting cells in these individual glands. The parotid glands are serous glands which secrete fluid devoid of mucin; the submandibular glands are of mixed type containing both serous and mucous cells; the sublingual contains mainly mucous cells.

Most saliva is secreted by the three pairs of large glands, the parotid, the submandibular and the sublingual. The relative volume of saliva secreted by the parotid and submandibular glands during different degrees of stimulation is shown in Table 3.1. In addition to the secretion produced by the three pairs of large glands, there is a contribution by the smaller glands of the oral mucosa, i.e. labial, lingual, buccal and palatal mucous glands. Their total relative contribution has been estimated as varying from about 30 to 53 per cent by volume (Schneyer, 1955). However, recently Dawes and Wood (1973) have reported that the contribution of the minor glands to whole saliva during rest and when stimulated with sour lemon drop was eight per cent and seven per cent respectively. The basic secretions of both the major and minor glands differ in composition, and their relative contribution to mixed saliva depends on various factors which affect salivary composition. Morphological changes observed during the secretory cycle are outlined in Chapter 2. Secretion is a complex process but at the present time a simplified view of the concept is as follows.

Table 3.1. *Approximate gland volume contribution* (%) *related to stimulation intensity* (*After Kerr, 1961*).

	Submandibular	Parotid
Minimal stimulation	66.6	33.3
Half maximal stimulation	50.0	50.0
Maximal stimulation	33.3	66.6

The salivary striated duct cells have a similar morphology to those associated with water transport in other parts of the body, e.g. kidney, and there is good evidence that the ducts do not play a passive role, but contribute to the composition of saliva (Henriques, 1961, 1962; Tandler, 1963; Junqueira, 1964; and Petersen, 1972). It has been shown that water and several electrolytes, calcium, chloride, bicarbonate, sodium and potassium, can be secreted and reabsorbed by the duct epithelium (Figure 3.1).

The fluid formation in salivary glands occurs in the acini. The acinar secretory process is an isotonic water transport in which the main active step is a sodium transport from the intracellular to the intercellular space. Sodium enters along the basal cell membrane down an electrochemical gradient as a result of an acetylcholine-induced enhanced permeability of the basal cell membrane to potassium and sodium that also changes the potential difference across this membrane. The result is the formation of an isotonic, high sodium and low potassium fluid that is modified in the duct system, mainly in the region of the striated ducts, by the reabsorption of sodium chloride in excess of water and in some glands by the secretion of potassium and bicarbonate. These transport processes are under the influence of the autonomic nervous system as are the acinar processes (Petersen, 1972).

One well-established physiological action of the duct epithelium is the concentration of iodide (Figure 3.2) and thiocyanate (Cohen, Logothetopoulos and Myant, 1955; Stephen et al, 1973). The nature and mode of action of the factors controlling the physiological action of the duct epithelium is not fully understood.

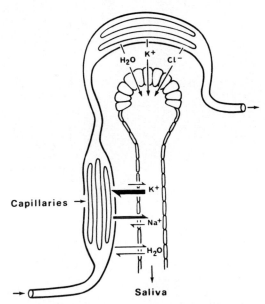

Figure 3.1. Diagrammatic representation of possible mechanisms underlying changes in concentration of salivary constituents (after Davenport, 1961).

A detailed account of the physiological mechanisms of salivary secretion of individual constituents is outside the scope of this book. For detailed information the reader is referred to the following reviews: Burgen and Emmelin (1961); Sreebny and Meyer (1964); Schneyer and Schneyer (1967); Emmelin and Zotterman (1972); Han, Sreebny and Suddick (1973); Thorn and Petersen (1974).

THE COMPOSITION OF SALIVA

Saliva consists of a complex mixture of inorganic and organic substances; these can be broadly subdivided into electrolytes, enzymes, other proteins, low molecular weight compounds and vitamins.

The final composition of saliva appears to be regulated by the autonomic nervous system as well as humorally. Salivary glands are innervated by parasympathetic a-sympathetic and β-sympathetic fibres. Both the parasympathetic and a-sympathetic fibres mediate their response by stimulation of guanyl cyclase activity in target tissues which leads to an increase in cyclic GMP. The difference in response between the parasympathetic and a-sym-

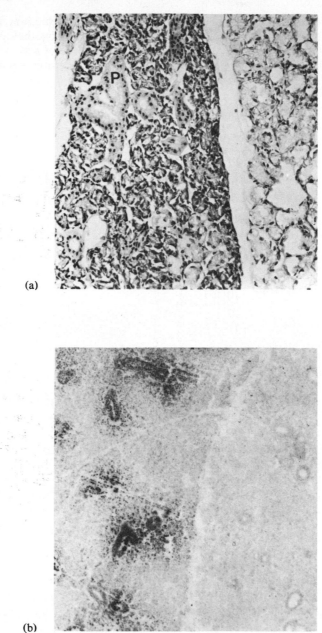

(a)

(b)

Figure 3.2. Adult male hamster. Submandibular gland tissue (left) and sublingual gland (right). a. H & E ($\times$ 88) Proximal duct (P) is shown. b. Autoradiograph—neutral red ($\times$ 60) showing ^{131}I concentration over proximal ducts in submandibular gland. There is little radioactivity over sublingual gland tissues.

pathetic systems is presumably related to different receptor sites in the various glandular constituents. β-sympathetic stimulation activates adenyl cyclase and thus increases the intracellular concentration of cyclic AMP.

The humoral control of saliva is less well understood. In addition to corticosteroids, both secretin and pancreozymin may alter salivary composition (Mulcahy, Fitzgerald and McGeeney, 1972). This latter action is probably brought about by regulation of the cyclic nucleotide concentrations.

A comprehensive summary of the constituents of mixed saliva, the individual gland secretions both stimulated and unstimulated, and gingival exudate is shown in Tables 3.2 to 3.7. These tables present the data, as far as possible, in the now internationally adopted S.I. units. A complete list of the numbered references in the tables is given in the reference list at the end of the chapter.

It must be stressed however that these tables have considerable limitations:
1. Although the initial impression is that voluminous data is available on the composition of saliva, with a few exceptions such as Shannon, Suddick and Dowd (1974), in most cases very few subjects have been studied, usually in undefined or unstandardised conditions.
2. Results even using similar assay methods vary from laboratory to laboratory. This means that although these tables give data showing differences in the magnitude of a particular parameter in the presence and absence of stimulation, if the two sets of data are from different laboratories, the 'apparent' difference may not in fact be real.
3. In the case of enzymes, the situation is further complicated by the wide range of assay methods used and also variations in the detailed assay procedure, and the units of activity selected. Hence it is particularly difficult to obtain comparative data on enzyme activities. Fortunately, the introduction of the S.I. system is likely to simplify this situation in the future.
4. A further complication in expressing the normal composition of saliva arises from a number of factors such as circadian variation.

Hence, any data presented in the tables can only be regarded as a general guide to the normal levels.

Another problem when studying secretions is the possibility of contamination from other sources, e.g. bacteria, exfoliated epithelial cells, etc. A list of enzymes found in mixed saliva but thought to be bacterial in origin is given in Table 3.8.

Considerably more information, using large numbers of samples collected in well-defined conditions and assayed by generally accepted procedures, is necessary before a more reliable picture of the composition of saliva can be obtained.

FACTORS AFFECTING COMPOSITION

The factors affecting the composition of saliva have been reviewed by Afonsky (1961), Burgen and Emmelin (1961), Jenkins (1966b) and Dawes (1970a). There are a number of important conclusions which can be drawn.

Table 3.2. *Composition of mixed saliva.*

Substance	Unstimulated Mean ± SD	Unstimulated Range	Stimulated Mean ± SD	Stimulated Range
Protein (g/l)		1.4–6.4[1]*	2.8*	1.8–4.2[31]
Total N$_2$ (g/l)			0.37[17] ± 1.12[8]	
Amino acids (mg/l)			40[31]	
Amylase (IU/l)	352 × 10^6 ± 242 × 10^6	73 × 10^6 –1 300 × 10^6 [17]		
Amylase (g/l)	0.38 ± 0.08[59](SEM) ± 0.32			
Lysozyme (mg/l)			108.9 ± 129.1	3.7–625[10]
Acid phosphatase (units[52]/l)			55.5 ± 31.9	5–130[10]
Acid phosphatase (SJR units[56]/l)	114 ± 69[48]			
Alkaline phosphatase (units[52]/l)			4.78± 2.7	0.25–11.1[10]
Alkaline phosphatase (SJR units[56]/l)	24 ± 21[48]			
Non-specific esterase (units[51]/l)			38.3 ± 18.3	1–75[10]
α-L-fucosidase (units/l)			520 ± 220[43]	
β-N-acetyl-D-glucosaminidase (units/l)			9580 ± 3100[43]	
Pseudo cholinesterase (units[46]/l)			0.56 ± 0.55	0–2.21[10]
α-D-mannosidase	Present[43]		Present[43]	
Glutamate oxaloacetate transaminase (units[18]/l)			27 500 ± 20 200[18]	
Glutamate pyruvate transaminase (units[18]/l)			12 500 ± 9900[18]	
Carbonic anhydrase (K/l)[36]			2100[45]	
Lipase (units[51]/l)			11.8 ± 5.75	2.0–27[10]
Sulphatase (units[51]/l)			1.91 ± 1.06	0.25–4.65[10]
Peroxidase (mg/l)	1.82 ± 1.07	0.38–3.50[21]	2.79 ± 1.16	1.10–4.68[21]
IgA (mg/l)	194.0[7]			
IgG (mg/l)	14.4[7]			
IgM (mg/l)	2.1[7]			
Kallikrein (units[64]/l)			777 000 ± 456 000	33 000 – 174 000[64]
Glucose (mmol/l)	0.055 ± 0.048[9]		0.056	0.02–0.17[31]
Lactate (mmol/l)				0.1–0.06[31]
Citrate (mmol/l)			0.004	0–0.1[1]
Ammonia (mmol/l)	3.22 ± 2.5[14]		4	0.6–7.1[31]
Urea (mmol/l)	0.09	2.33–12.5[1]	2.17	0.1–4.8[1]
Uric acid (mmol/l)	0.09	0.03–0.17[20]	0.18	0.06–1.25[31]
Creatinine (mg/l)	0.2	0.04–0.18[1]		
Cholesterol (mg/l)		0.07–1.3[31]		0.06–0.18[1]

Histamine (mg/l)	0.15			0—100[10]
Ascorbic acid (μmol/l)	10.8 ± 4.3[29]	4	0.11—0.18[49]	
Aneurin HCl (μg/l)	7[31]	16		6—36[20]
Choline (μg/l)	50[31]			
Riboflavin (μg/l)	30[31]	115		23—409[20]
Nicotinic acid (μg/l)	600[31]	6		1—17[31]
Pyridoxin HCl (μg/l)	0.1[31]	24		3—75[31]
Folic acid (μg/l)	80[31]	88		12—190[20]
Pantothenic acid (μg/l)	7[20]			2—14[20]
Thiamine (μg/l)				
Biotin (μg/l)	0.8[31]			
Cobalamin (Vitamin B_{12}) (μg/l)		3.3		1.5—5.0[20]
Vitamin K (μg/l)	15[31]			
Sodium (mmol/l)	6.2 ± 0.46(SEM)[14]	26.4 ± 11.8[61]		
Potassium (mmol/l)	21.6 ± 1.20(SEM)[14]	19.7 ± 3.9[61]		
Thiocyanate (mmol/l) { Smokers	1.3		0.83—1.94[37]	
non-smokers	0.35		0.17—0.50	
Calcium (mmol/l)	1.56 ± 0.06(SEM)[27]	1.48 ± 0.04(SEM)[27]		
Phosphate (mmol/l) (inorganic)	6.14 ± 0.61(SEM)[27]			
Phosphate (mmol/l) (total)	6.2[26]			
Magnesium (mmol/l)	0.21 ± 0.01t(SEM)[28]	0.15 ± 0.04(SEM)[28]		0.01—0.09[20]
Chloride (mmol/l)	17.40 ± 1.40(SEM)[14]	29.0 ± 8.8[61]		
Bromide (mmol/l)				1—3[20]
Iodide (μmol/l)	0.8		0—3[20]	0.25—1.2[21]
Fluoride (μmol/l)	15 ± 0.68	0.56 ± 0.25	0.5—3[31]	1.6—7.5[20]
Copper (μmol/l)	5.03 ± 2.4[17]	4.1		0—2.1[20]
Cobalt (μmol/l)		0.41		
Gold (μmol/l)	0.003 ± 0.001[32]			
Sulphur (g/l)	0.76[20]			
Total solids (% w/v)	6	0.53		0.41—0.72[31]
pH		7.08 ± 0.312	3—8[1]	6.20—7.60[19]
Nitrogen (vol. %)	2.5[20]			
Oxygen (vol. %)	1.0[20]			
CO_2 (ml/l)	15.0		8.2—25.3[20]	190—500[20]

The superscript numbers in this and the following tables refer to references; see end of chapter.
*Lowry method.[61]

SEM = Standard error of mean.

Table 3.3. *Composition of parotid saliva.*

Substance	Unstimulated Mean ± SD	Unstimulated Range	Stimulated Mean ± SD	Stimulated Range
Protein (g/l)	2.35 ± 3.87*		1.64 ± 0.51**	0.15—2.64[13]
Total N$_2$ (g/l)	0.586 ± 2.23[35]			
Carbohydrate (total) (g/l)			0.245 ± 0.058	0.154—0.334[15]
Precipitable carbohydrate (protein bound) (g/l)			0.213 ± 0.075	0.132—0.304[13]
Supernatant carbohydrate (free) (g/l)			0.026 ± 0.008	0.014—0.04[13]
Lipid (g/l)	0.028 ± 0.013[39]†			
Amylase (g/l)	1.03 ± 0.11(SEM)[50]		0.95 ± 0.15(SEM)	
Amylase (units[58]/l)	2912 × 10³ ± 593 × 10³ [55]		4010 × 10³ ± 2062 × 10³ [3 54]	
Lysozyme (mg/l)			23.1 ± 14.3	4.5—80[31]
Acid phosphatase (units[52]/l)	5.0 ± 2.1[55]		2.0 ± 1.2[54]	
Acid phosphatase (SJR units[56]/l)	14 ± 7[48]			
Alkaline phosphatase (SJR units[56]/l)	94 ± 44[48]			
Protease			Absent[57]	
Non-specific esterase (units[51]/l)			0.65	0.49—1.01[11]
Pseudo-cholinesterase (units[46]/l)			0.64	0.11—1.31[11]
Acid ribonuclease (units[22]/l)			251 000	170 000—420 000[22]
Alkaline ribonuclease (units[22]/l)			285 000	240 000—370 000[22]
Lactate dehydrogenase (units[27]/l)				2—12[27]
a-L-fucosidase (units[43]/l)			230 ± 170[43]	
β-N-acetyl-D-glucosaminidase (units[43]/l)			5070 ± 2930[43]	
a-D-mannosidase	Absent[43]		Absent[43]	
Carbonic anhydrase (K/ml)[26]	1.6[48]		2.2[48]	
Albumin (mg/l)			2.8	
IgA (mg/l)			39.5 ± 13.7	17—63[5]
IgG (mg/l)			0.36 ± 0.3	0—0.9[5]
IgM (mg/l)			0.43 ± 0.36	0.1— [5]
Secretory piece (mg/l)		0—20[6]		0—20[6]
Kallikrein (units[64]/l)			420 000 ± 251 000	180 000—910 000[54]
Lactoferrin (mg/l)		5—20[6]		5—20[6]
Glucose (mmol/l)	0.042 ± 0.038[55]		0.008 ± 0.003[54]	
Hexosamine (mg/l) (protein bound)			120 ± 62[40]	

Table 3.3—*continued.*

Constituent			
Fucose (mg/l) (protein bound)		96 ± 54[40]	
Sialic acid (mg/l)		10.5 ± 5.3[54]	
Pyruvate (mmol/l)			0.01—0.1[34]
Lactate (mmol/l)			0.2—0.5[34]
Citrate (mmol/l)		0.008	0—0.1[1]
Ammonia (mmol/l)	0.3[38]	0.6 ± 0.3[54]	
Urea (mmol/l)	3.0[38]	4.64	3.2—7.1[63]
Uric acid (mmol/l)	0.57 ± 0.25[55]	0.17 ± 0.05[54]	
Creatinine (mg/l)		0.01 ± 0.004[54]	
Free 17-hydroxycorticosteroids (mg/l)		2.06 ± 0.74[54]	
cAMP (nmol/l)		4.6 ± 1.4	1.5—6.3[33]
cGMP (nmol/l)		2.3 ± 1.8	0.2—6.2[33]
Sodium (mmol/l)	2.6 ± 2.00[53]	54.9 ± 16.91[54]	
Potassium (mmol/l)	36.7 ± 12.5[53]	16.0 ± 2.65[54]	
Thiocyanate (mmol/l) smokers	5.47 ± 3.2[54]		
non-smokers		3.2 ± 1.77[54]	
Calcium (mmol/l)	0.75 ± 0.25[53]	0.82 ± 0.55[54]	
Phosphate (mmol/l) (inorganic)	3.40 ± 1.40[53]	3.27 ± 2.60[24]	
Phosphate (mmol/l) (total)		5.60 ± 2.57[34]	
Magnesium (mmol/l)	0.10 ± 0.05[55]	0.02 ± 0.13[54]	
Chloride (mmol/l)	24.8 ± 7.6[53]	33.3 ± 13.4[54]	
Iodide (µmol/l)	4.2 ± 0.61[59]	1.4 ± 0.24[59]	
Fluoride (µmol/l)	1 ± 0.2[54]	1 ± 0.2[54]	
Bicarbonate (mmol/l)	0.85 ± 0.65[55]	29.8 ± 9.2[54]	
Total solids (%w/v)	0.72 ± 0.24[55]	0.92 ± 0.26[54]	
pH	5.92 ± 0.51[55]	7.67 ± 0.18[54]	
Specific gravity	1.0033 ± 0.0011[55]	1.0060 ± 0.0030[54]	
Molarity (mosmol/kg)	73.6 ± 14.5[55]	127.2 ± 34.95[54]	
Viscosity (centipoises)	1.082 ± 0.053[55]	1.20 ± 0.10[54]	

*Biuret method.
**‡Lowry method[61].
†Flow rate not stated.

Table 3.4. *Composition of submandibular saliva.*

	Unstimulated		Stimulated	
	Mean ± SD	Range	Mean ± SD	Range
Protein (g/l)	1.14 ± 0.58[25]		0.77 ± 0.36	0.32—1.43[44]
Total N₂ (g/l)	0.36 ± 0.20[25]			
Carbohydrate (total) (g/l)	0.084 ± 0.035[25]		0.104 ± 0.05	0.04—0.19[44]
Precipitable carbohydrate (protein bound) (g/l)			0.09 ± 0.049	0.02—0.16[44]
Supernatant carbohydrate (free) (g/l)			0.014 ± 0.01	0.00—0.04[44]
Lipid (g/l)	0.020 ± 0.015[39]*			
Amylase (g/l)	0.25 ± 0.06(SEM)[50] ± 0.24			
Lysozyme (mg/l)			15.0 ± 9.2**	5.0—42.0[30]
Acid phosphatase (units[52]/l)			5.5	1.9—12.8[11]
Protease			Present[57]	
Non-specific esterase (units[51]/l)			1.18	0.59—4.55[11]
Pseudo-cholinesterase (units[46]/l)			0.45	0.00—1.66[11]
Acid ribonuclease (units[22]/l)			121 000	40 000—160 000[22]
Alkaline ribonuclease (units[22]/l)			150 000	60 000—230 000[22]
α-L-fucosidase (units[43]/l)			280 ± 230**[43]	
β-N-acetyl-D-glucosaminidase (units[43]/l)			423 ± 257**[43]	
α-D-mannosidase	Absent[43]		Absent[43]	

Table 3.4—*continued.*

Carbonic anhydrase (K/l)[26]	2.0[48]		
IgA (mg/l)	15.9 ± 10.9[65]		
Kallikrein (units[64]/l)		422 000 ± 256 000[64]	110 000—1 080 000[64]
Hexosamine (mg/l) (protein bound)		60 ± 21[40]	
Fucose (mg/l) (protein bound)		46 ± 20[40]	
Sialic acid (mg/l)	0.5[38]	21 ± 12[40]	
Ammonia (mmol/l)	1.75[38]	0.05[38]	
Urea (mmol/l)		3.2	1.8—5.4[63]
Uric acid (mmol/l)	33 ± 4.6[42]	13 ± 1.2[42]	
Sodium (mmol/l)	2.6 ± 2.7[15]	54.8 ± 11.5[15]	
Potassium (mmol/l)	14.4 ± 2.2[15]	13.7 ± 3.6[15]	
Calcium (mmol/l)	1.56 ± 0.45[15]	2.13 ± 0.26[15]	
Phosphate (mmol/l) (inorganic)	3.6 ± 0.7[15]	1.57 ± 0.32[15]	
Phosphate (mmol/l) (total)	7.92 ± 6.50[25]		
Magnesium (mmol/l)	0.07 ± 0.028[15]	0.036 ± 0.012[15]	
Chloride (mmol/l)	11.9 ± 2.3[15]	32.2 ± 10.2[15]	
Bicarbonate (mmol/l)	2.2[15]	35.5[15]	
pH	6.73 ± 0.45[25]		

*Flow rate not stated.
**Combined submandibular and sublingual.

Table 3.5. *Composition of sublingual saliva.*

Substance	Unstimulated		Stimulated	
	Mean ± SD	Range	Mean ± SD	Range
Amylase (g/l)	0.26 ± 0.08(SEM)[50] ± 0.32			
a-D-mannosidase	Absent[43]		Absent[43]	
Sodium (mmol/l)			32.7 ± 10.4	21.6—55.0[25]
Potassium (mmol/l)			13.2 ± 2.0	9.8—17.3[25]
Calcium (mmol/l)			2.1 ± 0.4	1.7—3.0[25]
Phosphate (mmol/l) (inorganic)			1.4 ± 0.3	0.8—1.7[25]
Chloride (mmol/l)			26.2 ± 9.6	11.6—37.6[25]
Bicarbonate (mmol/l)			10.9 ± 3.6	4.5—16.5[25]

Table 3.6. *Composition of minor gland secretions.*

Substance	Unstimulated		Stimulated	
	Mean ± SD	Range	Mean ± SD	Range
Protein (g/l)	2.96 ± 1.02*	1.45–5.60[16]	2.58 ± 0.72*	1.45–3.55[16]
Amylase (IU/l)	903 × 10³ ± 790 × 10³	170 × 10³–2900 × 10³ [62]		
a-D-mannosidase	Present[43]		Present[43]	
Urea (mmol/l)	4.7			
Sodium (mmol/l)	13.9 ± 12.0	2.8–5.8[16]	37.3 ± 22.7	11.0–97.7[16]
Potassium (mmol/l)	19.3 ± 4.9	10.0–29.4[16]	17.3 ± 3.9	10.7–24.9[16]
Calcium (mmol/l)	2.29 ± 0.47	1.60–3.20[16]	2.03 ± 0.38	1.64–2.48[16]
Phosphate (mmol/l) (inorganic)	0.62 ± 0.23	0.25–1.07[16]	0.45 ± 0.11	0.21–0.61[16]
Magnesium (mmol/l)	0.65 ± 0.25	0.41–1.22[16]	0.54 ± 0.14	0.38–0.80[16]
Chloride (mmol/l)	31.4 ± 14.0	16.0–54.3[16]	56.5 ± 29.7	19.0–109.5[16]
Bicarbonate (mmol/l)	<3[16]		<3[16]	

*Lowry method.[61]

49

Table 3.7. *Composition of gingival exudate.*

	Mean ± S.D.
Protein (g/l)	68.3 ± 12.6[2]
Lysozyme (mg/l)	{ 24.4 ± 18.79*[5a] { 48.2 ± 16.02**[5a]
Acid phosphatase (units/ml)	119.6 ± 31.6[59a]
Lactate dehydrogenase	Present[60a]
Albumin ⎤ Fibrinogen ⎟ IgA ⎬ IgM ⎟ IgG ⎦	Concentrations similar to those in plasma[5b]
Sodium (mmol/l)	{ 88.3 ± 31.4[33a] {137.8 ± 42.6*[33a]
Potassium (mmol/l)	{ 17.4 ± 9.0[33a] { 17.5 ± 5.3*[33a]
Calcium (mmol/l)	{ 4.9 ± 1.8[33a] { 9.9 ± 4.9*[33a]

*Gingivitis.
**Periodontitis.

Table 3.8. *Bacterial contaminants of mixed saliva.*

β-N-acetyl-D-glucosaminidase*[43]
Acid phosphatase*[25]
Alkaline phosphatase*[35]
a-L-fucosidase*[43]
a-D-galactosidase[17]
β-D-galactosidase[17, 25]
β-D-glucuronidase[17, 25]
a-D-glucosidase[17]
β-D-glucosidase[17]
L-glutamate dehydrogenase[57]
Hyaluronidase[25]
Lactate dehydrogenase[57]
Lipase[25]
Malate dehydrogenase[57]
Neuraminidase[17, 58, 59]
Non-specific esterase*[25]
Pseudo-cholinesterase*[25]
Succinic dehydrogenase[57]

*Some activity in mixed saliva is salivary in origin.

Flow rate

Variation in flow rate has a marked effect on the concentration of various components in saliva. In general, as the flow rate of parotid saliva is increased slightly above the unstimulated rate, sodium, bicarbonate and pH increase; whereas potassium, calcium, phosphate, chloride, urea and protein decrease. At higher flow rates, sodium, calcium chloride, bicarbonate, protein and pH increase; whereas phosphate decreases and potassium shows little further change (Shannon and Prigmore, 1960; Dawes, 1969).

Diurnal variation

Unstimulated saliva shows significant circadian rhythms with regard to flow rate and in the concentrations of sodium and chloride, but not in the concentrations of protein, potassium, calcium, phosphate and urea (Dawes, 1972). The effect of such rhythms on salivary flow rate and composition must influence the concept of normal values. In any study on salivary constituents, therefore, the time of day when sampling is carried out could have an important bearing on the results.

Age

Saliva can be detected in babies soon after birth (Hymanson and Davidson, 1923; Lourie, 1943). Parotid saliva has been observed in the new-born and it appears that the flow rate of total saliva increases thereafter with age. By 3 to 5 years of age, the parotid resting flow rate is about 0.14 ml/min but decreases sharply over the next few years. Lourie (1943) suggested that this change is related to maturation of a central control mechanism. By 8 to 10 years, the parotid resting flow rate has fallen to a steady value that is at least as low as the average flow rate in the adult. There is a moderate increase in the flow rate of mixed saliva between the ages 8 and 29, and thereafter a slow decrease (Becks and Wainwright, 1943). This slow but steady decrease after 29 years of age may be due to the combined effects of atrophy of the acinar cells and progressive replacement of salivary gland tissue by fat (Chapter 13).

Little is known about the relationship between age and individual salivary constituents, although Becks (1943) demonstrated slight increase in the concentration of calcium and phosphorus in unstimulated total saliva of humans with age.

Sex

It has been claimed that in adult human beings resting and stimulated salivary flow rates are lower in females than in males (Shannon and Prigmore, 1958). It is possible that this difference may be due to a general sexual variation in the weight of the salivary glands, although there is no evidence for this. On the other hand the difference may be due to some other factor; for example, various changes in salivary electrolyte concentration have

51

been described in pregnancy (Marder, Wotman and Mandel, 1972) and during the menstrual cycle (Puskulian, 1972), but no detailed investigations have been carried out to investigate sexual differences in the composition of saliva. It is likely that any differences which do exist are of a subtle nature, and unless great care is exercised in controlling experiments, the differences could be obscured by the large number of other factors which affect salivary composition.

Drugs

The effects of drugs on salivary glands and their secretions have been reviewed by Burgen and Emmelin (1961) and Emmelin (1967). A drug may have no effect on salivary secretion or it may stimulate or suppress the secretion of saliva. In this way salivary composition may be altered by virtue of change in concentration of those constituents which are flow-rate dependent. Drugs may exert their effects by reflex action, by action on the central nervous system, through ganglionic action, via transmitter releasing drugs, cholinesterase inhibitors, parasympathomimetic or parasympatholytic agents and a- and β-sympathomimetic or sympatholytic agents. Many of the experiments which describe the action of drugs on salivary gland secretions were carried out on animals, and the results cannot be directly applied to the human situation. Much has still to be discovered about the effect of drugs on salivary flow rate, and also the effect on the composition of saliva.

The practical importance of the knowledge which we have is that care should be taken in the interpretation of results from patients who are undergoing therapy with drugs known to have an effect on the salivary glands or their secretions (Chapter 8).

Source of saliva

At the present time there are at least three types of cell capable of contributing to the composition of saliva, namely the serous and mucous acinar cells and the lining cells of the ducts. Although the compositions of the mucous and serous acinar secretions differ qualitatively and quantitatively, both are concerned with the transportation of electrolytes from serum to saliva, and synthesise amylase and a variety of mucoid substances. Saliva derived from the different groups of salivary glands varies in composition and the relative contribution of each group to mixed saliva may vary considerably. For instance, parotid saliva is relatively low in calcium when compared with submandibular secretions and most of the salivary amylase is derived from the parotid gland (Dawes, 1965). It is interesting to note that the main anion in the minor mucous gland secretions of the human is chloride (Wood and Dawes, 1968) and that no amylase and very little bicarbonate or phosphate is found in these secretions. Because of the low bicarbonate and phosphate concentrations, the lip mucous gland secretions are poorly buffered. Blood group substances are secreted in much higher concentrations than those present in submandibular saliva.

Considerable species variation may be found with certain constituents. An excellent example of this is provided by the salivary iodide concentration which varies markedly from animal to animal, as shown in Table 3.9, after Cohen and Myant (1959).

Table 3.9. *$S:P$ ^{132}I concentration ratios for mixed saliva and for saliva from separate salivary glands of ten species.* (*Cohen and Myant, 1959.*)

Species	Mixed	Parotid	Submandibular	Sublingual	Residual
Cat	+ +	0	0	+	+ +
Dog	+ + +	+ + +	0 to +	0 to +	+ to + +
Rabbit	+	+	−	−	+
Guinea-pig	+ + +	+ + +	+	+	+
Cotton-rat	+ + +	+ +	+ +	+ +	+
Rat	0	0	0	0	+
Mouse	+ + +	+	+ + +	0	+
Hamster	+ + +	+	+ + +	0	0
Mastomys	+ +	−	+ +	−	−
Man	+ + +	+ + +	+ + +	−	−

$0 = <1, + = 1\text{-}5, + + = 5\text{-}10, + + + = >10.$

Rest transients

A complication associated with the collection of saliva is the possible occurrence of 'rest transients'. It was observed that the concentration of potassium in saliva secreted at the start of a period of stimulation was greater than the concentration found after secretion had continued for a minute or two (Kestyüs and Martin, 1937). This phenomenon has been demonstrated for potassium and iodide in the dog submaxillary gland (Burgen and Seeman, 1958). Burgen (1956) suggested that a reasonable explanation of 'rest transients' is that at the beginning of stimulation the duct cells release their store of potassium into both blood and saliva, until some equilibrium is reached, depending on the strength of the stimulus. The practical importance of 'rest transients' is that if the effect of rate of flow on potassium concentration is studied by taking small samples at each rate, the concentration does appear to be dependent on the flow rate. Rest transients are masked if much larger volumes of saliva are collected at each flow rate (Jenkins, 1966c).

Diet

Dawes (1970a) reviewed the literature dealing with the effects of diet on salivary composition and stressed the difference between the immediate local reflex effect of diet on salivary flow rate, e.g. the relatively high flow rates elicited by highly flavoured diets or diets which require considerable mastication and systemic effects which may take some time to develop. He concluded that there is little evidence that differences in diet can exert systemic effects on salivary flow rate and composition, although high protein diets increase blood urea which, in turn, tend to maintain relatively high salivary urea levels. There is some evidence that the size and activity of the salivary glands is to some extent determined by the degree of functional activity. A regular diet which requires considerable mastication may increase the normal resting salivary flow.

Most mammals which ingest starch in their diet, including man, have the enzyme *a*-amylase in the saliva (Jacobsen, Melvaer and Hensten-Pettersen, 1972). The concentration of salivary amylase is not related to flow rate and appears to be under both neural and humoral control (Newbrun, 1962; Dawes and Jenkins, 1964). The effect of diet upon salivary composition has been examined by several workers and the consensus of opinion is that a high carbohydrate diet leads to elevated amylase levels, whereas a diet rich in protein promotes low amylase concentrations (Squires, 1953; Blumberger and Glatzel, 1963; Hall, Merig and Schneyer, 1967; Wesley-Hadzija and Pigon, 1972; Behall et al, 1973). Bates (1962) however, failed to detect any effect of dietary carbohydrates upon salivary amylase in man. The phenomenon of lower amylase with protein ingestion has been explained by a negative feedback system operating through gastrin (M. M. Ferguson, personal communication, 1974). It is also possible that other gastrointestinal hormones may influence salivary amylase levels (Mulcahy, Fitzgerald and McGeeney, 1972).

Duration and type of stimulus

Dawes (1969, 1970b) has shown that when the flow rate of stimulated parotid saliva is maintained constantly for several minutes, the composition of saliva changes considerably. Total protein, calcium, bicarbonate concentrations and pH increase with duration of stimulation, whereas the chloride concentration decreases. In recent studies (Caldwell and Pigman, 1966; Dawes, 1970c), in which flow rate, duration of stimulation and time of day were standardised, it was found that the nature of the stimulus decidedly influenced the protein concentration of both parotid and submandibular secretions. Other studies have shown that the composition of saliva varies with electric, pharmacological and gustatory stimuli (Dische et al, 1962; Dawes, 1966; Mandel et al, 1968).

Hormones

The sodium concentration of saliva is influenced by several corticosteroids as well as adrenocorticotropic hormone, although the mineralocorticoids, e.g. aldosterone, have been found to exert a more profound effect than glucocorticoids in the respect (Grad, 1952; White et al, 1955; Martin, 1958; Blair West et al, 1967). 17-hydroxycorticosteroids are present in parotid saliva and reflect plasma levels fairly accurately (Shannon et al, 1959; Shannon and Katz, 1964; Shannon, Prigmore and Beening, 1964; Shannon, Prigmore and Gibson, 1964). However, there is a greater ratio of cortisone to cortisol in saliva, as compared with plasma, and this is presumably effected by the presence of 11β-hydroxysteroid dehydrogenase activity in salivary glands (Katz and Shannon, 1964; Ferguson and MacPhee, in press; MacPhee and Ferguson, in press). This particular enzymic activity is found in the salivary ducts (Ferguson, 1967; Ferguson, Glen and Mason, 1970). Other steroids present in parotid saliva include aldosterone, oestradiol-17β and Δ^2-androstenedione (Katz and Shannon, 1964).

Recently, Puskulian (1972), in an investigation into the salivary changes during the normal menstrual cycle, has shown a decrease in the calcium and sodium concentration and an increase in the potassium concentration of submaxillary saliva at the time of ovulation, compared with the time of menstruation. It was suggested that a hormone, probably oestrogen, may be directly or indirectly responsible for the changes in salivary composition.

Size of salivary gland

The most accurate method of expressing salivary flow rate would be ml/min/g of gland, since variation in salivary composition may be due to variation in salivary gland weight. The great difficulty is to assess the weight of the salivary glands. However, Ericson (1970), using a radiographic and statistical method of estimating parotid gland size, has shown the size to be the most important cause of individual differences in the amount of stimulated parotid saliva secreted.

Plasma levels

The salivary concentration of some constituents, for example iodide, calcium and bicarbonate, is dependent on their plasma concentration (Mason, Harden and Alexander, 1966). Salivary levels can be interpreted therefore only if the plasma level is known. For example, as the concentration of iodide rises in plasma, the concentration of iodide in saliva also rises, but the saliva/plasma iodide ratio remains relatively constant.

MEASUREMENT OF SALIVARY CONSTITUENTS

It will be evident, from the above reviews of salivary composition and the factors which may influence it, that the conditions under which saliva is collected must be known before meaningful interpretations of the concentration of a single constituent can be made. This point will be re-emphasised in Chapter 8, where changes in salivary composition in disease are considered. A consequence of multifactorial variation is that a large normal range is quoted for some salivary constituents (Tables 3.2 to 3.6).

PROTECTIVE AND ANTIBACTERIAL FUNCTIONS OF SALIVA

It is probable that the layer of salivary mucus protects the underlying mucosa from the harmful effects of noxious stimuli, microbial toxins and minor trauma. Salivary mucins are basically glycoprotein in nature, and although the carbohydrate side chains comprise quite a large part of the molecule, they show some properties normally associated with polysaccharides. It is the properties of this group of glycoproteins which give saliva its lubricating properties. Salivary mucus coats foodstuffs with a lubricant layer which assists chewing and swallowing. Similarly, the surfaces of the tongue, oral mucosa and teeth have a lubricant coating in order that the complex interactions of these tissues involved in the production of speech can occur. The precise nature and composition of this continuous mucous coat, or sheath as it is sometimes termed, is unknown. The mucus in direct contact with the superficial epithelial cells of the oral mucosa is most likely derived from the secretions of the minor salivary glands, whose ducts open onto the mucosal surface. Recently, Adams (1973) in an investigation of the relationship of saliva and the surface of the oral mucosa, described the development and appearance of a 'fuzzy' coat on the outermost surface of oral epithelial cells. This layer contained mainly acidic mucopolysaccharide (glycosaminoglycan) and appeared to consist of two components; the first and innermost component being derived from microgranules within the cell, and the outer component from salivary mucopolysaccharides and glycoproteins. It has also been shown that the survival rate of Hela cells, which are subjected to changes in osmotic pressure, is enhanced if the cells are protected by a 'coat' of mixed saliva (Adams, 1973). The salivary layer is not stagnant but is constantly renewed by secretions from both minor and major salivary glands. Bloomfield (1921, 1922) has shown that salivary mucus takes a direct and relatively constant course along specific routes towards the oropharynx and is finally swallowed. Microorganisms and foreign particles are 'trapped' in the mucus and eventually destroyed by the gastric juice. This mechanical washing action is probably an important factor in limiting the microbial population of the mouth and preventing primary infection of the oral mucosa.

The antibacterial activity of saliva has been investigated by Bibby, Hine and Clough (1938), Van Kestern, Bibby and Berry (1942) and Kerr and Wedderburn (1958) and reviewed by Burnett and Scherp (1968) and MacFarlane and Mason (1972). Human saliva consists of a number of potential antimicrobial components such as lysozyme, the antilactobacillus thiocyanate-dependent factors, Green's factor, lactoferrin, salivary immunoglobulins and fluoride.

Lysozyme

Salivary lysozyme, first described by Fleming (1922) is derived from a number of sources; from the parotid, submandibular and sublingual glands (Hoerman, Englander and Shklair, 1956), from the gingival exudate (Brandtzaeg and Mann, 1964) and from the lysosomes of the salivary leucocytes. Jolles (1967) has shown that lysozymes from different sources have qualitatively the same biological activity, but different primary structure and specific activities. Salivary lysozyme is therefore not homogeneous in nature, but a mixture of different but closely related substances, and consequently its specific antimicrobial activity is not easily assessed. Inhibition between lysozyme and some constituents of saliva appears to occur in vivo, since Hoerman, Englander and Shklair (1956) described a mucopoly-saccharide present in submandibular-sublingual saliva which selectively inhibited the action of parotid lysozyme. It would appear that lysozyme has little inhibitory effect on the oral commensal flora (Gibbons, De Stoppeller and Harden, 1966), but appears to play a role in preventing non-commensal bacteria from colonising the oral cavity.

It is interesting to note, however, that lysozyme combined with complement and colostral IgA was able to lyse *E. coli* (Adinolfi et al, 1966). There is doubt as to whether this system could function in the mouth due to the anti-complementary nature of saliva, but it is possible that similar interactions may have a protective function in the gingival crevice.

Thiocyanate dependent-factors

It has been suggested by Dogon and Amdur (1970) that two thiocyanate-dependent factors are present in human parotid saliva. The first consists of thiocyanate and an as yet unidentified salivary protein component (Dogon and Amdur, 1965). The second system consists of a peroxidative enzyme, probably lactoperoxidase, thiocyanate and hydrogen peroxide (Klebanoff and Luebke, 1965). These antimicrobial factors are effective only on actively growing micro-organisms, killing them by inhibiting some essential growth factor (Zeldow, 1961). Much of the experimental work into the nature and activity of these factors has been carried out using parotid saliva, although anti-lactobacillus activity has been demonstrated using mixed saliva. The antibacterial activity of Klebanoff's factor in vivo is uncertain, since catalase which is produced by oral micro-organisms and by the cellular activities of the host is known to inhibit its action. The antibacterial effect of the thiocyanate-dependent factors on lactobacilli has been fully demonstrated, but the effect on the other oral commensal bacteria is unknown. There is some evidence that *E. coli*, and perhaps other coliform bacilli, are inhibited by thiocyanate-dependent factors (Klebanoff, Clem and Luebke, 1966).

Green's factor

The bacteriolytic factor described by Green (1959, 1966) in the saliva of caries-free individuals was believed to be important in protecting them against dental caries. However, there has been no evidence to suggest that the factor had any role to play in the general defence of the oral mucosa. Since Geddes (1972), in a reassessment of Green's work, was unable to demonstrate the factor in caries-free parotid saliva, the importance of Green's Factor is in considerable doubt.

Lactoferrin

Lactoferrin is an iron-binding protein normally present in milk. Masson, Heremans and Dive (1966) described lactoferrin in human saliva, other body fluids and in the lysosomes of polymorphonuclear leucocytes. It has been suggested that the iron-binding properties of this protein are of importance in protecting mucosal surfaces against infection. The precise way in which lactoferrin accomplishes its protective role is unknown. However, iron is essential for bacterial growth and if the host can deny iron to a potentially pathogenic bacterium, infection by that bacterium may be prevented. It is likely, therefore, that due to its strong iron-binding activity lactoferrin has an important role to play in the host defence to bacterial infection. There is at the moment no experimental work dealing with the antibacterial activity of lactoferrin on the commensal oral flora, although it is known that *Staph. aureus* and *P. aeruginosa* are inhibited (Masson et al, 1966).

Hydrogen ion concentration and buffering capacity

The pH of mixed saliva varies widely in any one individual; the normal range is 5.6 to 7.0 with an average value of 6.7. Many factors affect the pH and buffering capacity of saliva; the more important factors being salivary flow rate and the duration of stimulation. Although bicarbonate is the most important buffer in saliva, phosphate probably plays a small part (Lilienthal, 1955). The pH and buffering capacity of saliva may protect the oral tissues in two ways. Firstly, since many bacteria require specific pH conditions for maximal growth, saliva may deny such conditions and thereby prevent potential pathogens from colonising the mouth. It is of interest to note that the carrier rate of *C. albicans* in healthy young adults with a salivary pH 5.0 to 5.5 was 90 per cent compared with a carrier rate of 56 per cent in subjects with a pH of 6.5 to 7.0 (Young, Resca and Sullivan, 1951). Secondly it is possible that a relatively steady pH of about 6.7 is necessary for maximal activity of salivary antimicrobial agents and microbial antagonisms.

THE IMMUNOGLOBULINS

Salivary immunoglobulins have been reviewed by Brandtzaeg (1972). In terms of their protective function human salivary glands have a local immunological system which comprises largely secretory IgA with small amounts of IgG and IgM. Secretory piece which is glycoprotein in nature is conjugated with IgA in the secretory cells of the salivary glands and confers chemical stability on the IgA molecule, thereby increasing IgA's resistance to degradation in the very changeable environment of the mouth. Mixed saliva also receives variable amounts of IgG, IgA, and IgM from crevicular exudate (Brandtzaeg, 1965). Although the exact details of the in vivo function of salivary immunoglobulins are not known, a number of possible functions have been suggested. The oral tissues are covered with a coat of mucus, and present in this layer is secretory IgA, which has a well-developed agglutinating capacity (Newcomb and de Vald, 1969). It is probable that antigens in the form of bacteria and viruses are trapped in the mucous coat, are transported by the mechanical washing action of saliva to the stomach and are there inactivated by gastric juice. The mechanical washing action of saliva would similarly dispose of clumps of bacteria, agglutinated by IgA. It has also been suggested that IgA may complex with the protein covering of the oral epithelium and teeth, thus giving rise to a protective immunoglobulin coat (Heremans, Crabbie and Masson, 1966). The incorporation of IgA into the dental pellicle could perhaps give some protection against plaque formation. However, in contrast to this it is just as likely that IgA, due to its agglutinating activity, may participate in plaque formation by assisting in the formation of bacterial aggregates on the teeth. Oral bacteria which are coated with IgA are more easily phagocytosed by leucocytes and possibly more actively destroyed than bacteria coated with IgG and IgM. Although phagocytosis may occur in the gingival crevice and within the oral tissues, it is unlikely to occur to any extent in saliva or the epithelial surface.

The relationship of salivary immunoglobulins and oral disease has been investigated by a number of workers. There is evidence which suggests that the synthesis of salivary IgA antibodies can be specifically stimulated by micro-organisms proliferating in the oral cavity. Lehner, Cardwell and Clarry (1967) and Zengo et al (1971) found increased amounts of IgA in patients with a high resistance to dental caries, but Shklair, Rovelstad and Lamberts (1969) found no difference. It has been shown in primates, however, that a combination of intravenous injection and oral infection with live streptococci can inhibit the development of dental caries (Bowen, 1969). An increase in salivary IgA, IgM and IgG has been reported in patients with periodontitis when compared with normal individuals (Brandtzaeg, Fjellanger and Gjeruldsen, 1970) and raised titres of salivary immuno-globulins have been reported by Lehner (1965) in the saliva of patients with oral candida infections. IgA cannot fix complement and as a result a direct bacteriolytic effect has not been found. In combination with complement and lysozyme, however, human colostral IgA was able to lyse *E. coli.* Since saliva is anti-complementary it is unlikely that this system functions in the oral cavity, although it may act in the gingival crevice. It is notable that secretory IgA decreases with increase in flow rate and it may be that the high concentration of secretory IgA occurring in saliva secreted when there is minimal stimulation, e.g. during sleep, confers a protective antibacterial activity (Mandel and Khurana, 1969).

Although it is well known that immunoglobulins are present in saliva, there is no direct evidence that they can influence the development or course of dental disease in man. Brandtzaeg, Fjellanger and Gjeruldsen (1970) reported that there was no apparent increase in the incidence or severity of caries or gingival inflammation in the few patients with hypogammaglobulin-aemia whom they had studied.

BLOOD GROUP FACTORS

Approximately 80 per cent of individuals secrete their ABO blood group substances in high concentration in saliva. By definition, all secretors secrete H substance, while individuals of groups A, B and AB also secrete the group substances corresponding to their group. In forensic science, determination of the secretor status of a stain may be of importance. Since saliva contains amylase in high concentration the starch-iodide reaction or the use of starch agar plates are useful tests which act as a guide in determining whether or not a stain is of salivary origin. The secretor status of dried saliva stains may be established either by indirect inhibition methods or the newer direct techniques of mixed agglutination (Coombs and Dodd, 1961) and absorption-elution (Nickolls and Pereira, 1962). It is worthy of note that H substance is not evenly distributed throughout the stain but tends to be concentrated in the inner part, so that unless sampling is adequate a secretor may be missed (Pereira, 1967). It is also of interest that the concentration of blood group substances appear especially high in minor gland secretion (Milne and Dawes, 1973) and sublingual saliva (Wolf and Taylor, 1964). Blood group activity is negligible in parotid saliva, and sublingual and minor gland secretions contribute about 70 per cent of the blood group substances in whole saliva (Milne and Dawes, 1973). The high levels of activity in saliva from the labial salivary glands may be of value to forensic scientists in the detection of blood group substances on cigarette paper. It should be noted that if saliva in sufficient quantity can be obtained from a bite mark or any object which has come into contact with the mouth, then it may be possible to determine the blood group of the subject who made it. However, contamination of saliva in bite marks by various animal and vegetable substances may confuse results. Furthermore, following a bite, the subsequent bleeding into the wound might wash away the saliva. It is clear that from a forensic point of view no conclusion can be reached if blood groups of victim and suspect are identical. A comprehensive review of the role of saliva in forensic odontology has been published recently (Clift and Lamont, 1974).

It has been shown that salivary protein concentrations vary markedly according to an individual's blood group, tending to be high in subjects of group A. Furthermore, saliva IgA concentrations tend to be higher in ABH secretors than in non-secretors (Waissliluth and Langman, 1971). The relationship of blood group substances, secretor status and dental caries is conflicting. Witkop, Barros and Hamilton (1962) found no difference among the divisions of ABO groups and caries prevalence, whereas Aitchison and Carmichael (1962) found a greater liability to caries in blood group A. It would appear that if significant differences in blood group distribution among caries-resistant and caries-susceptible individuals exist, they are more likely to reflect genetic differences rather than the blood group factor glycoproteins directly affecting dental caries activity (Mandel, 1974).

PAROTIN

In 1954, Ito reported the extraction of a protein from bovine parotid gland which he named parotin. This substance was considered to function as a salivary gland hormone and when injected into rabbits had the effect of reducing blood calcium, increasing leucocyte count and enhancing the calcification of incisor dentine. A similar active substance was found in bovine submandibular gland and in human saliva and urine, and the calcium lowering action suggested as a bio-assay for the hormone (Ito, 1960). Effects on enamel, developing bone, ovary and testis after injection of parotin in mice have also been reported (Fleming, 1960). Although blood calcium reduction following parotin injection has been confirmed by Lazarus and Shepherd (1969), these workers strongly suggest that the effect is due to fasting, since control fasting animals also displayed reduced blood calcium. The status of parotin as a hormone is very much in doubt, although further investigations are warranted (Jenkins, 1966e).

NERVE GROWTH FACTOR

Extracts of mouse submandibular gland have been shown to markedly increase the growth of sympathetic ganglia and sensory nerves (Levi-Montalcini and Cohen, 1960). The active substance, termed nerve growth factor (NGF) has also been detected in mouse sarcomas, snake venoms and in neuroblastoma and sympathetic chain tissue in man.

Purification of mouse NGF has established it as a protein having a molecular weight of 28 000 to 30 000 Daltons. The active factor comprises two similar subunits with similar amino-acid compositions which can be dissociated. Similar structural and functional properties have been observed in NGF and insulin (Frazier, Angeletti and Bradshaw, 1972). Anti-serum to NGF has been produced (Cohen, 1960) which destroys nerve cells of the sympathetic ganglion when injected into newborn mice and rats. It has been reported by Burdman and Goldstein (1961) that children with neuroblastomas have higher serum concentrations of NGF than normal. Recently, the production of human NGF in a patient with a liposarcoma has been reported (Waddell et al, 1972). Blood and tumour tissue from this patient and the growth media of cultured tumour cells contained NGF by biological assay. Most interestingly, also, this patient developed an overgrowth of nerve tissue, presumably secondary to humoral stimulation, at the site of a cholecystectomy. The discovery of NGF has been an exciting one and a great deal remains to be learned about its primary site of production and how it acts.

Immuno-sympathectomised animals provide ideal material on which to test current theories on the role of the sympathetic nervous system and the way in which structures innervated by it can be affected by drugs (Zaimis, 1972; *Lancet*, 1972).

EPIDERMAL GROWTH FACTOR

Epidermal growth factor is an extract of male mouse submandibular salivary gland (Cohen, 1962). When injected into newborn mice it has the effect of increasing tooth eruption and eyelid opening. Enhanced epithelial keratinisation is observed in skin, whilst epithelial thickening of the lining of the oral cavity, oesophagus and stomach occurs (Cohen and Elliott, 1963; Cohen, 1964). The active component of epidermal growth factor is an antigenic protein which may be inactivated by heating in acid or alkali and by

61

proteolysis. The biological effect of the growth factor is observed when doses of 1 to 8 ug/1.5 g body weight per day are injected into newborn mice. Angeletti et al (1964) have shown the epithelial cell hyperplasia to be associated with an increase in protein and nucleic acid content and phosphatase, histidase and lactate dehydrogenase activity. From tissue culture experiments evidence has been provided that epidermal growth factor acts directly on skin and that the presence of dermis is not necessary for the biological effect (Cohen, 1964).

OTHER GROWTH FACTORS

Since the finding of nerve growth factor, subsequent studies have led to the isolation from mouse submandibular gland of other extracts which have a profound effect upon the growth of specific cells. Factors influencing the growth of chick cardiac cells (Bast and Mills, 1963), neural tube cells in organ culture (Adler and Narbaitz, 1965), and mesenchymal cells (Attardi et al, 1967) have been described. In addition, a thymocyte-transforming factor (Hoffman et al, 1967) and a fibroblast growth factor (Green, Tomita and Varon, 1971) have also been reported. Several of these factors are intimately associated with active esteropeptidases (Martinez-Hernandez, Nakane and Pierce, 1972).

REFERENCES

Adams, D. (1973) *Saliva, the Mucus Barrier and the Health of the Oral Mucosa.* Ph. D. Thesis, University of Wales.

Adinolfi, M., Glynn, A. A., Lindsay, M. & Milne, C. M. (1966) Serological properties of gamma A antibodies to *E. coli* present in human colostrum. *Immunology,* **10,** 515.

Adler, R. & Narbaitz, R. (1965) Action of rat submaxillary gland extracts on neural tube growth in organ culture. *Journal of Embryology and Experimental Morphology,* **14,** 281.

Afonsky, D. (1961) *Saliva and its Relation to Oral Health.* Birmingham: University of Alabama Press.

Aitchison, J. & Carmichael, A. F. (1962) The relationship between ABO blood mutations and dental caries. *Dental Practitioner and Dental Record,* **13,** 94.

Angeletti, P. U., Gandini-Attardi, D., Toschi, G., Salvi, M. L. & Levi-Montalcini, R. (1964) Azione dell' "epidermal growth factor" sulla sintesi di acidi nucleici e proteine dell' epitello cutaneo. *Experientia,* **20,** 146.

Attardi, D. G. R., Levi-Montalcini, R., Wenger, B. S. & Angeletti, P. U. (1967) Submaxillary gland of the mouse: effects of a fraction on tissues of mesodermal origin in virto. *Science,* **156,** 1253.

Bast, E. M. & Mills, K. S. (1963) Mouse submaxillary gland extract as a growth stimulator and orientor of chick cardiac cells in vitro. *Growth,* **27,** 295.

Bates, J. F. (1962) Some observations on the relationship between the concentration of parotid amylase and dietary carbohydrate in human subjects. *British Dental Journal,* **112,** 114.

Becks, H. (1943) Human saliva. XIV. Total calcium content of resting saliva of 650 healthy individuals. *Journal of Dental Research,* **22,** 397.

Becks, H. & Wainwright, W. W. (1943) Rate of flow of resting saliva of healthy individuals. *Journal of Dental Research,* **22,** 391.

Behall, K. M., Kelsay, J. L., Holden, J. M. & Clark, W. M. (1973) Amylase and protein in parotid saliva after load doses of different dietary carbohydrates. *American Journal of Clinical Nutrition,* **26,** 17.

Bibby, B. G., Hine, M. K. & Clough, O. W. (1938) The antibacterial action of human saliva. *Journal of the American Dental Association,* **25,** 1290.

Blair-West, J. R., Coglan, J. P., Denton, D. A. & Wright, R. D. (1967) Effect of endocrines on salivary glands. In *Handbook of Physiology Section 6, Alimentary Canal, Vol. II. Secretion,* (Ed.) Code, C. F. pp. 639-640. Washington, D.C.: American Physiology Society.

Bloomfield, A. L. (1921) Dissemination of bacteria in the upper air passes. 1. The circulation of foreign particles in the mouth. *American Review of Tuberculosis and Pulmonary Diseases* (Baltimore), **5,** 903.

Bloomfield, A. L. (1922) Dissemination of bacteria in the upper air passages. II. The circulation of bacteria in the mouth. *Johns Hopkins Hospital Bulletin,* **33,** 145.

Blumberger, W. & Glatzel, H. (1963) The variability of saliva secretion and saliva quality of a healthy man and its relation to the type of diet. *Deutsche Zeitschrift für Verdauungs- und Stoffwechselkrankheiten,* **23,** 210.

Bowen, W. H. (1969) A vaccine against dental caries. A pilot experiment in monkeys (Macaca irus). *British Dental Journal,* **126,** 159.

Brandtzaeg, P. (1965) Immunochemical comparison of proteins in human gingival pocket fluid, serum and saliva. *Archives of Oral Biology,* **10,** 795.

Brandtzaeg, P. (1972) Local formation and transport of immunoglobulins related to the oral cavity. In *Host Resistance to Commensal Bacteria,* (Ed.) MacPhee, T. Edinburgh: Churchill Livingstone.

Brandtzaeg, P. & Mann, W. V. (1964) A comparative study of the lysozyme activity of human gingival pocket fluid, serum and saliva. *Acta Odontologica Scandinavica,* **22,** 441.

Brandtzaeg, P., Fjellanger, I. & Gjeruldsen, S. T. (1970) Human secretory immunoglobulins. I. Salivary secretions from individuals with normal or low levels of serum immunoglobulins. *Haematology,* Supplementum 12, 1.

Burdman, J. A. & Goldstein, M. N. (1961) Long term tissue culture of neuroblastomas. III. In vitro studies of a nerve growth-stimulating in sera of children with neuroblastoma. *Journal of the National Cancer Institute,* **33,** 123.

Burgen, A. S. V. (1956) The secretion of potassium in saliva. *Journal of Physiology,* **132,** 20.

Burgen, A. S. V. & Emmelin, N. G. (1961) *Physiology of the Salivary Glands.* pp. 72-93, 144, 218. London: Arnold.

Burgen, A. S. V. & Seeman, P. (1958) The role of the salivary duct system in the formation of saliva. *Canadian Journal of Biochemistry and Physiology,* **36,** 119.

Burnett, G. W. & Scherp, H. W. (1968) *Oral Microbiology and Infectious Disease.* 3rd edition. pp. 309-324. Baltimore: Williams and Wilkins Company.

Caldwell, R. C. & Pigman, W. (1966) Changes in protein and glycoprotein concentrations in human submaxillary saliva under various stimulatory conditions. *Archives of Oral Biology,* **11,** 437.

Chauncey, H. H., Shannon, I. L. & Feller, R. P. (1967) Effect of oral and nasal chemoreception on parotid gland secretions. In *Secretory Mechanisms of the Salivary Glands,* (Eds.) Schneyer, L. H. & Schneyer, C. A. p. 351.

Clift, A. & Lamont, C. M. (1974) Saliva in forensic odontology. *Journal of the Forensic Science Society,* **14,** 241.

Cohen, B., Logothetopoulos, J. H. & Myant, N. B. (1955) Autoradiographic localisation of iodine-131 in the salivary glands of the hamster. *Nature (London),* **176,** 1268.

Cohen, B. & Myant, N. B. (1959) Concentration of salivary iodide, a comparative study. *Journal of Physiology,* **145,** 595.

Cohen, S. (1960) Purification of a nerve growth-promoting protein from the mouse salivary gland and its neurocytotoxic antiserum. *Proceedings of the National Academy of Sciences of the United States of America,* **46,** 302.

Cohen, S. (1962) Isolation of a mouse submaxillary gland protein accelerating incisor eruption and eyelid opening in the new-born animal. *Journal of Biological Chemistry,* **237,** 1555.

Cohen, S. (1964) Isolation and biological effects of an epidermal growth-stimulating protein. In *Metabolic Control Mechanisms in Animal Cells. National Cancer Institute Monographs,* **13,** 13.

Cohen, S. & Elliott, G. A. (1963) The stimulation of epidermal caratinization by a protein isolated from the submaxillary gland of the mouse. *Journal of Investigative Dermatology,* **40,** 1.

Coombs, R. R. A. & Dodd, B. (1961) Possible application of the principle of mixed agglutination in the identification of blood stains. *Medicine, Science and the Law,* **1,** 357.

Davenport, H. W. (1961) *Physiology of the Digestive Tract.* Chicago: Year Book Medical Publishers Incorporated.

Dawes, C. (1965) Some characteristics of parotid and submandibular salivary proteins. *Archives of Oral Biology,* **10,** 269.

Dawes, C. (1966) The composition of human saliva secreted in response to a gustatory stimulus and to pilocarpine. *Journal of Physiology,* **183,** 360.

Dawes, C. (1969) The effects of flow rate and duration of stimulation on the concentration of protein and the main electrolytes in human parotid saliva. *Archives of Oral Biology,* **14,** 277.

Dawes, C. (1970a) Effect of diet on salivary secretion and composition. *Journal of Dental Research,* **49,** 1263.

Dawes, C. (1970b) The approach to plasma levels of the chloride concentration in human parotid saliva at high flow rates. *Archives of Oral Biology,* **15,** 97.

Dawes, C. (1970c) Effects of different stimuli on the protein content of human parotid saliva. *IADR (North American Division),* Abstract No. 498.

Dawes, C. (1972) Circadian rhythms in human salivary flow rate and composition. *Journal of Physiology,* **220,** 529.

Dawes, C. & Jenkins, G. N. (1964) The effects of different stimulation on the composition of saliva in man. *Journal of Physiology,* **119,** 153.

Dawes, C. & Wood, C. M. (1973) The contribution of oral minor mucous gland secretions to the volume of whole saliva in man. *Archives of Oral Biology,* **18,** 337.

Dische, Z., Pallavicini, C., Kavasaki, H., Smirnow, N., Cizak, L. J. & Chien, S. (1962) Influence of the nature of the secretory stimulus on the composition of the carbohydrate moiety of glycoproteins of the submaxillary saliva. *Archives of Biochemistry and Biophysics,* **97,** 459.

Dogon, I. L. & Amdur, B. H. (1965) Further characterization of an antibacterial factor in human parotid secretions active against *Lactobacillus casei. Archives of Oral Biology,* **10,** 605.

Dogon, I. L. & Amdur, B. H. (1970) Evidence for the presence of two thiocyanage-dependent antibacterial systems in human saliva. *Archives of Oral Biology,* **15,** 987.

Ellison, S. A. (1967) Proteins and glycoproteins of saliva. In *Handbook of Physiology, Section 6, Alimentary Canal, Vol. II: Secretion,* (Ed.) Code, C. F. pp. 531-559. Washington, D. C.: American Physiology Society.

Emmelin, N. (1967) Pharmacology of salivary glands. In *Handbook of Physiology, Section 6, Alimentary Canal, Vol. II: Secretion,* (Ed.) Code, C. F. pp. 665-678. Washington, D.C.: American Physiology Society.

Emmelin, N. & Zotterman, Y. (1972) *Oral Physiology.* Oxford: Pergamon Press.

Ericson, S. (1970) The normal variation of the parotid size. *Acta Otolaryngologica,* **70,** 294.

Ericson, S. (1971) The variability of the human parotid flow rate on stimulation with citric acid, with special reference to taste. *Archives of Oral Biology,* **16,** 9.

Ferguson, M. M. (1967) Utilization of 11β-hydroxysteroids by the salivary gland ducts. *Histochemie,* **9,** 269.

Ferguson, M. M. & MacPhee, G. B. (1974) Kinetic study of 11β-hydroxysteroid dehydrogenase in rat submandibular salivary gland. *Archives of Oral Biology* (in press).

Ferguson, M. M., Glen, J. B. & Mason, D. K. (1970) Cortisol utilization by salivary gland, kidney and adrenal cortex. *Journal of Endocrinology,* **47,** 511.

Fleming, A. (1922) On a remarkable bacteriolytic element found in the tissues and secretions. *Proceedings of the Royal Society,* **B93,** 306.

Fleming, H. S. (1960) The effect of parotin in mice. *Annals of the New York Academy of Sciences,* **85,** 313.

Frazier, W. A., Angeletti, R. H. & Bradshaw, R. A. (1972) Nerve growth factor and insulin. Structural similarities indicate an evolutionary relationship reflected by physiological action. *Science,* **176,** 482.

Geddes, D. A. (1972) Failure to demonstrate the antibacterial factor of Green in caries-free parotid saliva. In *Host Resistance to Commensal Bacteria,* (Ed.) MacPhee, T. pp. 84-89. Edinburgh: Churchill Livingstone.

Gibbons, R. J., De Stoppellar, J. D. & Harden, L. (1966) Lysozyme insensitivity of bacteria indigenous to the oral cavity of man. *Journal of Dental Research*, **45,** 877.

Grad, B. (1952) The influence of ACTH on the sodium and potassium concentration of human mixed saliva. *Journal of Clinical Endocrinology and Metabolism*, **12,** 708.

Green, G. E. (1959) A bacteriolytic agent in salivary globulin of caries-immune human beings. *Journal of Dental Research*, **38,** 262.

Green, G. E. (1966) Properties of a salivary bacteriolysin and comparison with serum beta lysin. *Journal of Dental Research*, **45,** 882.

Greene, L. A., Tomita, J. T. & Varon, S. (1971) Growth stimulating activities of mouse submaxillary esteropeptidases on chick embryo fibroblasts in vitro. *Experimental Cell Research*, **64,** 385.

Hall, H. D., Merig, J. J. & Schneyer, C. A. (1967) Metrecal-induced changes in human saliva. *Proceedings of the Society for Experimental Biology and Medicine*, **124,** 532.

Henriques, B. L. (1961) Acinar duct transport in dogs' submaxillary salivary gland (Abstract). *Journal of Dental Research*, **40,** 719.

Henriques, B. L. (1962) A technique of studying salivary gland function. *American Journal of Physiology*, **203,** 1086.

Heremans, J. F., Crabbie, P. A. & Masson, P. L. (1966) Biological significance of exocrine gamma-A-immunoglobulin. *Acta Medica Scandinavica*, **179** (Supplement 445), 84.

Hoerman, K. C., Englander, H. R. & Shklair, I. L. (1956) Lysozyme: its characteristics in human parotid and submaxillo-lingual saliva. *Proceedings of the Society for Experimental Biology and Medicine*, **92,** 875.

Hoffman, H., Naughton, M. A., McDougall, J. & Hamilton, E. A. (1967) Nerve growth factor and a thymus inhibitor, separation by tissue culture on acrylamide gel. *Nature*, **214,** 703.

Hymanson, A. & Davidsohn, H. (1923) The saliva of the nursling. *American Journal of Diseases of Children*, **25,** 302.

Ito, Y. (1954) Biochemical studies on salivary gland hormone. *Endocrinologia Japonica*, **1,** 1.

Ito, Y. (1960) Parotin: A salivary gland hormone. *Annals of the New York Academy of Sciences*, **85,** 228.

Jacobsen, N., Melvaer, K. L. & Heristen-Pettersen, A. (1972) Some properties of salivary amylase: A survey of the literature and some observations. *Journal of Dental Research*, **51,** 381.

Jenkins, G. N. (1966a) *The Physiology of the Mouth.* 3rd edition. p. 328. Oxford: Blackwell Scientific Publications.

Jenkins, G. N. (1966b) *The Physiology of the Mouth,* 3rd edition. pp. 305-319. Oxford: Blackwell Scientific Publications.

Jenkins, G. N. (1966c) *The Physiology of the Mouth.* 3rd edition. pp. 306-307. Oxford: Blackwell Scientific Publications.

Jenkins, G. N. (1966d) *The Physiology of the Mouth.* 3rd edition. pp. 290-291. Oxford: Blackwell Scientific Publications.

Jenkins, G. N. (1966e) *The Physiology of the Mouth.* 3rd edition. p. 344. Oxford: Blackwell Scientific Publications.

Jolles, P. (1967) Relationship between chemical structure and biological activity of hen egg-white lysozyme and lysozymes of different species. *Proceedings of the Royal Society*, **B167,** 350.

Junqueira, L. C. U. (1964) Studies on the physiology of rat and mouse salivary glands. III. On the function of the striated ducts of mammalian salivary glands. In *Salivary Glands and their Secretions*, (Eds.) Screebny, L. M. & Meyer, J. p. 123. Oxford: Pergamon Press.

Katz, F. H. & Shannon, I. L. (1964) Identification and significance of parotid fluid corticosteroids. *Acta Endocrinologica*, **46,** 393.

Kerr, A. C. (1961) The physiological regulation of salivary secretion in man. *International Series of Monographs on Oral Biology.* p. 9. Oxford: Pergamon Press.

Kerr, A. C. & Wedderburn, D. L. (1958) Antibacterial factors in the secretions of human parotid and submaxillary glands. *British Dental Journal*, **105,** 321.

Kestyüs, L. & Martin, J. (1937) Über den Einfluens von Chorda und sympathicus Reizung aus die Zurammensitzung des submaxillar Speichels. *Pflugers Archiv für die gesemte Physiologie des Menschen und der Tiere*, **239,** 408.

Klebanoff, S. J. & Luebke, R. G. (1965) The antilactobacillus system of saliva. Role of salivary peroxidase. *Proceedings for the Society for Experimental Biology and Medicine*, **118,** 483.

Klebanoff, S. J., Clem, W. H. & Luebke, R. G. (1966) The peroxidase-thiocyanate-hydrogen peroxide antimicrobial system. *Biochimica et Biophysica Acta* (Amsterdam), **117,** 63.

Klinkhammer, J. M. (1968) Quantitative evaluation of gingivitis and periodontal disease. *Periodontics,* **6,** 207.

Lancet (1972) Leading article—Nerve growth factor. *Lancet,* **ii,** 1375.

Lazarus, J. H. & Shepherd, J. B. (1969) The influence of parotin on serum calcium in rabbits. *Archives of Oral Biology,* **14,** 87.

Lehner, T. (1965) Immunofluorescent investigation of Candida albicans antibodies in human saliva. *Archives of Oral Biology,* **10,** 975.

Lehner, T., Cardwell, J. E. & Clarry, E. D. (1967) Immunoglobulins in saliva and serum in dental caries. *Lancet,* **i,** 1294.

Levi-Montalcini, R. & Cohen, S. (1960) Effects of the extract of the mouse submaxillary salivary glands on the sympathetic system of mammals. *Annals of the New York Academy of Sciences,* **85,** 324.

Lilienthal, B. (1955) An analysis of the buffer system in saliva. *Journal of Dental Research,* **34,** 516.

Lourie, R. S. (1943) Rate of secretion of parotid glands in normal children. *American Journal of Diseases of Children,* **65,** 455.

MacFarlane, T. W. & Mason, D. K. (1972) Local environmental factors in the host resistance to commensal microflora of the mouth. In *Host Resistance to Commensal Bacteria,* (Ed.) MacPhee, T. pp. 64-75. Edinburgh: Churchill Livingstone.

McKeown, K. C. & Dunstone, G. H. (1959) Some observations on salivary secretion and fluid absorption by mouth. *British Medical Journal,* **ii,** 670.

Mandel, I. D. (1974) Relation of saliva and plaque to caries. *Journal of Dental Research,* **53,** 246.

Mandel, I. D. & Khurana, H. S. (1969) The relation of human salivary γA globulin and albumin to flow rate. *Archives of Oral Biology,* **14,** 1433.

Mandel, I. D., Katz, R., Zengo, A., Kutscher, A. H., Greenberg, R. A., Katz, S., Sharf, R. & Pintoff, A. (1968) The effect of pharmacologic agents on salivary secretion and composition in man. Pilocarpine, atropine and anticholinesterases. *Journal of Oral Therapeutics and Pharmacology,* **4,** 192.

MacPhee, G. B. & Ferguson, M. M. (1974) 11β-Hydroxysteroid dehydrogenase in subcellular particulates of rat submandibular salivary gland. *Pharmacology and Therapeutics in Dentistry* (in press).

Marder, M. Z., Wotman, S. & Mandel, I. D. (1972) Salivary electrolyte changes during pregnancy. *Journal of Obstetrics and Gynecology,* **112,** 233.

Martin, J. A. (1958) Interet des dosages sodium et potassium salivaires pour l'exploration corticosurrenalienne. *Annales de Biologie Clinique,* **16,** 546.

Martinez-Hernandez, A., Nakane, P. K. & Pierce, P. K. (1972) The secretory granules of the acinar cells of the mouse submaxillary gland. *American Journal of Anatomy,* **133,** 259.

Mason, D. K., Harden, R. McG. & Alexander, W. D. (1966) Problems of interpretation in studies of salivary constituents. *Journal of Oral Medicine,* **21,** 66.

Masson, P. L., Heremans, J. F. & Dive, C. H. (1966) An iron-binding protein common to many external secretions. *International Journal of Clinical Chemistry,* **14,** 735.

Masson, P. L., Heremans, J. F., Prignot, J. J. & Wauters, G. (1966) Immunohistochemical localization and bacteriostatic properties of an iron binding protein and bronchial mucus. *Thorax,* **21,** 538.

Milne, R. W. & Dawes, C. (1973) Relative contributions of different salivary glands to the blood group activity of whole saliva in humans. *Vox Sanguinis,* **25,** 298.

Mulcahy, H., Fitzgerald, O. & McGeeney, K. F. (1972) Secretion and pancreozymin effect on salivary amylase concentrations in man. *Gut,* **13,** 850.

Newbrun, E. (1962) Observations on the amylase content and flow rate of human saliva following gustatory stimulation. *Journal of Dental Research,* **41,** 459.

Newcomb, R. W. & de Vald, B. L. (1969) Antibody activities of human exocrine γA diphtheria antitoxin. *Federation Proceedings,* **28,** 765.

Nickolls, L. C. & Pereira, M. (1962) A study of modern methods of grouping dried blood stains. *Medicine, Science and the Law,* **2,** 172.

Pereira, M. (1967) New techniques in forensic immunology. In *Modern Trends in Forensic Medicine,* (Ed.) Simpson, K. pp. 95-114. London: Butterworths.

Petersen, O. H. (1972) Electrolyte transports involved in the formation of saliva. In *Oral Physiology*, (Eds.) Emmelin, N. & Zotterman, Y. pp. 21-31. Oxford & New York: Pergamon Press.

Puskulian, L. (1972) Salivary electrolyte changes during the normal menstrual cycle. *Journal of Dental Research*, **51**, 1212.

Schneyer, L. H. (1955) Method for the collection of separate submaxillary and sublingual saliva in man. *Journal of Dental Research*, **34**, 257.

Schneyer, L. H., Pigman, W., Hanahan, L. B. & Gilmour, R. N. (1956) Rate of flow of human parotid, sublingual and submaxillary secretions during sleep. *Journal of Dental Research*, **35**, 109.

Schneyer, L. H. & Schneyer, C. A. (1967) Inorganic composition of saliva. In *Handbook of Physiology, Section 6, Alimentary Canal, Vol. II: Secretion*, (Ed.) Code, C. F. pp. 497-530. Washington, D.C.: American Physiology Society.

Screebry, L. & Meyer, J. (1964) *Salivary Glands and their Secretions*. Oxford: Pergamon Press.

Shannon, I. L. & Prigmore, J. R. (1958) Physiologic chloride and levels in human whole saliva. *Proceedings of the Society for Experimental Biology and Medicine*, **97**, 825.

Shannon, I. L. & Prigmore, J. R. (1960) Parotid fluid flow rate. Its relationship to pH and chemical composition. *Oral Surgery, Oral Medicine and Oral Pathology*, **13**, 1488.

Shannon, I. L. & Katz, F. H. (1964) Free 17-hydroxycorticosteroid concentration of parotid fluid following intra-venous administration of cortisol. *Oral Surgery, Oral Medicine and Oral Pathology*, **78**, 403.

Shannon, I. L., Prigmore, J. R. & Beering, S. C. (1964) Base line values for the intramuscular ACTH test based on parotid fluid free 17-hydroxycorticosteroid levels. *Journal of Clinical Endocrinology and Metabolism*, **23**, 1258.

Shannon, I. L., Prigmore, J. R., Brooks, R. A. & Feller, R. P. (1959) The 17-hydroxycorticosteroids of parotid fluid, serum and urine following intramuscular administration of repository corticotrophin. *Journal of Clinical Endocrinology and Metabolism*, **19**, 1477.

Shannon, I. L., Prigmore, J. R. & Gibson, W. A. (1964) Parotid fluid and urine 17-hydroxycorticosteroid levels following graded intramuscular doses of corticotrophin. *Archives of Oral Biology*, **9**, 87.

Shannon, I. L., Suddick, R. P. & Dowd, F. J. jr. (1974) *Saliva: Composition and Secretion*. Basel: S. Karger.

Shklair, I. L., Rovelstad, G. H. & Lamberts, B. L. (1969) A study of some factors influencing phagocytosis of cariogenic streptococci by caries-free and caries-active individuals. *Journal of Dental Research*, **48**, 842.

Squires, B. T. (1953) Human salivary amylase secretion in relation to diet. *Journal of Physiology*, **119**, 153.

Stephen, K. W., Robertson, J. W. K., Harden, R. McG. & Chisholm, D. M. (1973) Concentration of iodide, pertechnetate, thiocyanate and bromide in saliva from parotid, submandibular and minor salivary glands in man. *Journal of Laboratory and Clinical Medicine*, **81**, 219.

Tandler, B. (1963) Ultrastructure of human submaxillary gland. II. The base of the striated duct cells. *Journal of Ultrastructure Research*, **9**, 65.

Thorn, N. A. & Petersen, O. H. (1974) *Secretory Mechanisms of Exocrine Glands*. Copenhagen: Munksgaard.

Van Kestern, M., Bibby, B. G. & Berry, G. P. (1942) Studies on the antibacterial factors of human saliva. *Journal of Bacteriology*, **43**, 573.

Waddell, W. R., Goldstein, M. N., Bradshaw, R. A. & Kirsch, W. M. (1972) Production of human nerve-growth factor in a patient with a liposarcoma. *Lancet*, **ii**, 1365.

Waissliluth, J. G. & Langman, M. J. S. (1971) ABO blood groups, secretor status, salivary protein, and serum and salivary immunoglobulin concentrations. *Gut*, **12**, 646.

Wesley-Hadzija, B. & Pigon, H. (1972) Effect of diet in West Africa on human salivary amylase activity. *Archives of Oral Biology*, **17**, 1415.

White, A. G., Entmacher, P. S., Rubin, G. & Leiter, G. (1955) Physiological and pharmacological regulations of human salivary electrolyte concentrations: with a discussion of electrolyte concentrations of some other exocrine secretions. *Journal of Clinical Investigation*, **34**, 246.

Wilsmore, N. M. (1937) A consideration of the osmotic pressure and viscosity of saliva. *Australian Dental Journal*, **41**, 161.

Salivary Glands in Health and Disease

Witkop, C. J., Barros, L. & Hamilton, P. A. (1962) In *Public Health Reports* (Washington), **77,** 928.

Wolf, R. O. & Taylor, L. L. (1964) The concentration of blood group substance in the parotid, sublingual and submaxillary salivas. *Journal of Dental Research,* **43,** 272.

Wood, C. M. & Dawes, C. (1968) The composition of lip mucous gland secretions. *IADR (North American Division),* Abstract No. 100.

Young, G., Resca, H. G. & Sullivan, M. T. (1951) The yeasts of the normal mouth and their relation to salivary acidity. *Journal of Dental Research,* **30,** 426.

Zaimis, E. (1972) *Nerve Growth Factor and its Antiserum,* (Ed.) Zaimis, E. London: Athlone Press.

Zeldow, B. J. (1961) Studies on the antibacterial action of human saliva. *Journal of Dental Research,* **40,** 446.

Zengo, A. N., Mandel, I. D., Goldman, R. & Khurana, H. S. (1971) Salivary studies in human caries resistance. *Archives of Oral Biology,* **16,** 557.

REFERENCES FOR TABLES 3.2 TO 3.8

1. Afonsky, D. (1961) *Saliva and its Relation to Oral Health.* Birmingham, Alabama: University of Alabama Press.
2. Bang, J. S. & Cimasoni, G. (1971) *Journal of Dental Research,* **50,** 1683.
3. Beeley, J. A., unpublished data.
4. Beerstecher, E. & Altgelt, S. (1951) *Journal of Biological Chemistry,* **189,** 31.
5. Brandtzaeg, P., Fjellanger, I. & Gjeruldsen, S. U. (1970) *Scandinavian Journal of Haematology,* Suppl. 12, 1.
5a. Brandtzaeg, P. & Mann, W. (1964) *Acta Odontologica Scandinavica,* **22,** 441.
5b. Brandtzaeg, P. (1965) *Archives of Oral Biology,* **10,** 795.
6. Brandtzaeg, P. (1971) *Archives of Oral Biology,* **16,** 1295.
7. Brandtzaeg, P. (1972) In *Host Resistance to Commensal Bacteria* (Ed.) MacPhee, T. Edinburgh: Churchill Livingstone.
8. Brown, J. B. & Klotz, N. J. (1934) *Journal of Dental Research,* **14,** 435.
9. Campbell, M. J. A. (1965) *Archives of Oral Biology,* **10,** 197.
10. Chauncey, H. H., Lionetti, F., Winter, R. A. & Lisanti, V. F. (1954) *Journal of Dental Research,* **33,** 321.
11. Chauncey, H. H., Henriques, B. L. & Tanzer, J. M. (1963) *Archives of Oral Biology,* **8,** 615.
12. Chauncey, H. H., Feller, R. P. & Henriques, B. L. (1966) *Journal of Dental Research,* **45,** 1230.
13. Daniels, T. E. & Newbrun, E. (1966) *Archives of Oral Biology,* **11,** 1171.
14. Dawes, C. (1972) *Journal of Physiology,* **220,** 529.
15. Dawes, C. (1974) *Archives of Oral Biology,* **19,** 887.
16. Dawes, C. & Wood, C. M. (1973) *Archives of Oral Biology,* **18,** 343.
17. de Jorge, F. B., Canelas, H. M., Dias, J. C. & Cury, L. (1964) *Clinica Chimica Acta,* **9,** 148.
18. Driezen, S., Stone, R. E., Driezen, J. G. & Spies, T. D. (1959) *Proceedings of the Society for Experimental Biology,* **102,** 449.
19. Driezen, S., Goodrich, J. S. & Levy, B. M. (1968) *Archives of Oral Biology,* **13,** 229.
20. Eastoe, J. (1961) In *Biochemists Handbook* (Ed.) Long, C. London: Spon, p. 909.
21. Edgar, M. & Geddes, D. M. (1974) Personal communication.
22. Eichel, H. J., Conger, N. & Chernick, W. S. (1964) *Archives of Biochemistry and Biophysics,* **107,** 197.
23. Ferguson, D. B. (1968) *Archives of Oral Biology,* **13,** 583.
24. Ferguson, D. B. & Fort, A. (1973) *Caries Research,* **7,** 19.
25. Ferguson, D. B. & Fort, A. (1974) *Archives of Oral Biology,* **19,** 47.
26. Gloster, J. (1955) *British Journal of Ophthalmology,* **39,** 743.
27. Gow, B. S. (1965) *Journal of Dental Research,* **44,** 885.
28. Gow, B. S. (1965) *Journal of Dental Research,* **44,** 890.
29. Hess, W. C. & Smith, B. T. (1949) *Journal of Dental Research,* **28,** 507.
30. Hoerman, K. C., Englander, H. R. & Shklair, I. L. (1956) *Proceedings of the Society for Experimental and Biological Medicine,* **92,** 875.

31. Jenkins, G. N. (1970) *Physiology of the Mouth* 3rd edition (revised). Oxford: Blackwell Scientific Publications.
32. Kanabrocki, E. L., Case, L. F., Fields, T., Graham, L., Miller, E. B., Oester, Y. T. & Kaplan, E. (1965) *Journal of Nuclear Medicine,* **6,** 489.
33. Kanamori, T., Kuzuya, H. & Nagatsu, T. (1974) *Journal of Dental Research,* **53,** 760.
33a. Kaslick, R. F., Chasens, A. J., Mandel, I. D., Weinstein, D., Waldman, R., Pluhar, T. & Zazzara, R. (1970) *Journal of Periodontology,* **41,** 93.
34. Kelsay, J. L., McCague, K. E. & Holden, J. M. (1972) *Archives of Oral Biology,* **17,** 439.
35. Kostlin, V. A. & Rauch, S. (1957) *Helvetica Medica Acta,* **5,** 600.
36. Lowry, O. H., Rosebrough, N. J., Farr, A. L. & Randal, R. J. (1951) *Journal of Biological Chemistry,* **193,** 265.
37. Maliszewski, T. F. & Bass, D. E. (1955) *Journal of Applied Physiology,* **8,** 289.
38. Mandel, I. D. & Ellison, S. A. (1965) *Annals of the New York Academy of Sciences,* **131,** 802.
39. Mandel, I. D. & Eisenstein, A. (1969) *Archives of Oral Biology,* **14,** 231.
40. Mandel, I. W. & Thompson, R. H. (1967) *Journal of Periodontology,* **38,** 310.
41. Mason, D. K. (1966) *M.D. Thesis, University of Glasgow.*
42. Mason, D. K., Boyle, J. A., Harden, R. M., Duncan, A. M. & Greig, W. R. (1966) *Journal of Dental Research,* **45,** 1439.
43. Menguy, R., Masters, Y. F. & Desbaillets, L. (1970) *Proceedings of the Society for Experimental Biology and Medicine,* **134,** 1020.
44. Newbrun, E. (1967) *Archives of Oral Biology,* **12,** 1289.
45. Nijjar, M. S., Pritchard, E. T., Dawes, C. & Philips, S. R. (1970) *Archives of Oral Biology,* **15,** 89.
46. Ravin, H. H., Tsou, K. C. & Seligman, A. H. (1951) *Journal of Biological Chemistry,* **191,** 843.
47. Rutenburg, A. M., Cohen, R. B. & Seligman, A. M. (1952) *Science,* **116,** 539.
48. Saito, S. & Kizu, K. (1959) *Journal of Dental Research,* **38,** 500.
49. Sanders, S. G. (1955) *Journal of Oral Surgery,* **13,** 193.
50. Schneyer, L. H. (1956) *Journal of Applied Physiology,* **9,** 453.
51. Seligman, A. M. & Nachlas, M. M. (1950) *Journal of Clinical Investigation,* **29,** 31.
52. Seligman, A. M., Chauncey, H. H., Nachlas, M. M., Manheimer, L. H. & Ravin, H. A. (1951) *Journal of Biological Chemistry,* **190.** 7.
53. Shannon, I. L. (1966) *U.S.A.F. School of Aerospace Medicine,* Publication No. SAM-TR-66-52.
54. Shannon, I. L. (1973) *Journal of Dental Research,* **52,** 1157.
55. Shannon, I. L. (1974) Personal communication.
56. Shinowara, G. Y., Jones, L. M. & Reinhart, H. L. (1942) *Journal of Biological Chemistry,* **1142,** 921.
57. Soder, P.-O. (1972) *Journal of Dental Research,* **51,** 389.
58. Somogyi, M. (1938) *Journal of Biological Chemistry,* **125,** 399.
59. Stephen, K. W., Harden, R. McG. & Mason, D. K. (1971) *Archives of Oral Biology,* **16,** 581.
59a. Sueda, T., Cimasoni, G. & Held, A. J. (1967) *Archives of Oral Biology,* **12,** 1205.
60. Weinstein, E., Khurana, H. & Mandel, I. D. (1971) *Archives of Oral Biology,* **16,** 157.
60a. Weinstein, E., Khurana, H. & Mandel, I. D. (1972) *Archives of Oral Biology,* **17,** 375.
61. White, A. G., Entmacher, P. S. & Rubin, G. (1955) *Journal of Clinical Investigation,* **34,** 246.
62. Whitehead, P. H. & Kipps, A. E. *CRE Report No. 127.*
63. Wotman, S., Mandel, I. D., Thompson, R. H. & Laragh, J. H. (1967) *Journal of Oral Therapeutics & Pharmacology,* **3,** 239.
64. Wotman, S., Greenbaum, L. & Mandel, I. D. (1969) *Biochemical Pharmacology,* **18,** 1261.
65. Zengo, A. N., Mandel, I. D., Goldman, R. & Khurana, H. S. (1971) *Archives of Oral Biology,* **16,** 557.

PART II

Salivary Gland Disease

CHAPTER 4

History and Clinical Examination

HISTORY

Patients with salivary gland disease present with a limited number of complaints. These are swelling, pain, dryness of the mouth (xerostomia), bad taste and, less commonly, excessive secretion of saliva (sialorrhoea).

Swelling and pain

These two symptoms will first be considered together as this is the way they often present. In acute sialadenitis, and also where there is duct obstruction, pain and swelling usually appear and regress at the same time. In the case of duct obstruction, the symptoms are initiated by eating foods which particularly stimulate salivary secretion, e.g. fruit or sweets. An external salivary fistula may also be accompanied by painful swelling at meal times.

Tumours often present with painless or asymptomatic swelling, but they may also present as dull pain. This indeed may be the only early symptom of a carcinoma of the deep lobe of the parotid gland (Vandenberg et al, 1964; Ulin, 1967).

Painful, usually bilateral, parotid and submandibular gland swelling may also occur after excessive ingestion of iodide (Harden, 1968), starch (Silverman and Perkins, 1966), lead and mercury (Nash and Morrison, 1949), or as a reaction to certain drugs, e.g. phenylbutazone (Cohen and Banks, 1966), thiocyanate and thiouracil (Nash and Morrison, 1949). In some of these latter conditions an allergic reaction may be involved.

Swelling

Asymptomatic or painless swelling may arise from local causes such as tumours, cysts or mucoceles of major or minor gland and chronic sialadenitis. Sialosis, an asymptomatic bilateral parotid swelling, has been described in association with a number of systemic conditions such as chronic malnutrition (Gillman, Gilbert and Gillman, 1947; Katsilambros, 1961); cirrhosis of the liver (Rothbell and Duggan, 1957; Borsanyi and Blanchard, 1961); in diabetes mellitus (Lyon, 1943; John, 1963; Davidson, Leibel and Berris,

1969). Unilateral or bilateral salivary gland enlargement may also occur in early cases of Sjögren's syndrome. In diabetes and Sjögren's syndrome where salivary flow is reduced secondary infection may cause the swelling to become painful.

Dryness of the mouth

Xerostomia, or dryness of the mouth, is not infrequently encountered in dental practice. The symptom may on the one hand be the manifestation of a local factor, e.g. mouthbreathing, but on the other may represent the first symptom of serious systemic disease, e.g. Sjögren's syndrome. It is therefore important, where no obvious cause is apparent, that such a complaint is investigated with regard not only to local aetiological factors causing reduced salivary gland function, but also to any other manifestation which may be revealed by general history and examination such as conjunctivitis, arthritis or dehydration.

Dryness of the mouth may result from four basic causes:
1. Factors affecting the salivary centre
2. Factors affecting the autonomic outflow pathway
3. Factors reducing salivary gland function (organic disease)
4. Alterations in fluid and electrolyte balance.

Various causes of xerostomia in each of these categories are summarised in Table 8.1.

Drugs are an increasingly common cause of xerostomia. The groups of drugs which commonly produce xerostomia as a side effect are described in greater detail in Chapter 8.

Taste abnormalities

The commonest cause of bad taste is pus-producing inflammatory conditions of salivary glands or of teeth and their supporting structures. Another source of 'bad' taste may be gastric or oesophageal disease although bad taste is associated with sialadenitis which is usually unilateral and the patient often has difficulty in localising it to the area of the oral mucosa anterior or posterior, left or right, from which it arises.

Loss of taste sensation following nerve damage, as in lesions causing facial paralysis above the geniculate ganglion (Figure 4.1), is localised in the lateral half of the tongue on the same side. Taste abnormalities associated with psychiatric states and mood disorders such as acute anxiety, fear hypochondriasis and depression are generalised and may be associated with dryness of the mouth.

Excessive saliva

Although less common as a symptom than dryness of the mouth, sialorrhoea or excessive secretion of saliva can occur from many different causes. These can be grouped according to basic cause as follows:

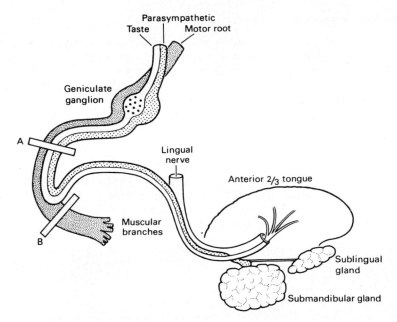

Figure 4.1. Distribution of facial nerve to anterior two-thirds of tongue and submandibular salivary glands. Damage at A leads to loss of taste sensation and gland function whilst at B this does not occur.

1. Factors affecting the higher central nervous system pathways or salivary centre directly
2. Local oral factors which reflexly stimulate salivary secretion.

The commonest cause of excessive salivation is acute inflammation of the oral cavity such as occurs with herpetic or aphthous ulceration, acute ulcerative gingivitis (Vincent's type), and ill-fitting dentures. It may also commonly occur in a variety of mental, psychiatric and neurological diseases: deteriorated schizophrenia, epilepsy, familial autonomic dysfunction and Parkinsonism, as well as cystic fibrosis of the pancreas, mercury poisoning, acrodynia and gastric and oesophageal disease.

From the foregoing the importance of adequate history-taking in the diagnosis and management of salivary gland disease is apparent. In the authors' experience, it is usually more informative than any other part of the clinical assessment of the patient.

CLINICAL EXAMINATION

Physical examination of the salivary glands involves examining the whole of the cervico-facial region. This should be carried out in a systematic way and involves inspection, and palpation both extra- and intra-orally, together with exploration of salivary duct orifices when indicated (Fast and Forest, 1968).

Inspection: extra-oral

The examiner should stand directly in front of and facing the patient about three to four feet away. He should examine for asymmetry, discolouration, visible pulsation and evidence of discharging sinuses.

Enlargement of salivary glands may be unilateral or bilateral and may involve one or all glands, major and minor. Usually, signs of parotid or submandibular gland enlargement are being sought.

Parotid

The classical sign of diffuse parotid salivary gland enlargement is shown in Figure 4.2 which demonstrates the swelling overlapping the tragus of the ear. While a localised swelling may be obvious if it is superficial, it may be entirely hidden if occurring deep in the gland tissues.

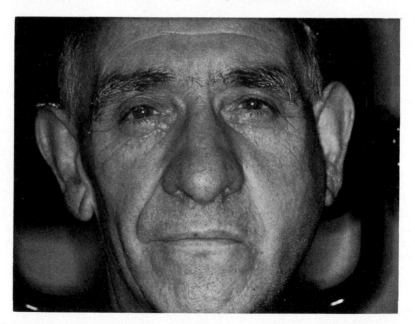

Figure 4.2. Left parotid enlargement. The swelling overlaps the tragus of the ear.

Submandibular

The classical signs of submandibular salivary gland enlargement are shown in Figure 4.3, which demonstrates the swelling just below and medial to the angle of the mandible. A frequent problem in the differential diagnosis of swellings in the parotid and submandibular regions is to distinguish between those of salivary and lymphatic gland origin. In general, those of salivary gland origin are single, larger, have a smoother surface and are often more

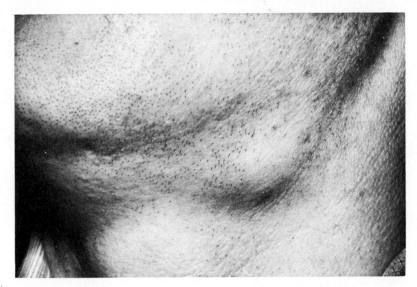

Figure 4.3. Left submandibular enlargement. The swelling is just below and medial to the inferior border of mandible.

deeply placed, but on some occasions it is not possible, on clinical examination, to make an accurate diagnosis and further tests of salivary gland function such as sialography, scintiscanning or scintigraphy may be helpful.

Inspection: intra-oral

This should include examination of salivary duct orifices and any evidence of occlusion, asymmetry, discolouration, visible pulsation and discharging sinuses.

Palpation

Palpation should be done with the palmar surface of the tips of the fingers, using a delicate but firm rotatory motion.

Extra-oral. Palpation of the face and neck, including salivary gland regions, should be carried out as shown in Figures 4.4 to 4.8. The examiner stands behind the patient whose head is inclined forward—this flexion of the neck relaxes the tissues in this region and in this way, the parotid and submandibular glands and any other neck swellings can be more easily palpated. It is necessary to determine whether the gland swelling is tender or non-tender, smooth or nodular, soft or firm, fixed or mobile, solid or cystic, fluctuant or tense, pulsatile or not. Swellings associated with the thyroid gland and larynx rise on swallowing, whereas those associated with salivary and lymph glands do not.

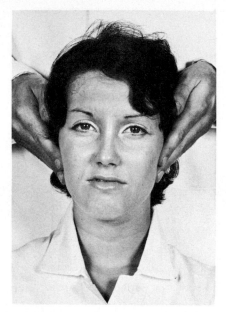

Figure 4.4. Bimanual palpation of the parotid glands.

Figure 4.5. Palpation of the L parotid gland.

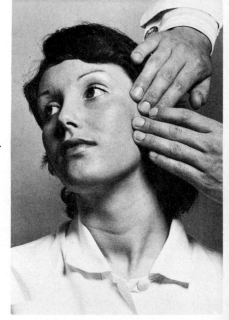

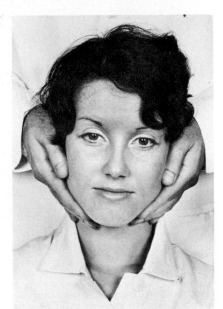

Figure 4.6. Bimanual palpation of the submandibular glands.

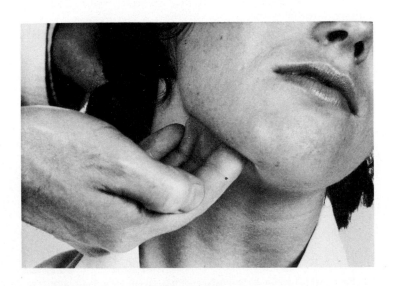

Figure 4.7. Palpation of the R submandibular tissues.

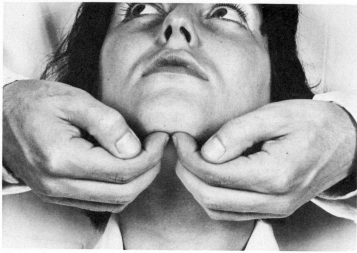

Figure 4.8. Palpation of the submental region.

Intra-oral. Intra-oral palpation is commonly employed in bimanual palpation of the submandibular glands and ducts, as shown in Figure 4.9, but
may also be used in bimanual palpation of labial or buccal minor salivary
glands and in the palpation of palatal glands by compressing them against
the underlying bone.

Auscultation

Auscultation may be helpful in identifying vascular swellings such as ectopic
thyroid tissue and haemangiomata.

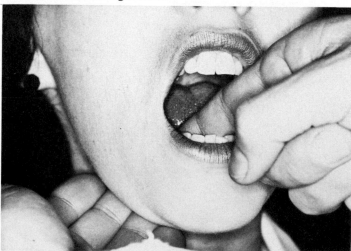

Figure 4.9. Bimanual palpation of right submandibular gland using both intra- and extra-oral
approaches.

Examination of salivary duct orifices

This may reveal important clinical information such as whether the duct orifices are patent or not. If pressure is exerted on the parotid or submandibular gland, it is possible to express some saliva from the duct orifice. The normal secretion is watery and crystal clear and easily expressed. In chronically inflamed states, it may contain debris, jelly-like blobs of mucus or frank pus. A lacrimal probe dilator (Figure 4.10) may be helpful in identifying the duct orifice and in the detection of a duct stricture or calculus.

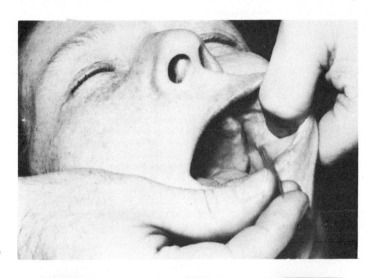

(a)

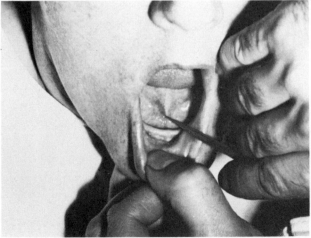

(b)

Figure 4.10. a. Location of L parotid duct orifice using lacrimal probe dilator. b. Location of R submandibular duct orifice using lacrimal probe dilator.

REFERENCES

Borsanyi, S. J. & Blanchard, C. L. (1961) Asymptomatic enlargement of the parotid glands in alcoholic cirrhosis. *Southern Medical Journal,* **54,** 678.

Cohen, L. & Banks, P. (1966) Salivary gland enlargement and phenylbutazone. *British Medical Journal,* **i,** 1420.

Davidson, D., Leibel, B. S. & Berris, B. (1969) Asymptomatic parotid gland enlargement in diabetes mellitus. *Annals of Internal Medicine,* **70,** 31.

Fast, T. B. & Forest, D. (1968) The importance of palpation; The examination of the salivary glands. In *Dental Clinics of North America: Symposium on Oral Medicine.* (Ed.) Mitchell, D. F. Philadelphia: W. B. Saunders Company.

Gillman, J., Gilbert, C. & Gillman, T. (1947) The Bantu salivary glands in chronic malnutrition with a brief consideration of the parenchyma-interstitial tissue relationship. *South African Journal of Medical Sciences,* **12,** 99.

Harden, R. McG. (1968) Submandibular adenitis due to iodide administration. *British Medical Journal,* **i,** 160.

John, J. H. (1963) Mikulicz's disease and diabetes. *Journal of the American Medical Association,* **101,** 184.

Katsilambros, L. (1961) Asymptomatic enlargement of the parotid glands. *Journal of the American Medical Association,* **178,** 513.

Lyon, E. (1943) Swelling of the parotid gland and diabetes mellitus. *Gastroenterologie (Basel),* **68,** 139.

Nash, L. & Morrison, L. F. (1949) Asymptomatic chronic enlargement of parotid glands; review and report of case. *Annals of Otology, Rhinology and Laryngology,* **58,** 646.

Rothbell, E. N. & Duggan, J. J. (1957) Enlargement of the parotid gland in disease of the liver. *American Journal of Medicine,* **22,** 367.

Silverman, M. & Perkins, R. L. (1966) Bilateral parotid enlargement and starch injection. *Annals of Internal Medicine,* **64,** 842.

Ulin, A. W. (1967) Surgical aspects of salivary gland disease. *American Journal of Gastroenterology,* **48,** 373.

Vandenberg, H. J. Jr, Kambouris, A., Pryzybylski, T. & Rachmaninoff, N. (1964) Salivary tumours, clinicopathologic review of 190 patients. *American Journal of Surgery,* **108,** 480.

CHAPTER 5

Developmental Anomalies

Developmental defects of the salivary glands are rare. When they occur they are generally associated with other facial abnormalities. It is clear that developmental anomalies of the salivary glands predispose to xerostomia and thus to sialadenitis and dental caries. Steggerda (1941) reported studies on a patient with absence of salivary glands from the standpoint of thirst production mechanism and water metabolism. The patient with xerostomia was required to drink a few mouthfuls of water every hour or so, presumably in response to the 'dry mouth reflex' (Cannon, 1937). However, the total fluid intake was 2783 ml/day compared with 2615 ml/day for a control. Other studies by Steggerda (1941) suggested that the salivary glands were not the sole factors in governing thirst; indeed the role of saliva in controlling thirst is very much in doubt (Jenkins, 1966).

Aplasia or agenesis, the congenital absence of the major salivary glands, is an uncommon occurrence. Any one of the glands or group of glands may be absent, unilaterally or bilaterally and the condition will give rise to xerostomia and an increased caries rate (Figures 5.1 and 5.2).

Familial agenesis of the parotid duct in three generations has been reported (Hughes and Syrop, 1959). In one case of those with hemifacial microstomia, parotid gland agenesis has been recorded (Entin, 1958). Agenesis of the parotid gland has also been noted in mandibulo-facial dysostosis (McKenzie and Craig, 1955). In 1943, Ashley and Richardson observed parotid agenesis in association with cleft palate and anophthalmia.

Atresia is the congenital occlusion or absence of one or more major salivary gland ducts and is exceedingly rare. Its presence may produce severe xerostomia and may lead to retention cyst formation (Beke, Tomaro and Stein, 1963). Orban (1957) has pointed out that this condition occurs more commonly in the floor of the mouth in association with sublingual and submandibular ducts.

Hypoplasia of the parotid gland in the Melkersson-Rosenthal syndrome may represent secondary atrophic changes to parasympathetic dysfunction (Rauch and Gorlin, 1970). Diverticuli, which probably represent a true

83

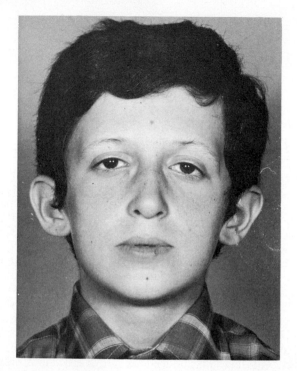

(a)

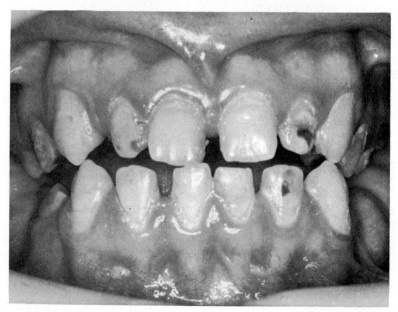

(b)

Figure 5.1. a. Extra-oral and b. intra-oral view of a 10-year-old boy with agenesis of major salivary glands.

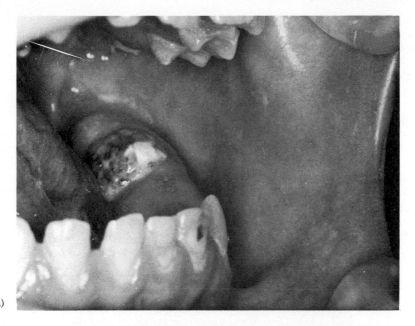

(a)

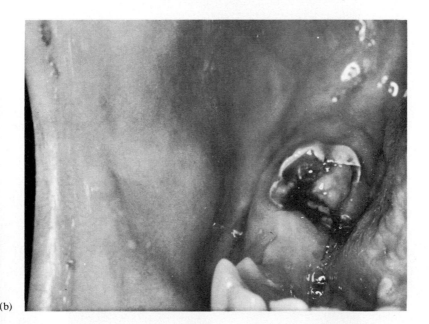

(b)

Figure 5.2. a. Severe dental caries, xerostomia and b. absence of parotid duct orifice in a 10-year-old boy with agenesis of major salivary glands.

malformation in the newborn or young, have been reported and this condition predisposes to recurrent sialadenitis (Pearson, 1935; Shulman, 1950).

Congenital fistula formation of duct system is generally associated with abnormal formation of branchial clefts (Rauch and Gorlin, 1970).

Aberrancy refers to the presence of salivary tissue at an abnormal site. An example is inclusion of salivary tissue within the ramus or body of the mandible. Usually an anatomical communication exists with normally situated gland tissue and may be considered an extreme example of developmental lingual mandibular salivary gland depression (Fordyce, 1956) (Figures 5.3 and 5.4). Salivary gland tissue has also been reported in the base of the neck, middle ear, mastoid bone and lymphoid tissue including the intra- or paraparotid lymph nodes (Rauch, 1959). It is important to note that such tissue may be the site of tumour formation.

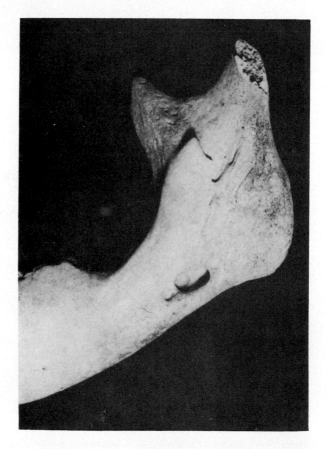

Figure 5.3. A deep mandibular defect near the lower border of the mandible.

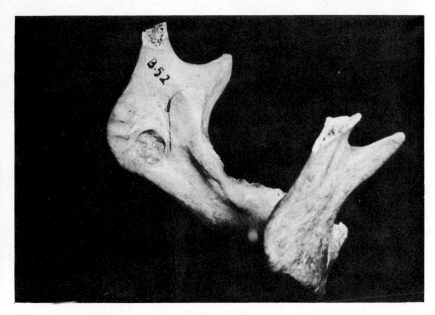

Figure 5.4. Deep mandibular defect in a mandible from 750 to 500 B.C.

Harvey and Noble (1968) published details of nine defects on the lingual surface near the angle in seven mandibles out of a series of over 950 examined. Previously Stafne (1942) had drawn attention to these defects or cavities by reporting 35 radiolucent areas near the angle of the mandible below the inferior dental canal. The lesions were more common in males and in all cases were asymptomatic. This was confirmed by Harvey and Noble (1968). Furthermore these investigators, in an extensive review of the literature, reported that of 20 clinical cases of defects below the mylo-hyoid line, salivary tissue was present in eleven. They drew attention, also, to five cases, four of which contained salivary tissue, that occurred anteriorly above the mylo-hyoid line and was thus related to the sublingual gland. Examples of the use of radiography and sialography to demonstrate the presence of such defects and their relation to salivary tissue are shown in Figures 5.5 and 5.6.

Microscopic examination of thin sections taken from such defects (Harvey and Noble, 1968) have excluded the possibility that the defects could have arisen as a result of the eruption to the surface of some earlier existing central conditions. Furthermore, this histological study also excluded the possibility that the growing mesoderm of the developing mandible could have enclosed a lobe of salivary gland during bone development. Surface bone resorption, by cause unknown, seems the probable explanation for these defects (Figures 5.7a and 5.7b).

The presence of salivary tissue, however, highlights the views of Fordyce (1956) and Seward (1960) that sialography may be helpful in the diagnosis

87

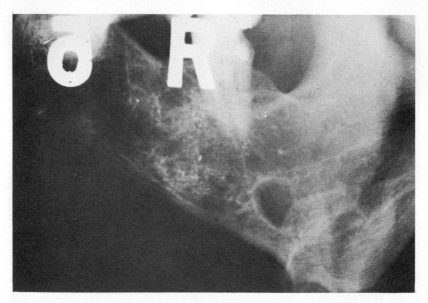

Figure 5.5. Radiography demonstrates a clear radiolucent area with sclerosed margins at angle of mandible.

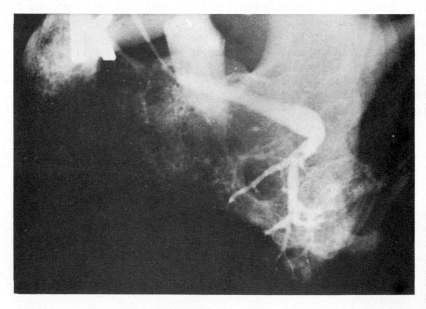

Figure 5.6. Sialography demonstrates the association of the submandibular duct system to the radiolucent lesion shown in Figure 5.5.

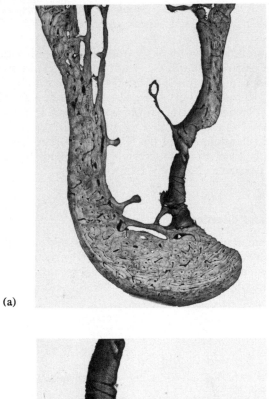

(a)

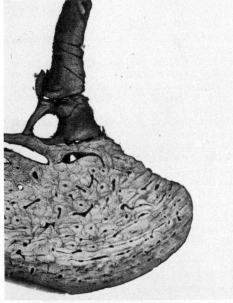

(b)

Figure 5.7. a. Coronal section through lower border of mandible showing defect ($\times$ 5). b. Lamellar bone formed by surface apposition on the lower border and haversian bone replacing it from within are interrupted by the resorbed surface of the defect. Normal bone bordering defect does not suggest interference during development ($\times$ 10).

89

(Figure 5.6). As mentioned earlier, neoplastic change may occur in these sites (Simpson, 1965; Silverglade, Alvares and Olech, 1968; Dhawan et al, 1970).

The following points are considered important in relation to developmental anomalies of the salivary glands. Aberrant salivary gland tissue found at distant sites probably relates to the fact that the entire ectodermal portion of the upper part of the foregut is capable of producing salivary tissue (Gardner, 1966). The primordia of salivary gland tissue formed during six to eight weeks of fetal life may lose their continuity with the oral mucosa and during subsequent development of the fetus may drift to their ectopic site. Aberrant glands appear to lack secretory ducts and at best form only rudimentary duct systems (Gardner, 1966).

Accessory ducts and diverticuli

It is of interest that Rauch (1959) found an accessory parotid duct in over half of a series of 450 salivary glands examined. Diverticuli, when present in the newborn or young child, probably represent true malformations. They may give rise to symptoms in adult life, being a predisposing factor to parotitis.

REFERENCES

Ashley, L. M. & Richardson, G. E. (1943) Multiple congenital anomalies in a stillborn infant. *Anatomical Record*, **86**, 457.
Beke, A. L., Tomaro, A. J. & Stein, M. (1963) Congenital atresia of sublingual duct with ranula. *Journal of Oral Surgery*, **21**, 427.
Cannon, W. B. (1937) *Digestion and Health*. London: Secker and Warburg.
Dhawan, I. K., Bhargava, S., Nayak, N. C. & Gupta, R. K. (1970) Central salivary gland tumors of the jaws. *Cancer*, **26**, 211.
Entin, M. A. (1958) Reconstruction in congenital deformity of the temporo-mandibular complex. *Plastic and Reconstructive Surgery and The Transplantation Bulletin*, **21**, 461.
Fordyce, G. L. (1956) The probable nature of so-called latent haemorrhagic cysts of the mandible. *British Dental Journal*, **101**, 40.
Gardner, A. F. (1966) *Diseases and Neoplasms of the Salivary Glands*. Chicago: Year Book Medical Publishers Inc.
Harvey, W. & Noble, H. W. (1968) Defects on the lingual surface of the mandible near the angle. *British Journal of Oral Surgery*, **6**, 75.
Hughes, R. D. & Syrop, H. W. (1959) A familial study of the agenesis of the parotid gland duct. In *Proceedings of the Tenth International Congress of Genetics*. p. 128. Montreal: University of Toronto Press.
Jenkins, G. N. (1966) *The Physiology of the Mouth*. p. 342. Oxford: Blackwell Scientific Publications.
McKenzie, J. & Craig, J. (1955) Mandibulo-facial dysostosis (Treacher-Collins syndrome). *Archives of Disease in Childhood*, **30**, 391.
Orban, B. J. (1957) *Oral Histology and Embroyology*. 4th Ed. St. Louis: C. V. Mosby Co.
Pearson, R. S. B. (1935) Recurrent swelling of parotid glands. *Archives of Disease in Childhood*, **10**, 363.
Rauch, S. (1959) *Die Speicheldrüsen des Menschen*. Stuttgart: Georg Thieme.
Rauch, S. & Gorlin, R. J. (1970) Diseases of the salivary glands. In *Thoma's Oral Pathology*, **2**, p. 969. (Ed.) Gorlin, R. J. & Goldman, H. M. St. Louis: C. V. Mosby Co.

Seward, G. R. (1960) Salivary gland inclusions in the mandible. *British Dental Journal,* **108,** 321.

Shulman, B. H. (1950) Acute suppurative infections of the salivary glands in the newborn. *American Journal of Diseases of Children,* **80,** 413.

Silverglade, L. B., Alvares, O. F. & Olech, E. (1968) Central mucoepithermoid tumors of the jaws. *Cancer,* **22,** 650.

Simpson, W. (1965) A Stafne's mandibular defect containing a pleomorphic adenoma—report of a case. *Journal of Oral Surgery,* **23,** 553.

Stafne, E. C. (1942) Bone cavities situated near the angle of the mandible. *Journal of the American Dental Association,* **29,** 1969.

Steggerda, F. R. (1941) Observations on the water intake of man with dysfunctioning salivary glands. *American Journal of Physiology,* **132,** 517.

CHAPTER 6

Sialadenitis

Inflammatory disorders of the major salivary glands which result from bacterial or viral infection are the most common salivary gland disease. On rare occasions an allergic reaction may result in a sialadenitis. Infection of the salivary glands is manifest by painful swelling of the affected gland with an alteration in salivary secretion rate and character. The flow rate is usually reduced to varying degree and the saliva becomes cloudy and thick. Mixed infections usually ascend from the mouth, whereas specific infections tend to be blood borne. Prompt and effective treatment is essential if recurrence is to be prevented.

BACTERIAL

Acute sialadenitis

Predisposing factors include reduction of salivary flow which may be a post-operative complication, especially of abdominal surgery when the patient is debilitated or dehydrated. Acute parotitis may follow the use of drugs such as phenothiazine and its derivatives which cause xerostomia and thus predispose to ascending infections (Banks, 1967). The condition may also represent an acute exacerbation of a low-grade chronic non-specific sialadenitis. Clinically, acute sialadenitis presents as a painful swelling accompanied by low-grade fever, elevated erythrocyte sedimentation rate, leucocytosis, general malaise and headaches. In addition to these features the overlying skin is reddened, trismus may be present, and oedema may involve the cheek, periorbital region and neck. A purulent discharge may be expressed from the affected duct by digital pressure. The micro-organisms involved include *Staphylococcus aureus, Staphylococcus pyogenes, Streptococcus viridans* and pneumococci. It is to be noted that the introduction of sulphonamides and antibiotics led to a marked reduction in the incidence of acute parotitis (Robinson, 1955). However, with the emergence of antibiotic-resistant *Staphylococcus aureus,* acute parotitis has become more prevalent again (Speirs and Mason, 1972). The treatment plan includes rest, antibiotic therapy and surgical drainage where necessary. The management of acute septic parotitis in hospital patients should consist of the following:

1. As soon as the possibility of acute septic parotitis is suspected, a specimen of pus should be obtained from the parotid duct orifice for a stained smear, bacteriological culture and antibiotic sensitivity. The specimen should be obtained by the doctor and not by a junior nurse or ward orderly who is unlikely to know the site of the parotid duct orifice. If no exudate can be milked out, the duct can be cannulated with a fine polythene catheter and irrigated to obtain a specimen for culture.

2. Blood cultures should be taken as septicaemia can predispose to, or result from, acute septic parotitis.

3. Antibiotic therapy should be begun as soon as the bacteriological specimens have been obtained. As infection is most likely to be caused by penicillin-resistant *Staph. aureus,* antibiotics of choice are likely to be cloxacillin, lincomycin or sodium fusidate (Fucidin). If a concomitant Gram-negative septicaemia is suspected, broad-spectrum antibiotics such as cephalothin, kanamycin or gentamicin could be used instead. Therapy can be altered if necessary when the bacteriology results are available. Antibiotics should be given by intramuscular or intravenous injection at least initially.

4. Supportive therapy, such as rehydration, oral hygiene, analgesics and avoidance of any drugs which reduce salivary flow, are important.

5. Surgical drainage may be required when acute septic parotitis is caused by *Staph. aureus.* It should be carried out early because of the rapidity of abscess formation which may occur in spite of the administration of antibiotics. The condition resolves or may become a low-grade chronic sialadenitis. Biopsy and sialography are contra-indicated in the acute stage, though the histological features would be those of acute inflammation (Figure 6.1).

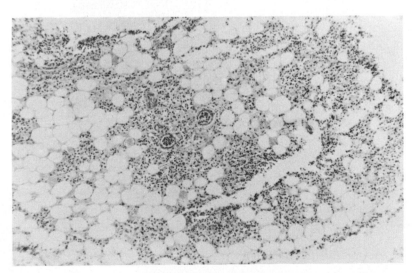

Figure 6.1. Acute parotitis. Acute inflammatory cell infiltrate is present throughout the fibro-adipose stroma. Polymorphonuclear leucocytes are present within duct lumens. ($\times$ 75.)

Chronic sialadenitis

As a complication of duct obstruction chronic sialadenitis is not uncommon, especially in the submandibular gland. In general, the aetiological factors are similar to those for acute sialadenitis. The condition usually is unilateral with pain and swelling in the pre-auricular, retromandibular or sub-mandibular region. On occasions there may be difficulty in distinguishing submandibular sialadenitis from sublingual or submandibular cellulitis due to other causes. However the affected duct orifice is reddened and a purulent, rather salty tasting discharge from the duct of the affected gland may be present. Salivary flow may be reduced and sialography (Figure 6.2) may show ductal dilatation. The histopathological features include hyper-plasia of duct epithelium, periductal lymphocytic infiltration, acinar atrophy and fibrosis leading to eventual disappearance of the acini.

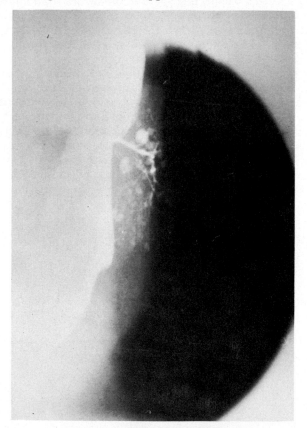

Figure 6.2. Globular sialectasis in L parotid chronic sialadenitis. Antero-posterior view.

Recurrent parotitis in childhood

Recurrent parotitis is a well-documented condition and occurs in both adults and children. The prevalence in adult life, however, is ten times greater

(Maynard, 1965). In children the ratio of affected males to females is of the order of 2:1 (Katzen and du Plessis, 1964). The attacks of parotitis consist of sudden pain and swelling in the region of one or both parotid glands usually lasting for a period of three to seven days. Beads of pus having a 'snow-storm' appearance may be expressed from the duct. Although the duct orifice is usually reddened, there is generally no erythema of the overlying skin. The systemic reaction varies from the trivial to severe. The affected gland may remain slightly enlarged between attacks which vary from one every few weeks to once or twice a year. Fortunately there is a marked tendency of the condition to resolve completely in children once puberty is attained. Those patients whose sialograms show little or no duct dilation and whose flow rates are within normal limits are more likely to recover spontaneously (Maynard, 1967). The aetiology of recurrent parotitis is uncertain (Katzen and du Plessis, 1964; Brook, 1969). Among the factors which have been considered are congenital obstruction, stagnation, disease of the duct wall as a result of allergy, auto-immune disease or infection either bacterial or viral. Maynard (1965) has suggested a possible sequence of events as follows: low secretion rate predisposes to retrograde infection and this gives rise to the symptoms. At this stage, duct proliferation will lead to recovery whilst irreversible disease tends to follow main duct changes. Katzen and du Plessis (1964) have suggested that hereditary, racial and hormonal factors may play a role in recurrent parotitis of childhood. In the management of recurrent parotitis culture of saliva or pus from Stensen's duct should be carried out so that appropriate antibiotic therapy may be instigated. Sialography should be performed to differentiate between those cases with or without main duct change (Figures 6.3 to 6.5). Stimulation of flow by chewing or massage prevents stagnation (Maynard, 1965). In view of frequent spontaneous recovery after puberty, surgical intervention should be avoided, if possible.

Specific bacterial sialadenitis and granulomatous disorders

The salivary glands are seldom involved in specific inflammatory disorders. On rare occasions, however, they may be the site of granulomatous disorders such as tuberculosis, syphilis and sarcoidosis (Rauch, 1959) and are affected as part of these systemic disease processes (Figure 6.6). The term Mikulicz's syndrome is often applied to the condition of bilateral salivary gland and lacrimal gland enlargement due to a known cause (Schaffer and Jacobsen, 1927), such as the specific granulomata as well as lymphoid neoplasia (Chapter 11). It is now known that uveoparotid fever or Heerfordt's syndrome is due to sarcoid involvement of the uveal tract, lacrimal and salivary glands. The minor salivary glands (Figure 6.7) may also be involved in this condition (Cahn, Eisenbud and Blake, 1964; Chisholm et al, 1971). It has been observed that salivary flow volumes and amylase content are reduced in mixed saliva (Bhoola et al, 1969) and parotid saliva (Chisholm et al, 1971) in patients with sarcoidosis. Kallikrein levels in saliva appear reduced in such patients (Bhoola et al, 1969). Actinomycosis of the parotid

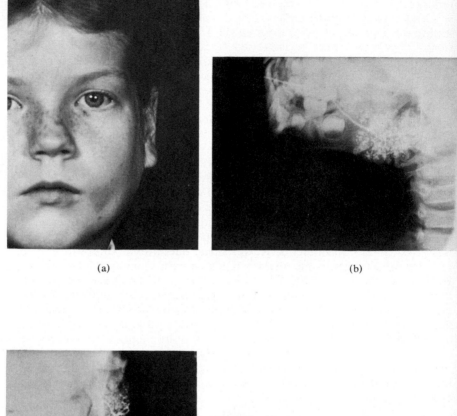

(a)   (b)

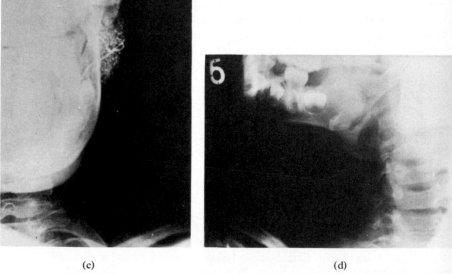

(c)   (d)

Figure 6.3. Recurrent parotitis in a 10-year-old girl. a. R parotid gland swelling. b. Lateral oblique sialogram showing globular sialectasis without duct dilation. c. Antero-posterior sialogram. d. Secretory phase sialogram showing no retention of medium.

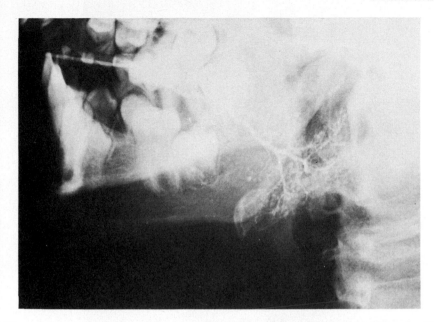

Figure 6.4. Lateral oblique sialogram showing globular sialectasis in a 12-year-old female with recurrent chronic parotitis.

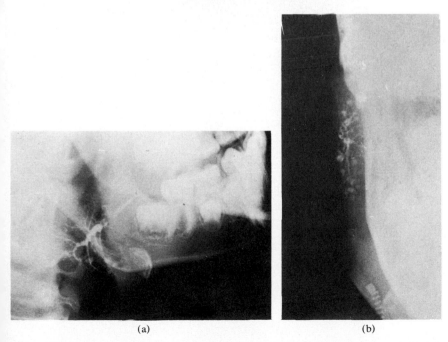

(a)   (b)

Figure 6.5. Chronic sialadenitis in an 11-year-old girl. a. Lateral oblique sialogram. b. Antero-posterior sialogram. Duct dilation and sialectasis is present.

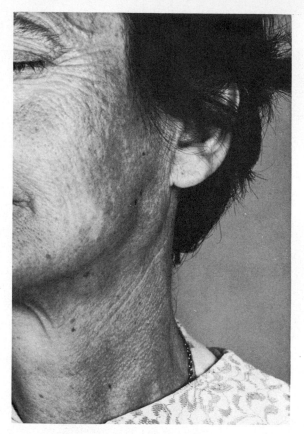

(a)

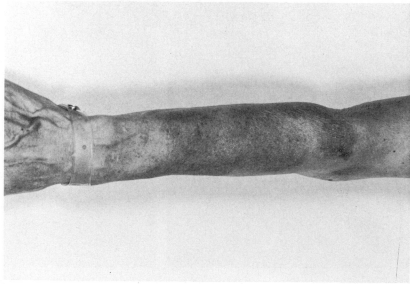

(b)

Figure 6.6. a. R parotid gland swelling in patient with sarcoidosis. b. Cutaneous lesions of sarcoidosis in patient illustrated in Figure 6.6a.

98

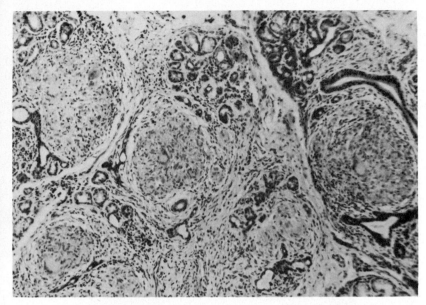

Figure 6.7. Multiple granulomas containing Langhan's type giant cells. Labial salivary glands in patients with Boeck's sarcoidosis. ($\times$ 126.)

gland has been reported but is exceedingly rare (Sazama, 1965; Hopkins, 1973). Resolution is usually achieved by appropriate treatment of the systemic disorder.

ALLERGIC SIALADENITIS

Salivary gland enlargement as a localised allergic reaction is rare (Pearson, 1961). Among the allergens reported are various foods, drugs such as chloramphenicol and oxytetracycline, various pollens and heavy metals. Allergic sialadenitis may be produced experimentally (Beutner et al, 1961; Chan, 1965; Sela et al, 1972) and the histopathological features include acute inflammation and parenchymal degeneration. It has been suggested that eosinophils in saliva and blood eosinophil count may be helpful diagnostically (Pearson, 1961). In the treatment of allergic sialadenitis antihistamines are of limited value (Cohen, 1965).

VIRAL SIALADENITIS

Mumps or epidemic parotitis

Mumps is an acute, infectious, viral disease that affects primarily the salivary glands, especially the parotids. It occurs in all areas of the world and is the most common of all salivary gland diseases. It is an endemic disease

99

throughout the year in temperate climates but there is usually a seasonal increase in late winter and spring. The disease affects both sexes equally, and is usually contracted by children and young adults. Mumps virus, which has an incubation period of two to three weeks, is transmitted by direct contact or in droplets of saliva. The onset is sudden with fever, headache and painful swelling of one or more salivary glands, more commonly the parotids, which are involved bilaterally in 70 per cent of cases (Figure 6.8). Classically, one gland is affected at first. The swelling reaches a maximum within two days and diminishes over an additional week.

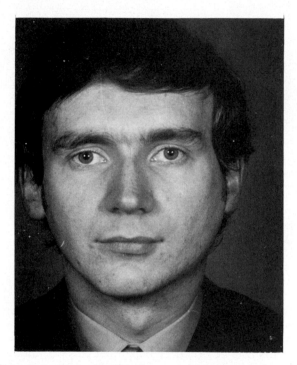

Figure 6.8. Bilateral parotid gland swelling in a case of mumps.

Adults who contract the disease may develop serious complications, such as orchitis and oöphoritis, although sterility is rare. Other organs which may be affected are the pancreas, liver, kidney or nervous system.

A durable immunity results from mumps and in adults is detected by their reacting to skin test antigen and by the presence of complement fixing antibodies. In serum, a rise in antibody titre, detected by complement fixation, occurs within a week. The virus may be detected by complement fixation in saliva two to three days before the onset of sialadenitis and for about six days afterwards. Treatment is usually symptomatic with isolation for six to ten days. Histologically a rather diffuse infiltration of the gland parenchyma by mononuclear cells and degeneration of acini is observed.

It is important to note that parotitis may be caused by other viruses such as Coxsackie virus type A, Echo virus, choriomeningitis virus and parainfluenza 1 and 3 viruses (Banks, 1968; Zollar and Mufson, 1970).

Salivary gland inclusion disease

This rare condition usually affects infants in the first few days of life. Infection occurs transplacentally without evidence of disease in the mother and debilitates the fetus, retards its development and gives rise to premature birth. There are no particular signs or symptoms. Hepatosplenomegaly, jaundice, thrombocytopenic purpura and involvement of the nervous system may be present. It has been reported that features of cytomegalic inclusion disease have been noted in 10 to 30 per cent of salivary glands of stillbirths, regardless of cause of death (Rauch, 1959). Adults are rarely affected, but in known cases there is association with severe debilitating diseases such as leukaemia or a terminal neoplasm. It is of interest that cytomegalo virus is associated with most cases of the post-perfusion syndrome, an atypical mononucleosis-like illness. The most frequent clinical manifestations are fever, hepatosplenomegaly and lymphocytosis and during the infection, immunological abnormalities may be induced (Kantor et al, 1970). Diagnosis depends on the detection of these characteristic cells in saliva, sputum or urine. Histologically, when the salivary glands are involved, numerous large doubly contoured inclusion bodies within the cytoplasm or nucleus of duct cells of parotid gland are observed (Figure 6.9).

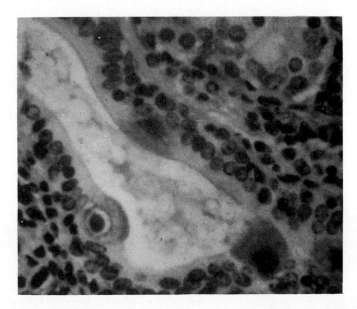

Figure 6.9. Inclusion bodies within epithelial duct cells of parotid gland in a case of cytomegalic inclusion disease. ($\times$ 240.)

101

Post-irradiation sialadenitis

A syndrome of acute swelling, tenderness and pain which subsides within a few days is a well-recognised sequel to irradiation of the major salivary glands (Bergonie and Speder, 1911; Ceresole, 1912; Desjardins, 1931; Kashima, Kirkham and Andrews, 1965). Xerostomia, gland tenderness and enlargement all appear invariably within 24 hours. Gland enlargement subsides without any specific therapy within three days (Kashima, Kirkham and Andrews, 1965). A significant finding in acute post-irradiation sialadenitis is the elevation of salivary amylase component of serum and urine. This hyperamylasaemia is directly related to the mass of salivary tissue irradiated, is a dose-related phenomenon and diminishes as the salivary glands are repeatedly irradiated. Histopathological changes in parotid and submandibular glands of patients who received a single therapeutic dose of radiation 24 hours prior to surgery include an acute inflammatory reaction associated with degenerative changes in serous cells and foci of necrosis in the gland parenchyma (Kashima, Kirkham and Andrews, 1965).

Studies of the reaction of the salivary glands of animals to irradiation have been confined largely to histological observations (English et al, 1955; Cherry and Glucksmann, 1959; Greenspan, Melamed and Pearse, 1964). In rats, the excretory ducts are least affected and the acini are most affected by irradiation. Initial degenerative changes are followed by regeneration when the dosage is low. Following high doses acinar regenerative activity is lost and duct proliferation becomes marked (Cherry and Glucksmann, 1959). Striking alterations in acid phosphatase and aminopeptidase appear early in rat salivary glands and precede morphological evidence of cell injury (Greenspan, Melamed and Pearse, 1964). A late histochemical change is an increase in alkaline phosphatase (Greenspan, Melamed and Pearse, 1964). The iodide trapping mechanism of the human parotid gland appears not to be affected by x-ray doses up to 3500 rad in 32 days (Awwad, 1959).

The ultrastructural appearance of rat parotid gland acinar cells following irradiation has been reported recently (Pratt and Sodicoff, 1972). Fine structure damage taking the form of cytolytic bodies composed of damaged cell organelles and vacuolation was evident as early as three hours following irradiation with 1600 rad. Maximal destructive change was observed at two days whilst evidence of damage was still present after eight days when vacuolation was severe.

The fundamental importance of salivary gland function in the prevention of dental defects has been demonstrated by Frank, Herdly and Philippe (1965). They have shown that, in patients receiving irradiation for carcinomas of the oral cavity, pharynx and larynx, acquired dental defects developed only in those patients in whom the salivary glands had been irradiated during treatment. These lesions developed whether or not the teeth had been inside or outside the field of irradiation.

A further route by which the salivary glands may be exposed to irradiation is the use of intravenous ^{131}I in the treatment of thyroid carcinoma. As a consequence of concentration in the salivary glands, salivary flow rates and amylase activity may be reduced in such cases. In these circumstances dental caries can be rampant (Schneyer and Tanchester, 1954).

Sialadenitis of minor glands

Inflammation of the minor salivary glands may occur as part of a local disease process or may reflect a generalised systemic disease. Earlier in this chapter attention was drawn to minor gland involvement in sarcoidosis with multi-organ involvement and, in Chapter 10, focal lymphocytic labial sialadenitis as a feature of connective tissue disorders such as Sjögren's syndrome will be described. Minor gland sialadenitis occurring as a local phenomenon is generally a secondary event following obstruction or trauma (Chapter 7). However, in the condition of stomatitis nicotina a striking clinical feature is the exaggeration of the duct orifices of the palatal salivary glands. These appear as red dots against the background of the pale mucosa (Figure 6.10). Histopathologically, squamous metaplasia of excretory duct epithelium is noted (Shafer and Waldron, 1961). Sialadenitis, marked duct dilation and mucous retention are other features of note (Thoma, 1941; Van Wyk, 1967). Duct changes in the palatal salivary glands of subjects with the habit of reverse smoking have recently been reported (Reddy et al, 1972). These workers described changes ranging from mild squamous metaplasia to marked dysplasia and indeed micro-invasive carcinoma in three of 135 cases. It is of interest that these changes occurred in the absence of marked duct dilation and prior to the leucoplakic change in the overlying palatal mucosa. Reddy et al (1972) observed duct dilation obstruction and acinar atrophy only in those cases where the reverse smoking habit was long standing. Furthermore, these workers make the interesting comment that the palatal duct orifice might form a portal of entry for tobacco pyrolytic products which may be carcinogenic.

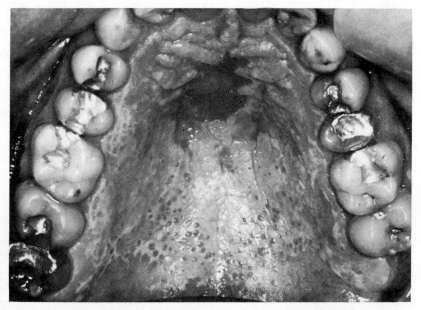

Figure 6.10. Stomatitis nicotina. Dilated duct orifices of palatal glands are clearly seen.

The condition of cheilitis glandularis apostomatosa, in which the lips, especially the lower, become swollen, is rare. The cause is unknown and the condition is painless and appears to affect males more than females. A thick viscid mucus can be expressed from the glands in the affected region. Although a labial sialadenitis is present, the underlying pathogenetic mechanism appears to be one of acinar and duct hypertrophy.

REFERENCES

Awwad, H. K. (1959) The influence of x-irradiation on the iodide-trapping mechanism of the human parotid gland. *British Journal of Radiology,* **32,** 376, 259.

Banks, P. (1967) Hypersensitivity and drug reactions involving the parotid gland. *British Journal of Oral Surgery,* **5,** 60.

Banks, P. (1968) Non-neoplastic parotid swellings: A review. *Oral Surgery, Oral Medicine and Oral Pathology,* **25,** 732.

Bergonie, J. & Speder, E. (1911) Sur quelques formes de réactions précoces après des irradiations Röntgen. *Archives d'Électricité Médicale,* **19,** 241.

Beutner, E. H., Djanian, A. Y., Geckler, R. C. & Witebsky, E. (1961) Serologic studies of rabbit antibodies to rabbit submaxillary glands. *Proceedings of the Society for Experimental Biology and Medicine (N.Y.),* **107,** 486.

Bhoola, K. D., McNicol, N. W., Oliver, S. & Foran, J. (1969) Changes in salivary enzymes in patients with sarcoidosis. *New England Journal of Medicine,* **281,** 877.

Brook, A. H. (1969) Recurrent parotitis in childhood. *British Dental Journal,* **127,** 271.

Cahn, L. R., Eisenbud, L. & Blake, M. N. (1964) Biopsies of normal-appearing palates of patients with known sarcoidosis. *Oral Surgery, Oral Medicine and Oral Pathology,* **18,** 342.

Ceresole, G. (1912) A la connaissance des reactions précoces après des irradiations Rontgen. *Archives d'Electricité Medicale,* **20,** 304.

Chan, W. C. (1964) Experimental sialo-adenitis in guinea pigs. *Journal of Pathology and Bacteriology,* **88,** 592.

Cherry, C. P. & Glucksmann, A. (1959) Injury and repair following irradiation of salivary glands in male rats. *British Journal of Radiology,* **32,** 596.

Chisholm, D. M., Lyell, A., Haroon, T. S., Mason, D. K. & Beeley, J. A. (1971) Salivary gland function in sarcoidosis. *Oral Surgery, Oral Medicine and Oral Pathology,* **31,** 766.

Cohen, L. (1965) Recurrent swelling of the parotid gland; report of a case due to allergy. *British Dental Journal,* **118,** 487.

Desjardins, A. U. (1931) Action of roentgen rays and radium on gastro-intestinal tract. *American Journal of Roentgenology, Radium Therapy, and Nuclear Medicine,* **26,** 151.

English, J. A., Wheatcroft, M. G., Lyon, H. W. & Miller, C. (1955) Long-term observations of radiation changes in salivary glands and general effects of 1,000 r to 1,750 r of x-ray radiation locally administered to heads of dogs. *Oral Surgery, Oral Medicine and Oral Pathology,* **8,** 87.

Frank, R. M., Herdly, J. & Philippe, E. (1965) Acquired dental defects and salivary gland lesions after irradiation for carcinoma. *Journal of the American Dental Association,* **70,** 868.

Greenspan, J. S., Melamed, M. R. & Pearse, A. G. E. (1964) Early histochemical changes in irradiated salivary glands and lymph-nodes of the rat. *Journal of Pathology and Bacteriology,* **88,** 439.

Hopkins, R. (1973) Primary actinomycosis of the parotid gland. *British Journal of Oral Surgery,* **11,** 131.

Kantor, G. L., Goldberg, L. S., Johnson, B. L., Derechin, M. M. & Barnett, E. V. (1970) Immunologic abnormalities induced by postperfusion cytomegalovirus infection. *Annals of Internal Medicine,* **73,** 533.

Kashima, H. K., Kirkham, W. R. & Andrews, J. R. (1965) Postirradiation sialadenitis: A study of the clinical features, histopathologic changes and serum enzyme variations following irradiation of human salivary glands. *American Journal of Roentgenology, Radium Therapy, and Nuclear Medicine,* **114,** 271.

Katzen, M. & du Plessis, D. J. (1964) Recurrent parotitis in cnildren. *South African Medical Journal,* **38,** 122.

Maynard, J. D. (1967) Recurrent parotid enlargement. *British Journal of Surgery,* **52,** 784.

Maynard, J. D. (1967) Parotid enlargement. *Hospital Medicine,* **1,** 620.

Pearson, R. S. B. (1961) Recurrent swellings of the parotid gland. *Gut,* **2,** 210.

Pratt, N. E. & Sodicoff, M. (1972) Ultrastructural injury following x irradiation of rat parotid gland acinar cells. *Archives of Oral Biology,* **17,** 1177.

Rauch, S. (1959) *Die Speicheldrusen des Menschen.* Stuttgart: George Thieme Verlag.

Reddy, C. R. R. M., Raju, M. V. S., Ramulu, C. & Reddy, P. G. (1972) Changes in the ducts of the glands of the hard palate in reverse smokers. *Cancer,* **30,** 231.

Robinson, J. R. (1955) Surgical parotitis, a vanishing disease. *Surgery,* **38,** 703.

Sazama, L. (1965) Actinomycosis of the parotid gland. Report of 5 cases. *Oral Surgery, Oral Medicine and Oral Pathology,* **19,** 197.

Schaffer, A. J. & Jacobsen, A. W. (1927) Mikulicz's syndrome: report of 10 cases. *American Journal of Diseases of Children,* **34,** 327.

Schneyer, L. H. & Tanchester, D. (1954) Some oral aspects of radioactive iodine therapy for thyroid disease. *New York Journal of Dentistry,* **14,** 308.

Sela, J., Ulmansky, M., Dishon, T., Rosenmann, E. & Bors, J. H. (1972) Experimental allergic sialoadenitis. I. Acute sialoadenitis induced by a local immune reaction. *Virchows Archiv für pathologische Anatomie und Physiologie und für klinische Medizin,* **355,** 213.

Shafer, W. G. & Waldron, C. A. (1961) A clinical and histopathologic study of leukoplakia. *Surgery, Gynecology and Obstetrics with International Abstracts of Surgery,* **112,** 411.

Speirs, C. F. & Mason, D. K. (1972) Acute septic parotitis: Incidence, aetiology and management. *Scottish Medical Journal,* **17,** 62.

Thoma, K. H. (1941) Stomatitis nicotina and its effect on the palate. *American Journal of Orthodontics,* **27,** 38.

Van Wyk, C. W. (1967) Nicotinic stomatitis of the palate—a clinicohistologic study. *Journal of the Dental Association of South Africa,* **22,** 106.

Zollar, L. M. & Mufson, M. A. (1970) Acute parotitis associated with parainfluenza 3 virus infection. *American Journal of Diseases of Children,* **119,** 147.

CHAPTER 7

Obstructive and Traumatic Lesions

Obstruction to the flow of saliva may follow lesions of the duct papilla, the presence of a salivary calculus (or sialolith) and pressure from lesions within and without the duct wall (Seward, 1968). Salivary fistula formation and Frey's syndrome may be complications of trauma to the parotid region. Mucoceles are common lesions and both traumatic and obstructive factors have been implicated in their formation. These various conditions are now described.

PAPILLARY OBSTRUCTION

The commonest cause of papillary obstruction is trauma, from, for example a sharp cusp of a tooth, faulty restorations, projecting clasps, over extended denture flanges and dentures with high occlusal planes. Alternatively, a soft tissue lesion such as an ulcer may lead to acute papillary obstruction. In this instance the onset is sudden although the symptoms are of short duration, resolving as the ulcer heals (Figure 7.1). Repeated trauma, however, will give rise to chronic papillary obstruction which may result in stenosis. Chronic papillary obstruction may lead to recurrent gland swelling especially at mealtimes. Ascending infection of the gland is common and will give rise to sudden, severe enlargement. Investigation of chronic papillary obstruction may be difficult especially if fibrosis has occurred. The duct opening may be difficult to locate and resist the insertion of a probe.

Sialography will demonstrate the degree of narrowing of the duct in the papillary region and dilation of the duct behind. The treatment of papillary obstruction includes removal of the cause. Where stenosis has occurred, then, papillectomy with careful suturing of the duct lining to the oral mucosa may be indicated.

DUCT OBSTRUCTION WITHIN THE LUMEN—SIALOLITHIASIS

Calcification within duct lumens leading to obstruction can be found in many organs of the human body, most often in the urinary tract, gall bladder and submandibular salivary gland. They may, however, also occur in the parotid, sublingual and minor salivary glands, pancreas and lungs. Salivary calculi

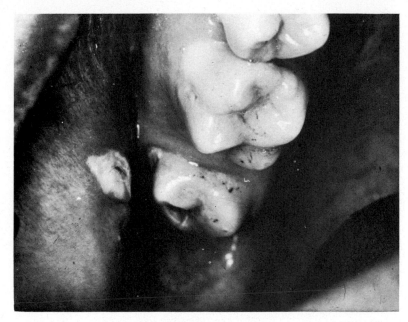

Figure 7.1. Traumatic ulceration around the orifice of the R parotid duct. The offending edge of a carious cavity can be seen.

are found in one per cent of subjects coming to autopsy (Rauch and Gorlin, 1970). Calculi are usually unilateral and round to oval in shape (Figure 7.2), have a smooth or irregular surface, vary in size from a small grain to the size of a peach stone, and are usually yellowish in colour. Calcium phosphates (74 per cent) and carbonates (11 per cent) comprise the major inorganic portion but iron oxide, sodium chloride, sodium or potassium thiocyanate and magnesium compounds may also be present (Wakeley, 1948; Rauch and Gorlin, 1970). Mucopolysaccharides, cholesterol and uric acid are generally present (Blatt, Mikkelsen and Denning, 1958; Mandel, 1971). The concept of initial organic nidus formation followed by deposition of inorganic material appears to be supported by ultrastructural study (Tandler, 1965). The various theories regarding the initial formation and subsequent enlargement of sialoliths have been well reviewed by Rauch and Gorlin (1970).

Parotid salivary constituents in patients with carbonate apatite sialoliths vary little from those of normal saliva (Blatt, Mikkelsen and Denning, 1958). However, the calcium/phosphorus ratio in submandibular saliva appears to be changed in patients with sialoliths (Schmidt-Nielsen, 1946; Blatt, 1964).

Adults are more commonly affected though sialolithiasis may occur in children, and the classical clinical signs and symptoms are those of pain and sudden enlargement of the affected gland, especially at mealtimes. Clinical diagnosis may be confirmed visually (Figures 7.3 and 7.4), by palpation (Figure 7.5) and plain radiographs (Figure 7.6). Treatment, depending on the site and clinical features, is by surgical removal of the calculus though in some cases removal of the gland may be necessary (Chapter 14). Histo-

107

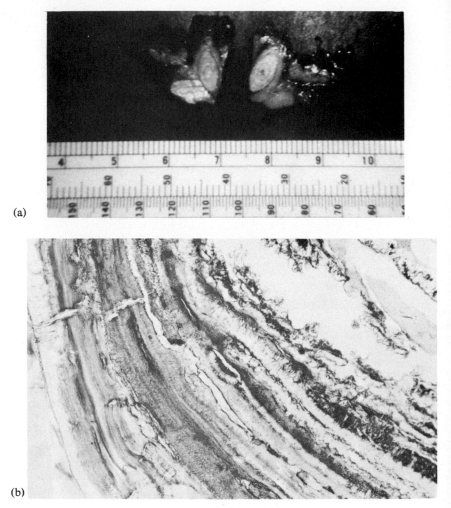

Figure 7.2. a. Gross specimen of laminated sialolith in submandibular duct within gland parenchyma. b. Portion of sialolith. Gelatin embedded, decalcified frozen sectioning shows laminated structure.

logically the affected gland will show the features of a chronic sialadenitis whilst within the affected duct calcified material is observed (Figure 7.7).

OBSTRUCTION DUE TO CAUSES IN OR AROUND THE DUCT WALL

Salivary duct obstruction may result from stricture especially following ulceration around a submandibular sialolith. Stricture may follow other traumatic injuries to the duct. These lesions are best treated by dilatation of the stricture with graduated sizes of urethral bougies, coated with lignocaine

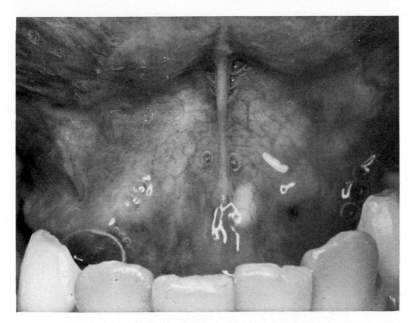

Figure 7.3. Sialolith present within the main duct of the L submandibular salivary gland.

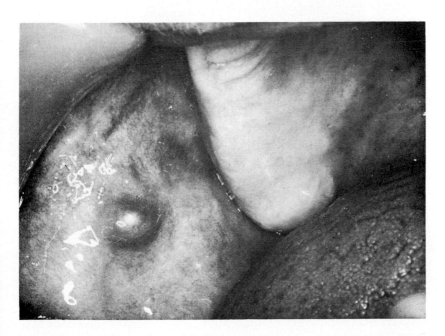

Figure 7.4. Sialolith obstructing the parotid duct at the orifice. The surrounding soft tissues are inflamed.

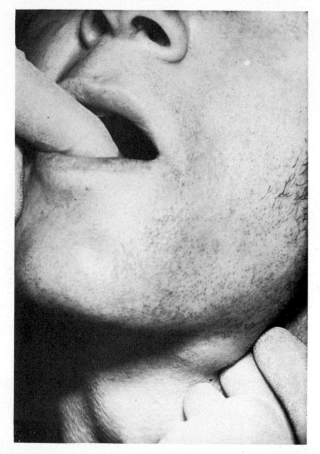

Figure 7.5. Bimanual palpation of L submandibular gland swelling caused by sialolith in main duct (see Figure 7.3).

urethral gel. Salivary ducts may be obstructed by pressure of tumours from without. Benign neoplasms simply compress the duct although malignant lesions may also infiltrate the duct wall.

SALIVARY DUCT FISTULA

A salivary duct fistula is defined as a communication between the duct system and the skin which allows secretion of saliva externally. Although uncommon, salivary duct fistula formation presents a troublesome and distressing condition for the patient. Internal fistulae may occur but since they drain into the oral cavity they are asymptomatic and therefore of little consequence. A salivary duct fistula may be congenital, although more commonly follows trauma—for example deep laceration of the cheek or as a complication of major gland surgery or result from ulceration and infection associated with

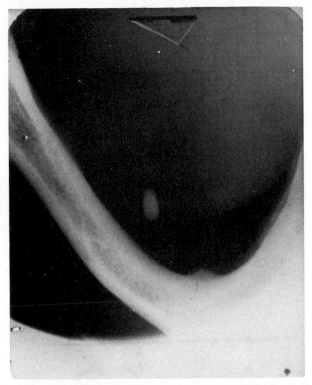

Figure 7.6. A right submandibular duct sialolith demonstrated by plain film radiography.

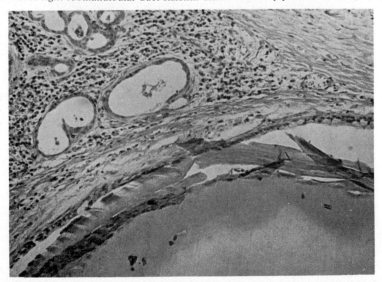

Figure 7.7. Laminated sialolith within the excretory duct of a minor salivary gland. Mucous metaplasia affects the lining epithelium and chronic inflammatory changes are present within adjacent salivary tissue. ($\times$ 100).

111

sialadenitis, large calculi or tumours (Hemenway and Bergenstom, 1971).

In clinical practice wound infection is common in cases of duct fistula and fibrous repair tissue may accumulate leading to the occlusion of the proximal duct so causing atrophy of the gland. More commonly an external fistulous tract is established (Figure 7.8). The site of duct involvement may be determined by sialography (Figure 7.9). Treatment and management is primarily by surgical repair (Lichenstein and Kopp, 1965; Hemenway and Bergenstrom, 1971).

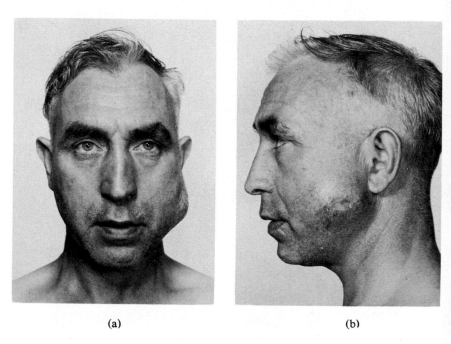

(a)   (b)

Figure 7.8. a, b. Parotid gland fistula in 46-year-old male, resulting as the complication of a parotid abscess.

FREY'S SYNDROME

In this unusual condition sweating and flushing of the skin over the distribution of the auriculo temporal nerve takes place following the stimulus to salivary secretion. The syndrome may follow parotid surgery, temporo-mandibular surgery or injuries and infections in this region. The condition is thought to arise following damage to the auriculo temporal nerve which contain post-ganglionic parasympathetic fibres from the otic ganglion. These damaged fibres then become united to sympathetic nerves from the superior cervical ganglion which supply the sweat glands of the skin. It is a distressing condition for the patient and difficult to treat (Chapter 14).

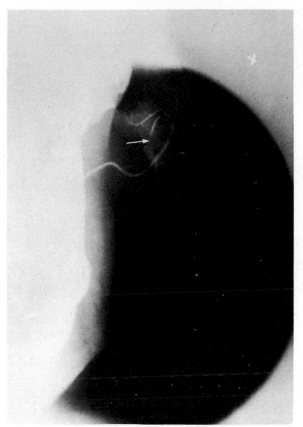

Figure 7.9. Salivary duct fistula demonstrated by sialography. Site of duct involvement is arrowed. Antero-posterior view.

MUCOCELE

Mucoceles may be superficial (Figure 7.10) or deep and may vary in size from a few millimetres to 1 cm in diameter. Those which are superficial have a bluish, translucent colour and rupture easily. Deeper seated mucoceles have the same colour as surrounding oral mucosa. Recurrence is common, especially of the superficial type of lesion.

Histologically mucoceles may be graded as a mucous extravasion cyst or a mucous retention cyst.

The cause of the mucous extravasation cyst is considered to be mechanical trauma of minor excretory ducts leading to severance of the duct, with resultant spillage of mucus into the connective tissue stroma. The mucous pool is localised or walled off by a condensation of connective and granulation tissue (Figure 7.11). A mucous retention cyst refers to a mucocele which results from a partial obstruction to the flow of saliva. As a consequence the duct dilates resulting in a cystic lesion lined by a simple columnar or pseudo-stratified squamous epithelium.

113

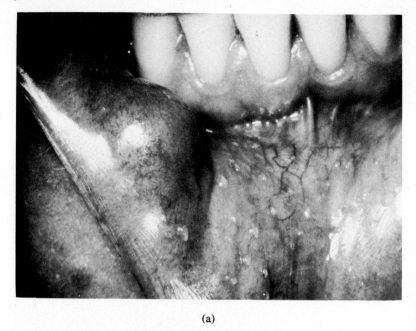

(a)

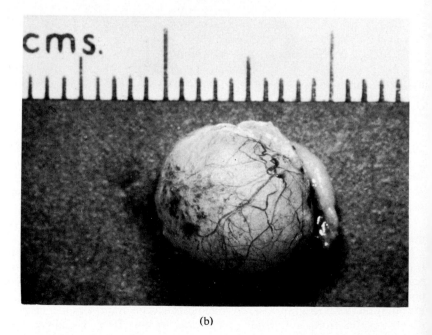

(b)

Figure 7.10. a. Mucocele affecting lower lip towards angle of mouth. b. Gross specimen.

114

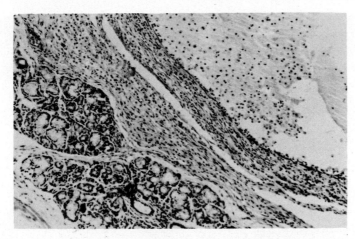

Figure 7.11. Granulation tissue lining of a mucous extravasation cyst (mucocele). ($\times$ 75.)

Mucoceles occur most commonly in the lower lip (Figure 7.10) followed by the buccal mucosa and floor of mouth. The palate and upper lip are rarely involved. A mucocele of anterior lingual salivary glands is often referred to as a cyst of Blandin-Nuhn.

Ranula is the name given to a form of mucocele which occurs in the floor of the mouth (Figure 7.12) and is associated with the ducts of the submandibular and the sublingual salivary glands. They are usually unilateral swellings, two to three cm in diameter which are soft and fluctuant with a bluish-violet colour. Although generally painless they may interfere with speech, mastication and swallowing. Histologically they have a simple cuboidal epithelial lining and probably arise as a result of partial obstruction to the flow of saliva. A rather rare lesion referred to as a deep ranula is one which extends through and below the mylo-hyoid muscle and may extend as far back as the base of skull or into the neck. This lesion may take its origin from the cervical sinus, normally obliterated during embryonic life. The 'true' cyst with a complete epithelial lining is usually small, about one cm in diameter, and located within the affected salivary gland. It is lined with stratified squamous epithelium. The treatment for all lesions is by surgical removal or by marsupialisation (Chapter 14).

Aetiology and pathogenesis

As mentioned previously in this chapter and as a consequence of experimental and clinical studies (Bhaskar, Bolden and Weinmann, 1956; Standish and Shafer, 1959; Robinson and Hjörting-Hansen, 1964; Sela and Ulmansky, 1969; de Araujo and Tomich, 1971), the main cause of mucoceles is thought to be rupture of a duct with resultant extravasation of mucus into the connective tissue stroma. Recent studies (Harrison and Garrett, 1972; Garrett and Harrison, 1972), however, have provided evidence for the view that complete ductal obstruction should not be disregarded as a possible

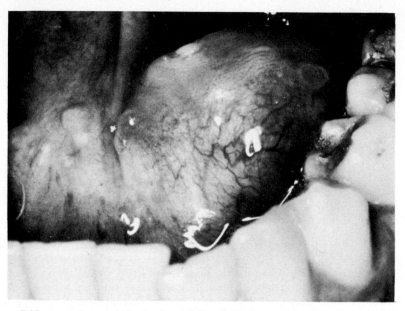

Figure 7.12. A ranula present in the floor of the mouth of a young patient.

aetiological factor in mucocele formation. These workers have shown that following duct ligation of the cat sublingual gland mucous extravasation could be produced in over half the glands studied whilst mucocele formation was present in one quarter. The critical factor appears to be avoidance of nerve involvement, such as the chorda, during the experimental procedure. Other important factors may be spontaneous secretion (Emmelin, 1961)—a feature of sublingual glands in the cat and human minor glands—the common site of the naturally occurring lesions; also, the presence of a capsule which has an inhibiting effect upon mucocele formation. Garrett and Harrison (1972) have shown, further, that lysosomal enzyme activity is increased in acinar cells in those glands undergoing atrophy. This was always associated with macrophage activity. Extravasated mucus in addition to inducing macrophage activity also causes a fibroblastic reaction with fibroblasts showing arylamidase activity—a feature of the healing process. These workers suggest that macrophage activity to remove mucus together with the fibroblastic healing processes would give rise to early pressure atrophy and thus inhibit mucocele formation. If these processes, however, do not contain extravasation in the early stage then a balance in time between secretion of fluid and its removal obtains and mucocele formation is established (Garrett and Harrison, 1972).

Minor salivary gland tissue which may be present in fibrous overgrowths resulting from trauma by ill-fitting dentures, shows sialadenitis, acinar atrophy and duct dilation (Arwill, Nilsson and Öberg, 1968). These workers suggest that trauma from the denture on the duct orifice leads to erosion with subsequent proliferation of the columnar duct epithelium to the oral mucosal surface.

Sialolithiasis of minor salivary glands

Minor gland sialolithiasis is rare, just over twenty cases having been reported In the literature (Lighterman, 1955; Chaudhry, Gorlin and Reynolds, 1960; Erickson and Hale, 1962; Holst, 1968; Eversole and Sabes, 1971). Males appear to be more commonly affected and the buccal mucosa seems to be the predominant site (Eversole and Sabes, 1971). Acinar and duct changes due to obstruction are similar to those reported in the major glands and are probably related to the duration, size and texture of the sialolith. Metaplastic changes range from the presence of ciliated pseudostratified columnar epithelium and mucous cell formation to squamous metaplasia of the excretory ducts. Acinar atrophy and intercalated and striated duct dilation are variable findings. Mucous retention appears to account for reactive oncocytic metaplasia (Eversole and Sabes, 1971) when it is observed histologically in lesions due to obstruction. The presence of a papilloma on the oral mucosa which coincidentally occludes a minor duct orifice may lead to secondary reactive duct hyperplasia. Eversole and Sabes (1971) suggest that this mechanism may give rise to the rare lesion ascribed the name intra-ductal papilloma (Castigiliano and Gold, 1954).

Experimental studies of rat submandibular gland recovery from obstruction at light and electron-microscopic levels have been undertaken recently (Tamarin, 1971a, b). Evidence of parenchymal cell death or mitotic activity was found to be extremely rare. Tamarin (1971a) suggests that gland recovery is the result of cell recovery and not the result of de novo cell differentiation. Secretory activity by acinar cells was observed to precede that in granular cells in the recovery phase. The fine structural characteristics of acinar secretory granules range from dense, crystaloid-like structures in the early phase to characteristic mature granules at the full recovery stage (Tamarin, 1971b).

REFERENCES

Arwill, T., Nilsson, B. & Oberg, G. (1968) Eversion of columnar epithelium in denture-induced hyperplasia of the oral mucous membrane of man. *Archives of Oral Biology,* **13,** 589.

Bhaskar, S. N., Bolden, T. E. & Weinmann, J. P. (1956) Pathogenesis of mucoceles. *Journal of Dental Research,* **35,** 863.

Blatt, I. M., Mikkelsen, W. M. & Denning, R. M. (1958) Studies in sialolithiasis. II. Uric acid calculus of the parotid gland: Report of a case. *Annals of Otology, Rhinology and Laryngology,* **67,** 1022.

Blatt, I. M. (1964) On sialectasis and benign lymphosialadenopathy. *Laryngoscope,* **74,** 1685.

Chaudhry, A. P., Gorlin, R. L. & Reynolds, D. H. (1960) Sialolithiasis of a minor salivary gland. *Oral Surgery, Oral Medicine and Oral Pathology,* **13,** 578.

de Araujo, N. S. & Tomich, C. E. (1971) Experimental production of mucus retention phenomenon in animals with isoproterenol. *Oral Surgery, Oral Medicine and Oral Pathology,* **31,** 849.

Emmelin, N. G. (1961) In *Physiology of the Salivary Glands.* (Eds.) Burgen, A. S. V. & Emmelin, N. G. pp. 96-97. London: Arnold.

Erickson, R. I. & Hale, M. L. (1962) Minor salivary gland sialolithiasis. *Oral Surgery, Oral Medicine and Oral Pathology,* **15,** 200.

Eversole, L. R. & Sabes, W. R. (1971) Minor salivary gland duct changes due to obstruction. *Archives of Otolaryngology,* **94,** 19.

Garrett, J. R. & Harrison, J. D. (1972) Histochemistry of mucocele formation induced by duct ligation of sublingual salivary glands in cats. *Histochemistry and Cytochemistry,* **110,** 401.

Harrison, J. D. & Garrett, J. R. (1972) Mucocele formation in cats by glandular duct ligation. *Archives of Oral Biology,* **17,** 1403.

Hemenway, W. G. & Bergenstrom, L. (1971) Parotid duct fistula: A review. *Southern Medical Journal,* **64,** 912.

Holst, E. (1968) Sialolithiasis of the minor salivary glands: Report of three cases. *Journal of Oral Surgery,* **26,** 354.

Lichtenstein, J. L. & Kopp, W. K. (1965) Closure of a parotid salivary fistula. *Journal of Oral Surgery,* **23,** 497.

Lighterman, L. (1955) Sialolithiasis of a minor salivary gland. *Oral Surgery, Oral Medicine and Oral Pathology,* **8,** 143.

Mandel, I. D. (1971) Composition of salivary gland stones. *I.A.D.R. North American Division,* Abstract No. 850.

Rauch, S. & Gorlin, R. J. (1970) In *Thoma's Oral Pathology.* Vol. 2, p. 692. St. Louis: C. V. Mosby.

Robinson, L. & Hjörting-Hansen, E. (1964) Pathologic changes associated with mucous retention cysts of minor salivary glands. *Oral Surgery, Oral Medicine and Oral Pathology,* **18,** 191.

Schmidt-Nielsen, B. (1946) The solubility of tooth substance in relation to the composition of saliva. *Acta Odontologica Scandinavica,* **7,** (Supplement 2), 1.

Sela, J. & Ulmansky, M. (1969) Mucous retention cyst of salivary glands. *Journal of Oral Surgery,* **27,** 619.

Seward, G. R. (1968) Anatomic surgery for salivary calculi. 1. Symptoms, signs and differential diagnosis. *Oral Surgery, Oral Medicine and Oral Pathology,* **25,** 150.

Standish, S. M. & Shafer, W. G. (1959) The mucus retention phenomenon. *Journal of Oral Surgery, Anesthesia and Hospital Dental Service,* **17,** 15.

Tamarin, A. (1971a) Submaxillary gland recovery from obstruction. I. Overall changes and electron microscopic alterations of granular duct cells. *Journal of Ultrastructure Research,* **34,** 276.

Tamarin, A. (1971b) Submaxillary gland recovery from obstruction. II. Electron microscopic alterations of acinar cells. *Journal of Ultrastructure Research,* **34,** 288.

Tandler, B. (1965) Electron microscopical observations on early sialoliths in a human submaxillary gland. *Archives of Oral Biology,* **10,** 509.

Wakeley, C. (1948) The surgery of the salivary glands. *Annals of the Royal College of Surgeons of England,* **3,** 289.

CHAPTER 8

Changes in Salivary Secretion and Composition in Disease

In this chapter, those factors and disease states which alter the rate of flow and composition of saliva are described.

FUNCTIONAL DISORDERS

The quantitative production of parotid saliva has been the subject of many studies (Schneyer and Levin, 1955; Schneyer, 1956; Kerr, 1961; Curry and Patey, 1964; Sewards, Hamilton and Patey, 1966; Shannon and Chauncey, 1967; Shannon, 1967; Mason et al, 1967; Ericson, 1968; Dawes, 1969). The conflicting results may be due to the variations in methods used and in the experimental conditions, and also to the fact that the secretion of saliva is affected by a number of psychological and environmental factors.

Factors influencing salivary flow rate

Some of the factors influencing salivary flow rate have already been referred to in Chapter 3. Those and other factors which may affect salivary flow rate will now be reviewed. In addition to organic disease of the salivary glands, mechanical stimulation, age, sex distribution and diet may lead to alterations in the rate of salivary flow (Jenkins, 1966; Bertram, 1967; Ericson, 1968; Brown, 1970; Dawes, 1970). Dehydration of the body (Winsor, 1930; Kerr, 1961) causes a diminution, and hyperhydration an increase (Shannon and Chauncey, 1967), in salivary secretion. Lower flow rates are also observed in hospitalised patients (Bertram, 1967). Mental stress, anxiety and psycho-pathological emotional states (Bates and Adams, 1968; Brown, 1970), fatigue (Nekrason and Chranilowa, 1933), infection (Krasnogorski, 1931), increased room temperature (Goldman et al, 1961), all lead to a diminution of salivary gland flow rate. Cigarette smoking has been shown to cause increase in salivary parotid flow rates (Barylko-Pikielna, Pangborn and Shannon, 1968). Recently, the effect of drugs, especially the tranquilliser and ganglion-blocking agents, has been shown to cause marked oral dryness (Scopp and Heyman, 1966; Bahn, 1972). Diurnal variation of salivary flow

(Hildes and Ferguson, 1958; Ferguson, Elliott and Potts, 1969; and Dawes, 1972) is a further important factor to be considered and therefore the time of collection (Zaus and Fosdick, 1943; Faber, 1943; Schneyer, 1956; Kerr, 1961) as well as the method of collection (Kerr, 1961) are important factors which influence the secretion of saliva. Body weight and other general body factors such as height, pulse rate, systolic and diastolic blood pressures, do not appear to influence salivary secretion (Kerr, 1961; Bertram, 1967; Brown, 1970). As Kerr (1961) has shown, the muscle activity involved in chewing on one side of the mouth leads to an increase in flow rate on that side. Recently, light deprivation has been shown to decrease salivary flow (Shannon and Feller, 1972).

Xerostomia

Xerostomia may be a sign or a symptom. It is a fairly common clinical complaint which can in some cases be extremely distressing to the patient. The incidence of xerostomia in patients attending the Glasgow Dental Hospital has been recorded (Lamb, A. B., personal communication, 1974). It is of interest that although xerostomia is a primary complaint in 1 in 1500 patients, on enquiry 1 in 10 patients had experienced dryness of the mouth as a regular symptom. It is useful to distinguish between true or primary xerostomia, where a pathological lesion is present in the salivary glands as a

Table 8.1. *Aetiology of xerostomia—Classification.*

1. Factors affecting the salivary centre, e.g:
   a) Emotions—fear, excitement, depression, etc.
   b) Neuroses—endogenous depression
   c) Organic disease—brain tumour
   d) Drugs (see Table 8.3)

2. Factors affecting the autonomic outflow pathway, e.g:
   a) Encephalitis
   b) Brain tumours
   c) Accidents
   d) Neurosurgical operations
   e) Drugs (see Table 8.3)

3. Factors affecting salivary gland function, e.g:
   a) Aplasia
   b) Sjögren's syndrome
   c) Obstruction
   d) Infection
   e) Irradiation
   f) Excision

4. Factors producing changes in fluid or electrolyte balance, e.g:
   a) Dehydration
   b) Diabetes insipidus
   c) Cardiac failure
   d) Uraemia
   e) Oedema

manifestation of either localised or generalised disease, and symptomatic or secondary xerostomia where no salivary lesion is present (Bertram, 1967). The effects upon the oral mucosa include epithelial atrophy, inflammation, fissuring and ulceration. In addition to xerostomia the patient may complain of a burning sensation, sore tongue, oral soreness and ulceration and difficulty with denture retention. Xerostomia, of whatever cause, predisposes to infection of the pharynx and salivary glands and to a marked increase in dental caries (Trimble, Etherington and Losch, 1938; Ericsson et al, 1954; Frank, Herdly and Philippe, 1965; Kapsinalis, 1966). The first case of persistent xerostomia was recorded by Hutchinson (1888).

The causes of xerostomia are numerous (Table 8.1) and have been reviewed by Faber (1943), Bertram (1967) and Brown (1970). As described earlier in this chapter, emotional and anxiety states and the effect of various drugs (Tables 8.2 and 8.3) such as tranquillisers, hypotensive agents and atropine-containing medications are implicated in symptomatic xerostomia. Other factors include pernicious anaemia, iron-deficiency anaemia, loss of fluid through haemorrhage, sweating, diarrhoea or vomiting, the polyuria of

Table 8.2. *Classes of drugs with xerostomic side effects.*

Analgesic mixtures
Anticonvulsants
Antiemetics
Antihistamines
Antihypertensives
Antinauseants
Antiparkinson
Antipruritics
Antispasmotics
Appetite suppressants
Cold medications
Diuretics
Decongestants
Expectorants
Muscle relaxants
Psychotropic drugs:
    CNS depressants
    Dibenzazepine derivatives
    Phenothiazine derivatives
    MAO inhibitors
    Tranquillisers—major and minor
Sedatives

From Bahn, S. L. (1972) Drug-related dental destruction. *Oral Surgery, Oral Medicine and Oral Pathology,* **33,** 49-54.

diabetes mellitis and diabetes insipidus and various vitamin and hormonal deficiencies. Primary xerostomia may be due to absence of salivary tissue, irradiation, glandular infection or obstruction and systemic disease such as Sjögren's syndrome in which the salivary glands are involved. Disease affecting nervous transmission, either the afferent or efferent portion of the reflex, will affect flow. The causes of xerostomia in 80 patients studied at the

Table 8.3. *Brand names of drugs with xerostomic side effects with relative xerostomic potential; evaluated from PDR.*

Acutuss—4[a]	Daricon—1
Akineton—1	Decadron—Questionable
Alased—1	Decagesic—Questionable
Aldoclor—3	Decholin—3
Aldomet—3	Dehist—2
Aludrox—2	Demazin—2
Aluscop—2	Demerol—3
Ambenyl expectorant—1	Demerol APAP—3
Amphaplex—1	Deprol—3
Anti-Nausea Supprettes—2	Desa Hist PFS—Questionable
Antrenyl—3	Diafen—3
Antrenyl-Phenobarbital—3	DIA-quel liquid—4
Antrocol—3	Didrex—4
Appetrol—2	Dimetane—3
Arco-Lase Plus—2	Dimetapp—2
Artane—1	Dimethacol—2
Atarax—3	Disipal—1
Ataraxoid—4	Disomer—Questionable
Atrocholin—4	Diupres—2
Aventyl HCl—3	Diutensen-R—2
Bamadex—2	Dolonil—1
B and O Supprettes—2	Dolophine HCl—2
Barbidonna—4	Donnagel—4
Bar-Tropin tablets—Questionable	Donnagesic—4
Belbarb—4	Donnalate—4
Belladenal—2	Donnasep—3
Bellergal—4	Donnatal—4
Benadryl Kapseals—2	Drilitol Spraypak—Questionable
Bendectin—2	Drize M capsules—3
Biphetamine—2	Dronactin—4
Bonine—4	Duovent—3
Bucladin Softab—3	Eldonal—4
Butibel—4	Enarax—1
Butibel-Zyme—4	Enduretrol—4
Butiserpazide 25/50 Prestabs—2	Enduron—4
Butiserpine—2	Enduronyl—4
Cantil—4	Esimil—3
Capla—4	Eskaserp—1
Caplaril—4	Estomul—2
Carrhist Forte—1	Etrafon—2
Chardonna—4	Eutonyl—3
Chlor-Trimeton—2	Eutron—3
Clistin—4	Exna-R—2
Cogentin—1	Festalan—Questionable
Colrex Decongestant—1	Flagyl—3
Combid—1	Forhistal—4
Compazine—3	Gemonil—Questionable
Consotuss—1	Gourmase PB—4
Convertin—4	Haldol—2
Converzyme—4	Hexadrol Phosphate—Questionable
Coplexen—3	Hispril—3
Coriforte—2	Histabid Duracap—2
Corilin—2	Histaspan—2
Cyclex—4	Histaspan D—2
Cydril—2	Histaspan Plus—2
Darbid—1	Hydergine—Questionable

[a] 1 = Most xerostomic, 4 = least xerostomic.

Table 8.3 (*continued*)

HydroDIURIL—Questionable
Hydromox—2
Hydropres—2
Ilocalm—3
Ionamin—2
Ismelin—3
Kanumodic—3
Kemadrin—1
Kolantyl—2
Largon—2
Levamine—4
Levoprome—3
Levsin—1
Librax—1
Mallenzyme—1
Marax—4
Marplan—1
Matulane—3
MCS Triaminic—Questionable
Mellaril—3
Mepergan—1
Matatensin—2
Metreton—2
Milpath—2
Monomeb—2
Murel—4
Naquival—2
Nembu-donna—2
Neo-Syncphrine—Questionable
Norflex—1
Norpramin—4
Nydrazid Injection—2
Obesa-Mead—1
Obetrol—1
Obotan—2
Olbese No. 1—1
Omni-Tuss—4
Ornade—4
Pamine—1
Panitol H.M.B.—3
Parest—2
Parnate—2
Pathibamate—1
Pathilon—1
Peganone—Questionable
Periactin—4
PERKÉ capsules—4
Permitil—4
Phantos—3
Phenergan—3
Pipanol—3
Piptal—4
Piptal PIIB—4
Placidyl—Questionable
Plegine—3
Plimasin—1
Polaramine—2

Preludin—3
Per-Sate—3
Pro-Banthine—1
Prolixin—2
Prolixin Enanthate—2
Prydonnal—2
Pyma timed capsules—2
Pymadex timed capsules—2
Pyribenzamine—1
Quaalude—2
Quadamine Granucaps—2
Quilene—1
Raudixin—3
Rau-Sed—2
Rautrax—3
Rauzide—3
Regroton—4
Rela—3
Renese—Questionable
Renese-R—2
Repoise—2
Rinohist—4
Robinul—4
Rynatuss—3
Salutensin—2
Sibena—2
Sidonna—2
Sinequan—4
Sinubid—4
Sinulin—4
Sinusule—4
Sinutab—Questionable
Softran Softab—3
Solacen—4
Solfo-Serpine—2
Solu-Cortef—Questionable
Somnafac—2
Sopor—4
Sorboquel—2
Span-RD—3
Sparine—2
Spasticol—4
Stelazine—3
Symmetrel—4
Tacaryl HCl—4
Talwin—4
Taractan—4
Teldrin—3
Telepaque—4
Temaril—3
Tenuate—3
Tepanil—3
Thora-Dex—3
Thorazine—3
Tindal—3
Tofranil—4
Torecan—4

Table 8.3 (*continued*)

Tral—2	Tussaminic—Questionable
Transentine HCl—1	Tuss—Ornade—3
Transentine phenobarbital—1	Tybatran—4
Trest—3	ULO—4
Triaminic—Questionable	Unitensen-R—2
Triavil—3	URI—2
Tridal—4	Uriplex—2
Trilafon—3	Ursinus—Questionable
Trisulfaminic—3	Vesprin—2
Tussagesic—Questionable	Vistaril—4

From Bahn, S. L. (1972) Drug-related dental destruction. *Oral Surgery, Oral Medicine and Oral Pathology*, **33**, 49-54.

Glasgow Dental Hospital are shown in Table 8.4. A striking feature is the high percentage (73 per cent) of patients in whom systemic factors were implicated as a cause of xerostomia.

Table 8.4. *Aetiology of xerostomia in 80 patients attending Glasgow Dental Hospital.*

Local	{ Candidosis	5 }	13%
	{ Miscellaneous	5 }	
Systemic	Sjögren's syndrome	30	
	Psychogenic + drugs	12	
	Drug induced	10	73%
	Anaemia	5	
	Endocrine	2	
Cause unknown		11	14%

Lamb. A. B. and Mason, D. K. (unpublished observations).

Treatment is aimed at seeking and removing the cause. The use of a glycerine and lemon mouthwash is helpful in alleviating the symptoms in most cases (for details see Chapter 10). The stimulation of salivary flow by pilocarpine has been used by some workers. The use of mouthwashes such as solutions containing sodium chloride and sodium bicarbonate may also be of value. Recently, synthetic saliva, containing carboxymethylcellose, sorbitol and optimal quantities of salts has been developed (Matzker and Schreiber, 1972; Gravenmade, Roukema and Panders, 1974) and appears promising. The use of trithioparamethoxyphenylpropene (Sulfarlem—Laboratoires Latéma) has been described by French workers (Deniker et al, 1970), but the authors have no experience of this drug. In the general management of xerostomia, strict attention to oral hygiene is essential and microbiological examination at regular intervals is of value if recurrent oral candidal infection is to be avoided (Chapters 10 and 20).

Sialorrhoea

Increased salivation (sialorrhoea or ptyalism) is relatively uncommon. The predisposing factors include acute inflammatory conditions leading to stomatitis, such as herpetic and aphthous ulceration. Increased salivation is commonly encountered during the period when teeth are erupting in young individuals. Patients with neurological disturbances such as mental retardation, Parkinsonism, schizophrenia and epilepsy are subject to sialorrhoea. Drooling or pooling of saliva in the mouth in these cases may be due to loss of muscle control or other factors rather than to increased flow rate per se (Wotman and Mandel, 1973). The rate of salivary flow may be increased in mercury poisoning, acrodynia and rabies. In familial dysautonomia, a syndrome thought to result from an inborn error in catecholamine metabolism, increased salivation, especially during excitement, is a frequent finding.

With regard to treatment, attention to the cause together with the use of bicarbonate mouthwashes are helpful for this distressing condition. The use of anti-cholinergic drugs having an atropine-like effect, duct reconstruction or nerve sectioning may be necessary in severe cases (Chapter 14).

CHANGES IN SALIVARY COMPOSITION IN DISEASE

Alterations of salivary composition have been reported in various disease states affecting salivary glands or other body tissues. With the advent of better methods for the collection of saliva and the availability of new analytical techniques there has been an increase in biochemical measurements of salivary constituents. Many of the changes in biochemical composition found merely reflect changes in blood, plasma or serum levels, and while they may be of research interest are not of diagnostic significance. The use of saliva may be advantageous when frequent monitoring of a constituent such as electrolytes and urea is required, thus avoiding repeated venepuncture. There are instances where changes in salivary composition have proved helpful in clinical assessment and diagnosis of patients.

Problems of the interpretation of studies on salivary constituents

When interpreting the significance of the concentration of a salivary constituent it is necessary to consider some of the factors which might influence it. These are numerous and have been described in detail in Chapter 3.

The influence of the following factors should be considered:

1. Species
2. Sex
3. Source of saliva
4. Nature of the stimulus
5. Duration of the stimulus
6. Rest transients
7. Flow rate
8. Plasma level
9. Diet
10. Hormones
11. Diurnal variation
12. Drugs

All or any one of these factors may affect the level of a particular salivary constituent (Figure 8.1). It is essential therefore to define the conditions under which a sample of saliva is obtained before any significance can be attributed to the results of its biochemical analysis.

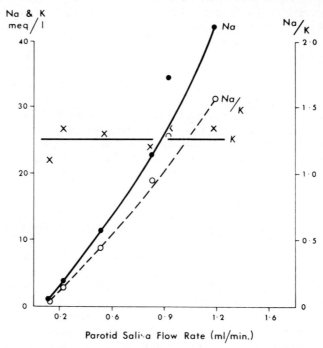

Figure 8.1. Sodium and potassium concentration in saliva and sodium/potassium ratio at varying salivary flow rates.

Diseases in which alterations in salivary composition occur

These diseases include fibrocystic disease, thyroid disease, sialosis, hypertension, adrenal disease, diabetes and connective tissue diseases, and are discussed below.

Fibrocystic disease

The exocrine glands, in particular the pancreas, salivary, sweat and bronchial glands, are affected in this condition. Marked changes occur in salivary composition. In parotid saliva there are elevated concentrations of sodium, calcium and phosphorus (Chauncey et al, 1962) and high levels of urea and uric acid have also been reported. In the submandibular saliva elevated protein, glycoproteins, calcium, phosphorus, sodium, chloride urea and uric acid have been reported (Mandel, 1967).

High calcium and phosphorus concentration in submandibular saliva in children with cystic fibrosis leads to calculus forming on teeth. However, it is of interest that it does not produce an increased incidence of salivary gland stones. Submandibular saliva in cystic fibrosis has been shown to contain preformed hydroxyapatite, yet despite this stones do not form (Henkin and Schecter, 1971).

Since Di Sant' Agnese's original observation that there was a raised sodium level in the sweat of patients with fibrocystic disease (Di Sant' Agnese et al, 1953), the measurement of sweat sodium after pilocarpine iontophoresis has been the standard diagnostic method. McGrady and Bessman (1955) and Johnston (1956) found raised parotid saliva sodium levels and Lawson (1967) and Saggers et al (1967) have suggested the use of salivary sodium measurements using a sodium responsive micro-electrode as a clinical test in the diagnosis of fibrocystic disease (Figures 8.2 and 8.3). They described in unstimulated parotid saliva of homozygote values above 10 meq per litre (range 10 to 50 meq per litre) as compared with a group of normals and heterozygotes (Figure 8.4). At first it was suggested that the sodium-responsive micro-electrode placed close to the orifice of the parotid duct was demonstrating an increase in parotid salivary sodium level, but it is likely that the electrode tip is in contact with mixed saliva derived from minor salivary glands as well as the parotid. While the sweat test is the more

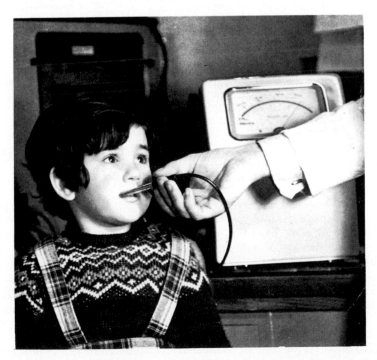

Figure 8.2. Screening test for fibrocystic disease. Use of sodium-responsive micro-electrode for measurement of salivary sodium level.

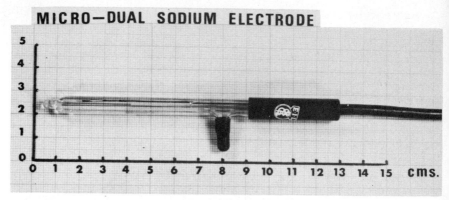

Figure 8.3. Sodium-sensitive micro-electrode which is used to monitor electrolyte levels in body fluids such as saliva.

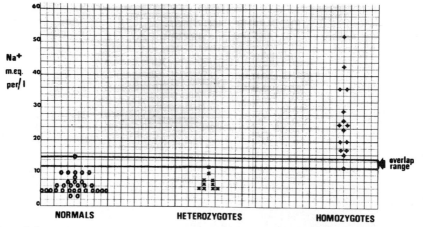

Figure 8.4. A comparison of the unstimulated parotid saliva pNa values; from normals, cystic fibrosis heterozygotes, and homozygotes using a micro-dual sodium electrode.

accurate diagnostic test, the use of the salivary sodium test in mass screening of four-month-old infants, has been suggested by Lawson, Westcombe and Saggers (1969). This screening technique is being evaluated at the present time and if successful will allow early diagnosis and treatment of this condition.

Since the salivary glands are affected generally in cystic fibrosis, then conceptually biopsy of the minor labial salivary glands should reflect the nature of the disease process and indeed this has been shown (Sweeney et al, 1967). Interstitial fibrosis, acinar atrophy and duct dilation are present together with the accumulation of eosinophilic plaque-like material within duct lumens. At an ultrastructural level, apart from more mucus being present, the cells of the labial salivary glands show little difference from the normal (Doggett, Bentinck and Harrison, 1971).

The treatment of cystic fibrosis involves attention to diet and the prevention of infection by antibiotic therapy.

Thyroid disease

The thyroid and salivary glands share a similar iodide-concentrating mechanism (Wolff, 1964). In the thyroid inorganic iodide is taken up from the plasma and is concentrated in the thyroid to many times the plasma level. It is then conjugated with protein and by a series of steps is transformed to the thyroid hormones triiodothyronine (T_3) and thyroxine (T_4) which are secreted. Similarly in the salivary glands the iodide is concentrated from the plasma but conjugation with protein does not occur, the inorganic iodide being secreted in the saliva. Measurement of the plasma inorganic iodide (PII) is of value in assessing thyroid disease such as non-toxic goitre and studying the action of anti-thyroid drugs (Wayne, 1967). Following a tracer dose of radioiodine, the PII may be determined by measuring the specific activity of salivary iodine. In normal individuals good correlation exists between PII concentration calculated from the specific activity of urinary and salivary iodine (Wayne, 1967). Advantages of obtaining saliva rather than urine samples are frequency of collection, avoidance of errors due to bladder emptying and absence of iodine in organic combination. A relatively low PII value, calculated from salivary activity, has been demonstrated in thyrotoxicosis (Alexander et al, 1966) and in dyshormonogenesis due to dehalogenase deficiency (Papadopoulos et al, 1966).

There is also a rare condition called the congenital iodide trapping defect in which iodide is not concentrated by thyroid and salivary glands (Stanbury and Chapman, 1960; Wolff, Thompson and Robbins, 1964). These patients present with hypothyroidism but they are difficult to diagnose from other forms of thyroid deficiency. If a congenital thyroid trapping defect is suspected it is easy to demonstrate the defect in the salivary iodide trap. In such a patient the saliva/plasma iodide ratio is less than one. Normally the saliva/plasma ratio is at least 10 and may be as high as 100 at resting salivary flow rates (Mason et al, 1967).

Sialosis

In this condition there is painless bilateral enlargement of the parotid glands (see Chapter 12). An increase in the parotid and submandibular potassium levels has been reported (Rauch, 1959) and may have diagnostic value.

Hypertension

In patients with essential or primary hypertension, decrease in sodium concentration with normal potassium concentration has been described and the sodium/potassium ratio has been suggested as a convenient screening test for aldosteronism and hypertension. Lawler, Hickler and Thorn (1962)

129

suggested ratios of 0.3 or below as diagnostic, below 0.5 as likely, and above 1.0 as excluding aldosteronism.

Adrenal disease

Patients with untreated Addison's disease were found to have a mean sodium/potassium ratio of 5.0. Wotman et al (1971) have suggested that raised potassium levels in submandibular saliva in pseudo-primary aldosteronism may be helpful in distinguishing this condition from primary aldosteronism. While these results are of interest they are dependent on accurate measurement of sodium and potassium concentration in saliva. The potassium level is relatively constant but the sodium is dependent on flow rate which in turn will alter the sodium/potassium ratio (Mason et al, 1967). For this reason blood and urine tests are preferred.

Other systemic diseases

As well as fibrocystic disease, abnormal salivary protein patterns have been associated with various pathological conditions. These include diabetes mellitus (Finestone, Schacterele and Pollack, 1973), and osteoporosis (Bonilla, Fuller and Stringham, 1968), connective tissue disorders (Chisholm, Beeley and Mason, 1973) and sarcoidosis (Beeley and Chisholm, unpublished observations).

The technique of isoelectric focusing separates proteins as a function of their isoelectric point in a pH gradient. The technique has high resolving power and will fractionate proteins which differ in their isoelectric points by only 0.02 pH unit. Separation of salivary proteins by isoelectric focusing in polyacrylamide gels from saliva of patients with Sjögren's syndrome, and from normal individuals, is shown in Figures 8.5 and 8.6. Only preliminary studies on the quantitative changes associated with pathological disorders have been made. These include a-amylase, kallikrein, lysozyme and albumin in sarcoidosis (Bhoola et al, 1969; Chisholm et al, 1971; Beeley and Chisholm, unpublished observations) and lysozyme in connective tissue disorders (Beeley, personal communication).

Recent studies designed to monitor salivary composition at the time of ovulation and also during pregnancy have shown submandibular calcium levels to be reduced during pregnancy (Mardar, Wotman and Mandel, 1972) and alkaline phosphatase to be raised in the pre-ovulatory period (Foster, Busse and Lorincz, 1971). Recently development of a whole saliva electrolyte determination has led to a test for a digitalis-toxic effect. Whole saliva has potassium and calcium concentration greatly elevated in patients who are digitalis toxic (Wotman and Mandel, 1973).

Dental disease

Saliva may theoretically affect the dental environment in several ways—by its mechanical cleansing action, by reducing enamel solubility, by buffering and

130

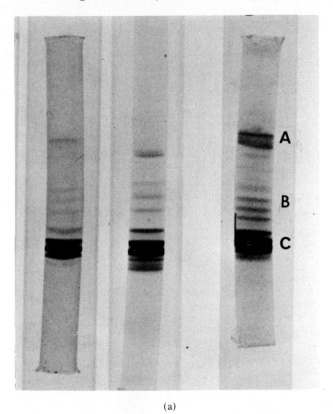

(a)

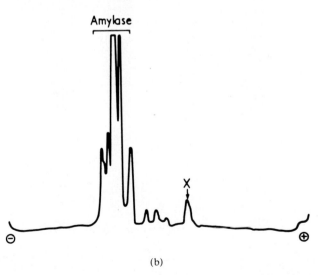

(b)

Figure 8.5. a. Iso-electric focusing on poly-acrylamide gels of parotid saliva from normal individuals. b. Densitometric tracing shows peak in 'X' region and corresponds to band A.

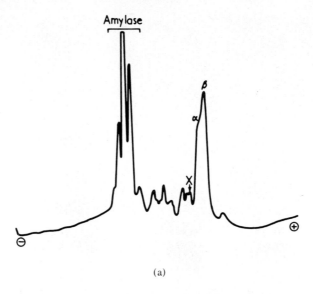

(a)

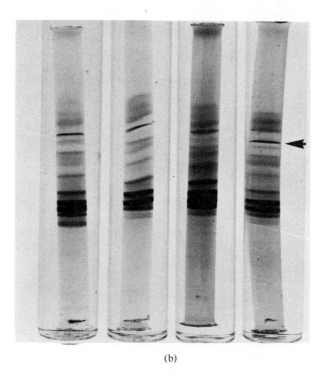

(b)

Figure 8.6. a. Densitometric tracing and b. acrylamide gels in parotid saliva from patients with Sjögren's syndrome. Arrow corresponds to a and β peaks.

neutralising acids produced by micro-organisms or diet, and by its probable antibacterial effect. Although markedly reduced flow rates, as may be found in pathological states, such as post-irradiation sialadenitis and Sjögren's syndrome, are associated with an increase in dental caries minor fluctuations in salivary flow rate and composition have not been clearly shown to have this association. Factors which have been studied include antisolubility factors, e.g. calcium and phosphate, antacid factors, e.g. pH, and antibacterial factors, e.g. lysozyme and IgA (Mandel, 1974). As far as the initiation of dental caries and gingivitis is concerned it appears that saliva will exert any effect it may have through dental plaque rather than by direct action on the tooth or gingival surface.

The secretion of drugs in saliva

The salivary glands are usually described as having an excretory function because of their handling and secretion of certain substances such as iodide, thiocyanate, mercury and lead. Of course if such a substance (e.g. iodide) is then swallowed and reabsorbed it cannot really be regarded as having been excreted from the body. Drugs or substances derived from them may be secreted in saliva; for example cough mixtures contain large amounts of iodide which after ingestion is secreted in saliva (Mason et al, 1967). Alkaloids such as morphine (Munch, 1934a, b), metronidazole, a drug used in the treatment of acute ulcerative gingivitis (Stephen et al, 1966) and ethyl alcohol have all been detected after their systemic administration.

Earlier reports have indicated that antibiotics were secreted in saliva (Bender, Pressman and Tashman, 1953) and it has been assumed that antibiotics secreted in saliva influence the oral flora and the antibiotic sensitivity of oral micro-organisms (*British Medical Journal,* 1971). More recently, Speirs et al (1971) studied levels of penicillin, ampicillin, cloxacillin and cephalexin in serum, parotid and mixed salivas up to six hours after oral drug administration but significant salivary antibacterial levels could not be found in spite of adequate serum levels. Further investigations with erythromycin stearate, sodium fusidate, tetracycline, pristinamycin and lincomycin have given similar results. With erythromycin estolate and spiramycin antibacterial activity was occasionally detected in parotid and mixed saliva but sulphadimidine, clindamycin and rifampicin consistently could be detected in mixed saliva and parotid saliva; the concentration in mixed saliva being greater (Stephen and Speirs, 1972). In an extension of this study (McFarlane et al, 1974) these workers have demonstrated that with tetracycline and erythromycin estolate antibacterial levels were found only in gingival fluid with no detectable activity in parotid, submandibular and labial minor gland secretions. However, with clindamycin and rifampicin antibacterial activity was found in parotid, submandibular and labial gland secretions as well as gingival fluid (Table 8.5). From associated laboratory studies using a water/octanal membrane transport model, it was concluded that to be secreted by salivary glands, a compound must have the right order of hydrophile-lipophile balance under existing serum and salivary pH conditions.

Table 8.5. *Mean concentration of antibiotics in gingival fluid (GF), parotid saliva (PAR), submandibular (SUB) and minor gland saliva (MIN) at 1 hour, 3 hours and 6 hours. The results are shown as a ratio with the serum level.*

	Ampicillin	Cephalexin	Tetracycline	Erythromycin estolate	Clindamycine	Rifomycin
			1 hour			
GF	10	31	26	25	42	63
PAR	—	—	—	—	2	21
SUB	—	—	—	—	8	30
MIN	—	—	—	—	8	24
			3 hours			
GF	7	4	17	14	66	74
PAR	—	—	—	—	3	47
SUB	—	—	—	—	—	54
MIN	—	—	—	—	8	38
			6 hours			
GF	54	—	—	—	57	73
PAR	—	—	—	—	—	58
SUB	—	—	—	—	—	69
MIN	—	—	—	—	—	39

There has been surprisingly little work carried out on the pharmacology of drugs secreted in saliva. The studies reported here indicate that this is an obvious area for reappraisal of previous work and for further research. The possibility of drugs entering mixed saliva from the gingival fluid as well as from separate gland secretions should be borne in mind.

REFERENCES

Alexander, W. D., Papadopoulos, S., Harden, R. McG., MacFarlane, S., Mason, D. K. & Wayne, E. (1966) The plasma inorganic iodine concentration in thyrotoxicosis. *Journal of Laboratory and Clinical Medicine,* **67,** 808.

Babkin, B. P. (1950) *Secretory Mechanism of the Digestive Glands.* New York: Paul B. Hoeber Inc. Medical Book. Department of Harper & Brothers.

Bahn, S. L. (1972) Drug-related dental destruction. *Oral Surgery, Oral Medicine and Oral Pathology,* **33,** 49.

Barylko-Pikielna, N., Pangborn, R. M. & Shannon, I. L. (1968) Effect of cigarette smoking on parotid secretion. *Archives of Environmental Health,* **17,** 731.

Bates, J. F. & Adams, D. (1968) The influence of mental stress on the flow of saliva in man. *Archives of Oral Biology,* **13,** 593.

Becks, H. & Wainwright, W. W. (1943) Rate of flow of resting saliva of healthy individuals. *Journal of Dental Research,* **22,** 391.

Beeley, J. A. (1974) Personal communication.

Beeley, J. A. & Chisholm, D. M. (1974) Unpublished observations.

Bender, I. B., Pressman, R. S. & Tashman, S. G. (1953) Studies on excretion of antibiotics in human saliva. I. Penicillin and Streptomycin. *Journal of the American Dental Association,* **46,** 164.

Bertram, U. (1967) Xerostomia. Clinical aspects, pathology and pathogenesis. *Acta Odontologica Scandinavica,* **25,** Suppl. 49, 1.

Bhoola, K. D., McNicol, N. W., Oliver, S. & Foran, J. (1969) Changes in salivary enzymes in patients with sarcoidosis. *New England Journal of Medicine,* **281,** 877.

Changes in Salivary Secretion and Composition in Disease

Blatt, I. M. (1962) Submaxillary salivary flow: A test of chorda tympani nerve function as a basis for surgical intervention in Bell's palsy. A study of 61 patients. *Transactions of the American Academy of Ophthalmology and Otolaryngology,* **66,** 723.

Bonilla, C. A., Fuller, G. & Stringham, R. M. Jr (1968) Electrophoretic patterns of osteoporotic saliva—a comparative study. *Journal of Oral Medicine,* **23,** 85.

British Medical Journal (1971) Leading article, **ii,** 63.

Brown, C. C. (1970) The parotid puzzle: A review of the literature on human salivation and its applications to psychophysiology. *Psychophysiology,* **7,** 66.

Brun, R. & Domine, E. (1958) Etude sur la transpiration. *Acta Dermatovenereologica,* **38,** 91.

Chauncey, H. H., Levine, D. M., Kass, G., Schwachman, H., Henriques, B. L. & Kuliczyeki, L. L. (1962) Parotid gland secretory rate and electrolyte concentration in children with cystic fibrosis. *Archives of Oral Biology,* **7,** 707.

Chisholm, D. M., Beeley, J. A. & Mason, D. K. (1973) Isoelectric focussing in polyacrylamide gels of saliva in Sjögren's syndrome and rheumatoid arthritis. *Oral Surgery, Oral Medicine and Oral Pathology,* **35,** 620.

Chisholm, D. M., Lyell, A., Haroon, T. S., Mason, D. K. & Beeley, J. A. (1971) Salivary gland function in sarcoidosis. *Oral Surgery, Oral Medicine and Oral Pathology,* **31,** 766.

Curry, R. C. & Patey, D. H. (1964) A clinical test for parotid function. *British Journal of Surgery,* **51,** 891.

Dawes, C. (1969) The effects of flow rate and duration of stimulation on the concentrations of protein and the main electrolytes in human parotid saliva. *Archives of Oral Biology,* **14,** 277.

Dawes, C. (1970) Effect of diet on salivary secretion and composition. *Journal of Dental Research,* **49,** 1263.

Dawes, C. (1972) Circadian rhythms in human salivary flow rate and composition. *Journal of Physiology,* **220,** 529.

Deniker, P., Colonna, L., Loo, H., Ackermann, R., Pompians-Miniac, L. & Predine, F. (1970) Traitement de la secheresse buccale produite par les medicaments psychotropes. *La Presse Medicale,* **53,** 2383.

Di Sant' Agnese, P. A., Darling, R. C., Perera, G. A. & Shea, E. (1953) Abnormal electrolyte composition of sweat in cystic fibrosis of the pancreas: Clinical significance and relationship to the disease. *Pediatrics,* **12,** 549.

Doggett, R. G., Bentinck, B. & Harrison, G. M. (1971) Structure and ultrastructure of the labial salivary glands in patients with cystic fibrosis. *Journal of Clinical Pathology,* **24,** 270.

Ericson, S. (1968) The parotid gland in subjects with and without rheumatoid arthritis. *Acta Radiologica,* Suppl. 275. Stockholm.

Ericsson, Y., Hellström, I., Jared, B. & Stjernström, L. (1954) Investigations into the relationship between saliva and dental caries. *Acta Odontologica Scandinavica,* **11,** 179.

Faber, M. (1943) The causes of xerostomia. *Acta Medica Scandinavica,* **113,** 69.

Ferguson, D. B., Elliott, A. L. & Potts, A. J. (1969) Variations in human parotid saliva over 24 hour periods. *Journal of Dental Research,* **48,** 1132.

Finestone, A. J., Schacterele, G. R. & Pollack, R. L. (1973) The comparative analysis of diabetic and non-diabetic saliva Study I: Protein separation by disc gel electrophoresis. *Journal of Periodontology,* **44,** 175.

Foster, R. O., Busse, W. F. & Lorincz, A. B. (1971) Salivary alkaline phosphatase levels during the menstrual cycle. Presented at *American College of Surgeons National Meeting, Washington, D.C.*

Frank, R. M., Herdly, J. & Philippe, E. (1965) Acquired dental defects and salivary gland lesions after irradiation for carcinoma. *Journal of the American Dental Association,* **70,** 868.

Goldman, A., Hanan, L., Rechtman, L. & Wagner, M. (1961) Variations of rate of parotid secretion in man with changes in environmental temperatures. *Alabama Dental Review,* **8,** 15.

Gore, J. T. (1938) Saliva and enamel decalcification—II. Saliva separator. *Journal of Dental Research,* **17,** 69.

Gravenmade, E. J. S., Roukema, P. A. & Panders, A. K. (1974) The effect of mucin-containing artificial saliva on severe xerostomia. *International Journal of Oral Surgery,* **3,** 32.

Henkin, R. I. & Schecter, P. J. (1971) Idiopathic hypogensia with Dysgensia, Hyposmia and Sysosmia: A new syndrome. *Journal of the American Medical Association,* **217,** 4.

Hildes, J. A. & Ferguson, H. (1958) The concentration of electrolytes in normal human saliva. *Canadian Journal of Biochemistry and Physiology,* **33,** 217.

135

Salivary Glands in Health and Disease

Holmes, J. H. (1964) Changes in salivary flow produced by changes in fluid and electrolyte balance. In *Salivary Glands and Their Secretions*. (Eds.) Sreebny, L. M. & Meyer, J. New York: Pergamon Press.
Hutchinson, J. (1888) A case of "dry mouth". *Transactions of the Clinical Society of London*, **21**, 180.
Jenkins, G. N. (1966) *The Physiology of the Mouth*, 3rd Ed. Oxford: Blackwell Scientific.
Johnston, W. H. (1956) Salivary electrolytes in fibrocystic disease of the pancreas. *Archives of Disease in Childhood*, **31**, 447.
Kapsinalis, P. (1966) Caries activity and saliva flow. *Journal of Oral Medicine*, **21**, 107.
Kerr, A. C. (1961) *The Physiological Regulation of Salivary Secretions in Man. A Study of the Response of Human Salivary Glands to Reflex Stimulation*. Oxford: Pergamon Press.
Korting, G. W. & Kleinschmidt, W. (1953) Veranderungen der speichelsekretion bei hautkrankheiten. *Dermatologische Wochenschrift*, **128**, 772.
Krasnogorski, N. I. (1931) Bedingte und unbedingte reflexe im kindesalter und ihre bedeutung fur die klinik. *Ergebnisse der innere Medizin und Kinderheilkunde*, **39**, 613.
Lawler, D. P., Hickler, R. B. & Thorn, G. W. (1962) The salivary sodium/potassium ratio. *New England Journal of Medicine*, **267**, 1136.
Lawson, D. (1967) Use of a micro-sodium electrode in the diagnosis of cystic fibrosis. In *Modern Problems in Pediatrics*. p. 273. Basle/New York: Karger.
Lawson, D., Westcombe, P. & Saggers, B. (1969) Pilot trial of an infant screening programme for cystic fibrosis: Measurement of parotid salivary sodium at 4 months. *Archives of Disease in Childhood*, **44**, 715.
Mandel, I. D. (1967) Diagnostic clues in saliva. *Diagnostica*, **4**, 11.
Mandel, I. D. (1974) Relation of saliva and plaque to caries. *Journal of Dental Research*, **53**, 246-266.
Marder, M. Z., Wotman, S. & Mandel, I. D. (1972) Salivary electrolyte changes during pregnancy. I. Normal pregnancy. *American Journal of Obstetrics and Gynecology*, **112**, 233.
Mason, D. K. (1966) *Studies in Salivary Glands and their Secretions in Health and Disease*. M.D. Thesis, University of Glasgow.
Mason, D. K., Harden, R. McG., Boyle, J. A., Jasani, M. K., Williamson, J. & Buchanan, W. W. (1967) Salivary flow rates and iodide trapping capacity in patients with Sjögren's syndrome. *Annals of the Rheumatic Diseases*, **28**, 95.
Matzker, J. & Schreiber, J. (1972) Synthetischer Speichel zur Therapie der Hyposialien, insbesondere bei der radiogenen Sialadenitis. *Zeitschrift für Laryngologie, Rhinologie, Otologie und ihre Grenzgebiete*, **51**, 422.
Munch, J. C. (1934a) Antidotes. *Journal of the American Pharmaceutical Association*, **23**, 91.
Munch, J. C. (1934b) Human toxicosis. *Journal of the American Medical Association*, **102**, 1929.
MacFarlane, C. B., McCrosson, J., Stephen, K. W. & Speirs, C. F. (1974) Physicochemical factors influencing the presence of antibiotics in salivary secretions. *Journal of Dental Research*, Supplement 53, 1081, Abstract 151.
McGrady, K. & Bessman, S. P. (1955) The detection of mucoviscidosis by the determination of saliva chloride. *American Journal of Diseases of Children*, **90**, 610.
Nekrasow, P. A. & Ghranilowa, N. W. (1933) Ueber den einfluss korperlicher arbeit den undebingten speichelreflex beim menschen. *Archivio di Scienze Biologiche*, **34**, 603.
Östlund, S. G. (1953) *Palatine Glands and Mucin*. Lund: Berlingska Boktryckeriet.
Papadopoulos, S., McFarlane, S., Harden, R. McG., Mason, D. K. & Alexander, W. D. (1966) Iodine excretion in urine, saliva, gastric juices and sweat in dehalogenase deficiency. *Journal of Endocrinology*, **36**, 341.
Rauch, S. (1959) *Die Speicheldrusen des Menschen*. Stuttgart: Georg Thieme Verlag.
Rauch, S. & Gorlin, R. J. (1970) In *Thoma's Oral Pathology*, Vol. II, (Eds.) Gorlin, R. J. & Goldman, H. M. p. 986. St. Louis: C. V. Mosby Co.
Saggers, B. A., Lawson, D., Stern, J. & Edgson, A. C. (1967) Rapid method for the detection of cystic fibrosis of the pancreas in children *Archives of Disease in Childhood*, **42**, 187.
Schneyer, L. H. (1956) Source of resting total mixed saliva of man. *Journal of Applied Physiology*, **9**, 1.
Schneyer, L. H. & Levin, L. E. (1955) Rate of secretion by individual salivary gland pairs in man under two conditions of stimulation. *Journal of Dental Research*, **35**, 725.
Scopp, I., Heyman, R., Goldberg, M. & Croy, D. (1965) Dryness of the mouth with use of tranquillizers: chlorpormazine. *Journal of the American Dental Association*, **71**, 66.

136

Sewards, H. F. G., Hamilton, D. I. & Patey, D. H. (1966) An investigation of the value in clinical practice of the Curry test for parotid function. *British Journal of Surgery,* **53,** 3.

Shannon, I. L. (1962) Parotid fluid flow rate as related to whole saliva volume. *Archives of Oral Biology,* **7,** 391.

Shannon, I. L. (1967) Physiological baselines for total protein in human parotid fluid collected without exogenous stimulation. *Journal of Oral Medicine,* **22,** 3.

Shannon, I. L. & Chauncey, H. H. (1967) Hyperhydration and parotid flow in man. *Journal of Dental Research,* **46,** 1028.

Shannon, I. L. & Feller, R. P. (1972) Light deprivation and parotid flow in the human. *Journal of Dental Research,* **51,** 6.

Speirs, C. F., Stenhouse, D., Stephen, K. W. & Wallace, E. T. (1971) Comparison of human serum, parotid and mixed saliva levels of phenoxymethylpenecillin, ampicillin, cloxacillin and cephalexin. *British Journal of Pharmacology,* **43,** 242.

Stanbury, J. B. & Chapman, E. M. (1960) Congenital hypothyroidism with goitre. Absence of an iodide concentrating mechanism. *Lancet,* **i,** 1162.

Stephen, K. W. & Speirs, C. F. (1972) Oral environmental source of any anti bacterial drugs— the importance of gingival fluid. In *Host Resistance to Commensal Bacteria.* (Ed.) MacPhee, T. p. 76. Edinburgh & London: Churchill Livingstone.

Stephen, K. W., McLatchie, M. F., Mason, D. K., Noble, H. W. & Stevenson, D. M. (1966) Treatment of acute ulcerative gingivitis (Vincent's type). *British Dental Journal,* **121,** 313.

Suhara, R. & Asakawa, H. (1959) On the composition of human parotid resting saliva and reflex. *Journal of Nihon University School of Dentistry,* **1,** 153.

Sweeney, L. R., Hedrick, M. C., Meskin, L. H. & Warwick, W. J. (1967) The involvement of the labial mucous salivary gland in patients with cystic fibrosis. II. The heterozygote state. *Pediatrics,* **40,** 421.

Trimble, H. C., Etherington, J. W. & Losch, P. K. (1938) Rate of secretion of saliva and incidence of dental caries. *Journal of Dental Research,* **17,** 299.

Wayne, E. J. (1967) The value of inorganic iodine studies in the clinical assessment of thyroid disease. *Journal of Clinical Pathology* (Supplement), **20,** 353.

Winsor, A. L. (1930) The effect of dehydration of parotid secretion. American Journal of Psychology, **42,** 602.

Wolff, J. (1964) Transport of iodide and other anions in the thyroid gland. *Physiological Reviews,* **44,** 45.

Wolff, J., Thompson, R. H. & Robbins, J. (1964) Congenital goitrous cretinism due to the absence of iodide-concentrating ability. *Journal of Clinical Endocrinology and Metabolism,* **24,** 699.

Wotman, S., Baer, L., Mandel, I. D. & Laragh, J. H. (1971) Submaxillary potassium concentration in true and pseudoprimary aldosteronism. *Archives of Internal Medicine,* **126,** 248.

Wotman, S. & Mandel, I. D. (1973) Salivary indications of systemic disease. *Postgraduate Medicine,* **53,** 73.

Zaus, E. A. & Fosdick, L. S. (1934) Effects of saliva upon gastric digestion. *Journal of Dental Research,* **14,** 1.

GORDON M. RICK, D.D.S.
DEPARTMENT OF ORAL PATHOLOGY
SCHOOL OF DENTISTRY
LOMA LINDA UNIVERSITY

CHAPTER 9

Neoplasms

Salivary gland tumours present problems of diagnosis to clinicians and pathologists alike. Differences of opinion have been expressed with regard to the histogenesis of these lesions. The nomenclature and classification of tumours have been based upon histological pattern and behavioural characteristics, although these may vary considerably. The incidence of salivary tumours, including sex distribution and regional variation, together with site and racial differences, are now considered.

Incidence

Salivary gland tumours are relatively uncommon, comprising fractionally more than three per cent of all tumours (Evans and Cruickshank, 1970). In general, the incidence shows little variation between Europe and the United States where the major studies have been undertaken. However, slight exceptions include Eskimos, who appear to be a high-risk group and, in the non-white populations of the United States and Africa, females are affected more commonly than males.

Site

The parotid glands are by far the most commonly affected and tumours at this site are approximately ten times more common than those in either the submandibular glands or the minor glands taken as a group (Thackray, 1968). Tumours of the sublingual salivary glands are even less common and therefore are extremely rare (Tables 9.1, 9.2). For intra-oral salivary gland tumours the palate is the commonest site followed by the upper labial glands and buccal glands (Ranger, Thackray and Lucas, 1956).

Race

It is of interest that certain racial groups show variation from this general situation. Amongst the Chinese in Malaya, for example, 30 per cent of salivary tumours occur in the submandibular glands, whilst in South Africa 29 per cent of tumours affect the palatal salivary glands.

138

Table 9.1. *Approximate percentage distribution of the main tumour types in salivary glands.*

	Parotid[a]	Submandibular[a]	Sublingual[b]	Minor[c]
Adenoma	74	64	—	54
pleomorphic				
monomorphic	8.6	2.4	—	2
Muco-epidermoid tumour	3.2	1.8	—	6
Acini cell tumour	2.3	0.3	—	—
Carcinoma	11.9	31.5	100	38
	100	100	100	100

From: [a]Thackray, A. C. and Lucas, R. B. (1974).
  [b]Foote, F. W. and Frazell, E. L. (1953).
  [c]Glasgow Dental Hospital.

It is worth noting that the light microscopic appearances of minor gland tumours closely resemble those of their major gland counterparts. However, in the minor gland tumours the myxochondroid or chondroid elements are less extensive, and the epithelial component predominates in pleomorphic adenomas of the palatal salivary glands. Differences in incidences, and histological variation in the stromal elements between major and minor salivary gland tumours, may be related to morphological differences between the various glands (Chapter 2).

Table 9.2. *Percentage of minor salivary gland neoplasms (Glasgow, 1955-1964).*

	Location			
Type	Palate	Buccal	Upper lip	Lower lip
Adenoma				
plcomorphic	30	12	10	2
monomorphic	—	2	—	—
Muco-epidermoid tumour	2	4	—	—
Acini cell tumour	—	—	—	—
Carcinoma	24	14	—	—

AETIOLOGY

There is no evidence, either clinical or experimental, to suggest that in the salivary glands a pre-existing inflammatory, obstructive or traumatic condition predisposes to malignant change (Evans and Cruickshank, 1970). There is evidence, however, that an association may exist between salivary gland carcinoma and breast cancer (Berg, Hutter and Foote, 1968). The association with blood group factors or secretors and non-secretors now appears unlikely (Garrett et al, 1971).

In experimental animals, salivary gland tumours may be induced by a variety of agents, including carcinogenic hydrocarbons (Bauer and Byrne, 1950; Cherry and Glücksman, 1965), ionising radiation (Glücksman and Cherry, 1962) and polyoma virus (Stewart, Eddy and Borgese, 1958; Dawe, Morgan and Slatick, 1966). Almost without exception the lesions have been duct carcinomas of the squamous cell type, although tumours with adeno-matous pattern have been produced on occasion (Friborsky, 1965). Carcino-genic co-factors such as Vitamin D deficiency (Rowe et al, 1970) may be important.

An origin of salivary gland tumours from epithelial cells appears to be the current majority view. Willis (1967) has suggested that neoplasia may occur simultaneously in duct and acinar cells in some tumours. Other workers have postulated the cell of origin to be an individual cell type, such as the myoepithelial cell (Hübner et al, 1971). Various tumours may arise from either intercalated or excretory ducts, and this theory (Eversole, 1971) is based upon salivary gland embryogenesis and the potential of duct epithelium during reactive processes. The varied stromal reaction in some salivary gland tumours may be explained by secretory activity of tumour cells or metaplasia.

The concept of a myoepithelial cell having the ability to produce stromal mucins in salivary pleomorphic adenomas has been advanced. Epithelial and connective tissue-type mucins have been distinguished histochemically in the stroma of pleomorphic adenomas (Azzopardi and Smith, 1959), and two entirely different amino sugar-containing compounds, characterised as epithelial and connective tissue mucin respectively, have been reported in the tumour (Quintarelli and Robinson, 1967). These latter investigators observed no changes suggesting transformation from epithelial mucin to connective tissue mucin, and could find no data to support the concept of an epithelial or myoepithelial cell modifying its biological characteristics to produce a mesenchymal mucin. However, the ability of epithelial cells to stimulate connective tissue stroma to proliferate in a myxomatous or chondroid direction, perhaps by an 'organiser' mechanism, seemed possible. The chondroid areas observed in some pleomorphic adenomas had been accounted for in terms of this 'organiser' activity of neoplastic epithelium (Yates and Paget, 1952). The myoepithelial cell is considered to play an important role in mixed tumours of skin and the essential criteria for the production of the mixed-type pattern of these skin tumours are thought to be myoepithelial proliferation, mucin secretion and slow growth. Lennox, Pearse and Richards (1952) suggested that in such skin appendage tumours a highly variable and labile epithelial mucin might be modified by contact with the stroma so that it acquires the histochemical properties and character-istics of a connective tissue mucin.

In salivary glands the presence of cells with characteristics of both epithelial and myoepithelial cells have been noted and regarded as being transitional forms in the transformation of secretory epithelial cells into myoepithelium (Tandler, 1965), and this concept is a key theme in a review of myoepithelial cells (Hamperl, 1970). There are close morphological and functional similarities between smooth muscle cells and myoepithelial cells and they have in common a closely related or identical protein which shows immuno-logical cross-reactivity with acto-myosin (Archer and Kao, 1968). The origin of the myoepithelial cell remains unknown (Chapter 2), but it is worth noting, however, that desmosomes are observed between myoepithelial and contiguous cells and that such connections, other than for endothelium, are not a feature of cells or mesenchymal derivation.

It is of interest that at an ultrastructural level a significant role in the histogenesis of certain tumours of human mammary glands has been postulated for myoepithelial cells (Murad and Haam, 1968). However, other workers (Sykes et al, 1968) do not share this view and in a comprehensive review of the ultrastructure of human mammary gland tumours no convincing evidence could be found to correlate mammary gland tumour cells with myoepithelium (Ozzello, 1971).

A cell line called Nagoya-78, from a human salivary gland mixed tumour has shown the cells to have epithelial characteristics and although many were described as being stellate in shape and resembling myoepithelial cells (Kondo, Muragishi and Imaizuma, 1971), myofilaments were not described in the ultrastructural studies of these cultured cells. It is to be noted that, in culture, epithelial cells may assume an elongated fibroblast-like appearance. In experimental salivary gland tumours, epithelial-mesenchymal interactions are well established and strong evidence, based on chromosome-marked cells, has been provided that such tumours with predominant connective tissue features actually arise from epithelial cells and that mesenchymal cells do not contribute neoplastic cells to the tumour (Dawe et al, 1971).

Electronmicroscopic studies have suggested that the myoepithelial cell plays an important role in the growth and development of pleomorphic adenoma, adenoid cystic carcinoma, adenolymphoma and oncocytoma (Hübner et al, 1971). Quantitative ultrastructural comparison, however, of the cells of pleomorphic adenomas and of normal salivary glands, show that differences in percentage volumes of individual cell types are highly significant (Table 9.3). In this study a higher proportion by volume of cells of

Table 9.3. *Stereological analysis using the method of point counting of 120 electronmicrographs from five normal human minor salivary gland lobules and 180 electronmicrographs from seven pleomorphic adenomas.*

	Duct-type cell	Myoepithe-lial-type cell	Acinar-type cell	Other-type cell	Total
Pleomorphic adenoma	16000 (61.5%)	1271 (4.9%)	1140 (4.4%)	7619 (29.2%)	26030 (100%)
Normal minor salivary gland	397 (2.6%)	469 (6.2%)	12092 (77.8%)	2074 (13.4%)	15532 (100%)

From Chisholm, D. M. et al (1974).

duct origin in pleomorphic adenoma indicates that this cell, rather than the myoepithelial cell, is the principal cell of this tumour (Chisholm et al, 1974). However, more information is required in respect of the origin, ultrastructure and possible transformation of parenchymal cells in neoplasia before firm conclusions can be drawn as to the cell of origin of salivary gland tumours. The application of the immunohistochemical method for identification of actomyosin in myoepithelium (Archer and Kao, 1968), to tumour material may be of considerable value.

NUCLEAR DNA CONTENT OF SALIVARY NEOPLASMS

Recently the nuclear DNA content of salivary epithelial tumour cells has been determined in tissue sections by microspectrophotometry (Kino, Richart and Lattes, 1973a, b; Eneroth and Zetterberg, 1973). Deviation from the normal number of chromosomes is a characteristic feature of most malignant tumours and they may cause quantitative changes in nuclear DNA content. An increase of 25 to 50 per cent above the normal value has been reported in malignant parotid tumours (Eneroth and Zetterberg, 1973). It is of much interest that nuclei of monomorphic adenoma cells have identical DNA values to normal control cells, whilst highly differentiated muco-epidermoid tumour cells exhibited higher DNA values (Eneroth and Zetterberg, 1973). This supports the concept that despite their high cellularity, monomorphic adenomas are benign lesions whilst muco-epidermoid tumours are best regarded as malignant. Nuclear DNA content of benign human tumours in general have shown a diploid to tetraploid distribution pattern, and this is true of benign salivary tumours and well-differentiated muco-epidermoid tumours (Kino, Richart and Lattes, 1973a). Adenoid cystic carcinomas also, have principally a diploid to tetraploid nuclear DNA pattern albeit with a relatively highly concentrated diploid mode (Kino, Richart and Lattes, 1973b). An aneuploid distribution in a benign neoplasm in man has not been reported. Poorly differentiated muco-epidermoid tumours showing frank malignant change, however, have an aneuploid nuclear DNA pattern without a clear peak (Kino, Richart and Lattes, 1973b).

CLASSIFICATION

In the past some salivary gland tumours have not only been given a variety of names but also these terms have been applied to quite separate and different lesions. Recently, however, the World Health Organisation International Centre for the Histological Classification of Salivary Gland Tumours has published a classification and concise description of salivary tumours, paying particular attention to the behavioural pattern of individual lesions (Thackray, 1972). Epithelial tumours of the salivary glands are divided into four broad categories—adenomas, muco-epidermoid tumour, unclassified tumours and allied conditions (Table 9.4). In the following account of these lesions, this recommended classification and terminology will be adopted. Comprehensive descriptions of the histological appearance of major gland neoplasms (Foote and Frazell, 1954; Evans and Cruickshank, 1970), minor gland neoplasms (Chaudhry, Vickers and Gorlin, 1961; Luna, Stimson and Bardwil, 1968) and clinico-pathological follow-up studies (Wyatt, Henry and Curwen, 1967; Morgan and MacKenzie, 1968) have been published and are recommended for detailed study.

Table 9.4. *Histological typing of salivary gland tumours.*

I. Epithelial tumours

A. *Adenomas*
  1. Pleomorphic adenoma (mixed tumour)
  2. Monomorphic adenomas
    (a) Adenolymphoma
    (b) Oxyphilic adenoma
    (c) Other types

B. *Muco-epidermoid tumour*

C. *Acinic-cell tumour*

D. *Carcinomas*
  1. Adenoid cystic carcinoma
  2. Adenocarcinoma
  3. Epidermoid carcinoma
  4. Undifferentiated carcinoma
  5. Carcinoma in pleomorphic adenoma (malignant mixed tumour)

  II. Non-epithelial tumours

  III. Unclassified tumours

  IV. Allied conditions

A. *Benign lympho-epithelial lesion*

B. *Sialosis*

C. *Oncocytosis*

From Thackray, A. C. (1972).

EPITHELIAL TUMOURS

Adenomas

Pleomorphic adenoma (mixed tumour)

This is the commonest type of salivary gland tumour and originates through neoplastic transformation of duct epithelium. The term mixed tumour was introduced to draw attention to the dual origin of the lesion from epithelial and mesenchymal elements (McFarland, 1943). At the present time, however, the majority view would indicate that the tumour is of epithelial origin entirely (Evans and Cruickshank, 1970). The term pleomorphic adenoma, which has descriptive rather than histogenetic significance, seems preferable and is recommended by the W.H.O. Pleomorphic adenomas are usually solitary, begin as a small, painless nodule and grow slowly in size without fixation to skin, mucous membranes or deeper structures (Figures 9.1 to 9.5). Recurrences, which are almost certainly due to incomplete removal, often manifest as multiple foci. The tumour is encapsulated and characterised histologically by the pleomorphic or 'mixed' appearance. Thus cuboidal, duct-like tumour cells proliferating in clumps, sheets and cords are observed within a connective tissue stroma which may show hyaline, myxoid or chondroid areas (Figures 9.5 to 9.8). It is of interest that many pleomorphic adenomas may be highly cellular, show cellular atypia or infiltration of the

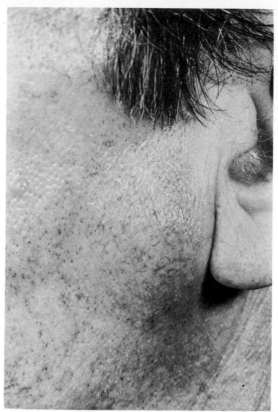

Figure 9.1. Pleomorphic adenoma of the superficial lobe of the L parotid gland.

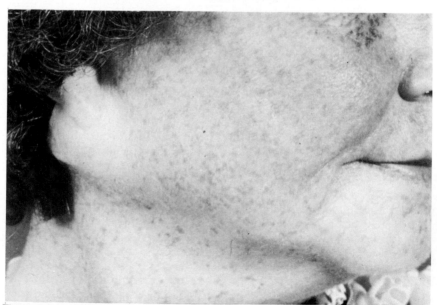

Figure 9.2. Pleomorphic adenoma of the R parotid gland.

144

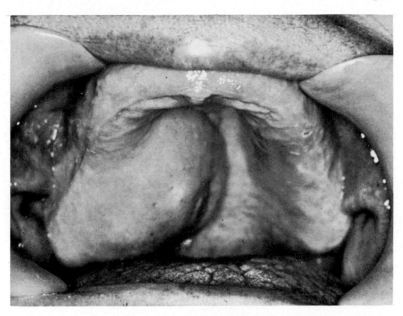

Figure 9.3. Palatal swelling with mucosal ulceration in a 45-year-old male patient. The lesion was slow growing, painless and histopathological examination showed the typical features of a pleomorphic adenoma.

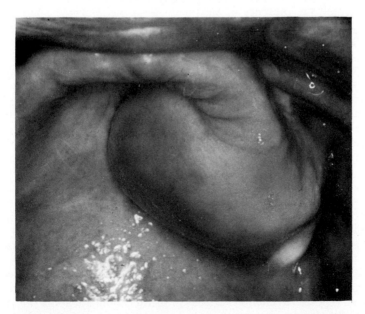

Figure 9.4. Firm swelling of palate and L tuberosity region. Histopathological examination showed a pleomorphic adenoma.

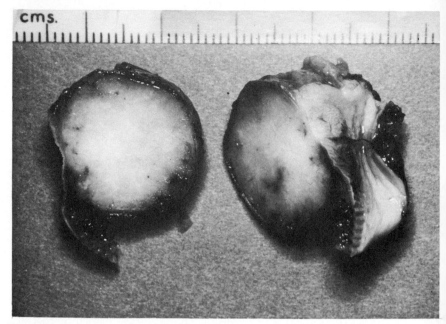

Figure 9.5. Gross appearance of pleomorphic adenoma from palate.

capsule and yet remain benign. Recently, Azzopardi and Zayid (1972) demonstrated the presence of elastic tissue in pleomorphic adenomas and this has been confirmed ultrastructurally (Allen, 1974). Ultrastructural study of pleomorphic adenomas of salivary gland have shown the presence of epithelial-duct and myoepithelial-type cells, and, in addition, a cell having characteristics of both duct and myoepithelial cells has been described and termed a transitional cell (Oota and Takahashi, 1958; Kierszenbaum, 1968) indeterminate cell (Welsh and Meyer, 1968) or an incompletely differentiated cell (Eneroth and Wersäll, 1966). Acinar-type cells (Eneroth and Wersäll, 1966) and stellate-shaped cells, considered to be 'compressed' duct cells, have also been described (Deppish and Toker, 1969) in the tumour. In addition to an amorphous ground substance, the following cell types have been noted in mucoid or myxomatous regions of the tumour: fibroblasts and endothelial cells (Kierszenbaum, 1968); indeterminate, duct and myoepithelial cells (Welsh and Meyer, 1968); and 'neoplastic' myoepithelial cells (Mylius, 1960). A region described as having a myoepithelial pattern at the light-microscopic level has been studied ultrastructurally (Welsh and Meyer, 1968) and the cell type present described as being 'not the same as myoepithelial cells seen at the periphery of the ductular epithelial formations' and thus termed an indeterminate cell. Cells described as being consistent with myoepithelium and considered to be mesenchymal in origin have been reported in chondroid areas of pleomorphic adenoma (Doyle et al, 1968). Cells considered to be true cartilage cells have been reported (Welsh and Meyer, 1968) in these regions. Nuclear inclusion bodies may be present in tumour cells of pleomorphic adenomas (Kierszenbaum, 1969), although their origin and significance is uncertain. Squamous metaplasia has also been reported (Chisholm et al, 1974). The ultrastructural characteristics of tumour cells from a pleomorphic adenoma are illustrated (Figures 9.9 to 9.12).

The tumour is relatively radio-resistant and careful local excision with a margin of normal tissue is the treatment of choice. Shelling-out procedures tend to result in recurrences because of tumour-cell infiltration of the capsule; although where recurrences do occur they remain benign.

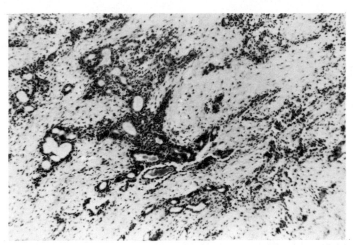

Figure 9.6. Clumps of epithelial tumour cells forming duct-like structures. The supporting stroma is fibro-myxoid in character. (× 75.)

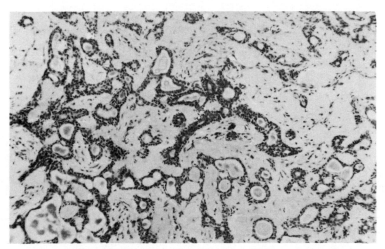

Figure 9.7. Pleomorphic adenoma showing tumour cells forming cords and clumps. Duct-like structures are present. (× 75.)

147

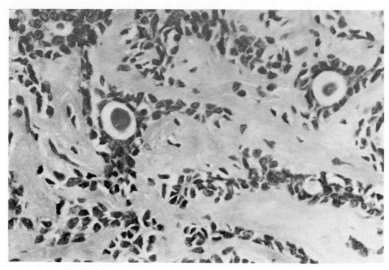

Figure 9.8. Pleomorphic adenoma. Duct-like structures are formed by the tumour cells. The stroma is hyalinised. (× 200.)

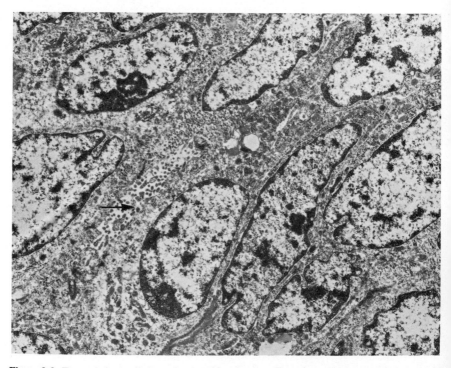

Figure 9.9. Tumour duct cells in a pleomorphic adenoma. Duct formation and the presence of micro villi are indicated. (× 6600.)

148

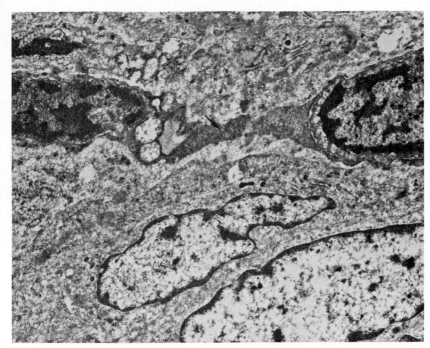

Figure 9.10. 'Indeterminate' cell in a pleomorphic adenoma. (× 7200.)

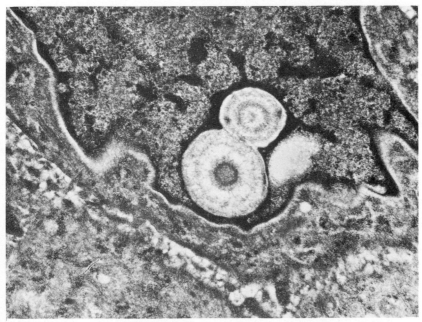

Figure 9.11. Intra-nuclear inclusion bodies in an epithelial tumour cell from a pleomorphic adenoma of palatal glands. (×15 000.)

149

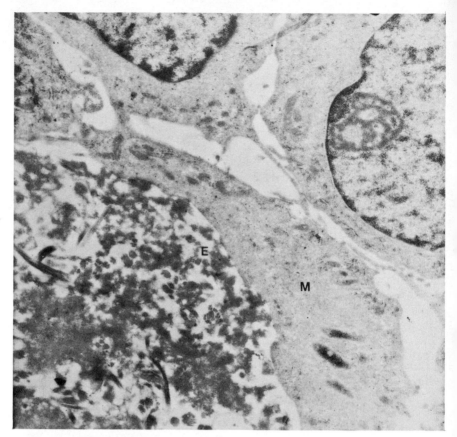

Figure 9.12. Elastic tissue (E) being formed within a pleomorphic adenoma. Myoepithelial cell (M) is present. ($\times$ 4800.)

Monomorphic adenomas

These benign tumours are characterised by the regularity of their cell structure and pattern.

Adenolymphoma

The adenolymphoma is a distinctive tumour which arises almost constantly in relation to the parotid gland in a superficial location especially at the lower pole. Commonly the lesions arise multifocally and a striking clinical feature is that bilateral gland involvement occurs in approximately 7 to 10 per cent of cases. The lesions are slow growing and males over 40 years of age are more commonly affected. Histologically, the tumour is composed of glandular and often cystic structures having a papillary cystic pattern, lined by columnar eosinophilic epithelial cells upon a less well-defined row of basal cells. The basal cells are cuboidal to polygonal in shape. A variable amount of lymphoid tissue with follicle formation characterises the stroma (Figures 9.13 to 9.14). Ultrastructurally the cytoplasm of the epithelial cell component is rich in mitochondria, many of which have an abnormal structure and thus resemble oncocytes (Tandler and Shipkey, 1964a, b; McGavran, 1965). The lymphoid component has the fine structural characteristics similar to those found in conditions produced by a cell-mediated immune mechanism of the delayed hypersensitivity type. It may be that this lesion represents a tissue reaction of the delayed hypersensitivity type initiated by metaplasia of striated duct epithelium, rather than a true neoplasm (Allegra, 1971). Of special interest is the fact that the adenolymphoma concentrates ^{99m}Tc pertechnetate to a much greater degree than normal salivary tissue so that scintiscanning is a most useful diagnostic test (Stebner et al, 1968). Malignant variants have been described but must be considered extremely rare (Pava et al, 1965; Little and Rickles, 1965). Rarely the tumour affects the minor salivary glands although in these cases the lymphoid element is usually absent (Bernier and Bhaskar, 1958; Veronesi and Corbetta, 1960). It seems most likely that the adenolymphoma arises from residues of salivary duct epithelium included within lymph nodes entrapped in the parotid due to the late encapsulation of the gland during development (Azzopardi and Hou, 1964).

The presence of sebaceous gland elements has been described in salivary glands (Hamperl, 1931; Meza-Chávez, 1949) and salivary gland tumours (Hartz, 1946; Lee, 1949; Rawson and Horn, 1959). It has been suggested that salivary duct epithelium possesses the ability to differentiate into sebaceous elements (Meza-Chávez, 1949). Salivary gland tumours composed predominantly of sebaceous gland elements in a lymphoid background (Figure 9.15) have been described and called sebaceous lymphadenomas (McGavran, Bauer and Ackerman, 1960). The nature and origin of these

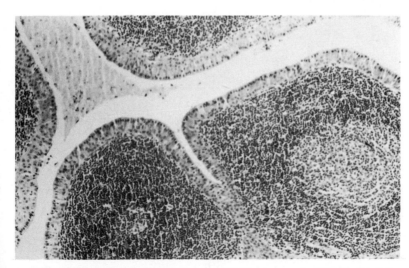

Figure 9.13. Adenolymphoma showing lymphoid infiltrate, germinal centre formation and typical epithelial layer. ($\times$ 110).

151

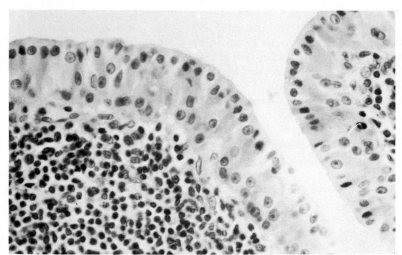

Figure. 9.14. Higher magnification showing double-layered epithelial lining to duct-like spaces. (× 250.)

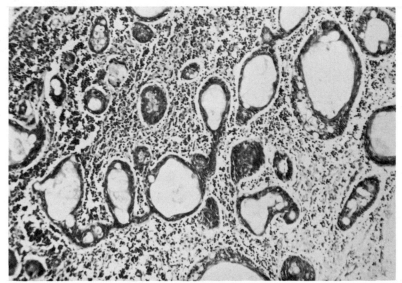

Figure 9.15. Adenolymphoma with sebaceous elements. (× 80.)

rare tumours is in many ways comparable to adenolymphoma (Evans and Cruickshank, 1970). Intra-oral lesions may occur (Epker and Henry, 1971) and malignant variants have been recorded (Silver and Goldstein, 1966).

Oxyphilic adenoma

This tumour is composed of large cells having a granular eosinophilic cytoplasm which are distributed throughout a scanty connective tissue

152

stroma. Many such lesions may in fact represent a severe degree of oncocytic hyperplasia rather than true neoplasia (Kleinsasser et al, 1966). The tumour cells closely resemble oncocytes which are cells rich in oxidative enzymes and derived from duct epithelium (Chapter 2). With increasing age oncocytes are increasingly present in normal salivary glands and this tumour has a pre-dilection for older females. The tumour has also been termed an oncocytoma (Ackerman, 1943). Ultrastructurally, the tumour cells are characterised by the presence within the cytoplasm of large, abnormal mitochondria. Malignant variants can occur but are extremely rare (Eneroth, 1965).

Basal-cell adenoma

Two further very rare types of monomorphic adenoma are the basal-cell adenoma and the clear-cell adenoma (Kleinsasser and Klein, 1967). In the basal-cell adenoma the type of cells and their arrangement closely resemble those of the basal-cell carcinoma of skin. In the clear-cell adenoma, duct-like structures surrounded by clear cells in the position normally occupied by the myoepithelial cells are observed. These tumours are so rare that their behaviour has not been fully assessed. The basal-cell adenoma arises most commonly in the parotid gland, though minor gland involvement has been reported (Christ and Crocker, 1972). This tumour appears to affect older individuals, is slow growing, encapsulated and benign. Fine structural study of the basal cell adenoma (Hübner, Kleinsasser and Klein, 1971) has shown the tumour cells to contain few organelles but many fine filaments, the origin and function of which remain unknown. These workers also described the presence of elastic-like tissue in relation to the tumour cells.

Muco-epidermoid Tumour

This tumour, considered to arise from duct epithelium, is characterised by the presence of squamous cells, mucus-secreting cells and cells considered to be of an intermediate type (Stewart, Foote and Becker, 1945; Foote and Frazell, 1954; Bhaskar and Bernier, 1962). Depending upon the relative pro-portion of individual cell types, the tumour may range from a solid variety to one in which cystic spaces lined by mucus-secreting cells predominate (Figures 9.16 to 9.18). Clear cells may be present but stromal changes characteristic of the pleomorphic adenoma such as mucoid and myxochon-droid metaplasia are absent. The amount of mucin present varies consider-ably, individual cell keratinisation is common and sebaceous elements and oncocytes may be present. Ultrastructural studies (Hübner and Kleinsasser, 1970) have demonstrated the presence of glycogen-rich cells, cells containing numerous tonofilaments and mucus-secreting cells. The so-called intermedi-ate cells displayed no uniform structural organisation and myoepithelial cells did not occur. The tumour is non-encapsulated and generally slow growing. However, the clinical features and behaviour of the lesion are difficult to predict. Muco-epidermoid tumours account for 3 to 9 per cent of all salivary tumours and 60 to 70 per cent occur in the parotid. Intra-oral tumours

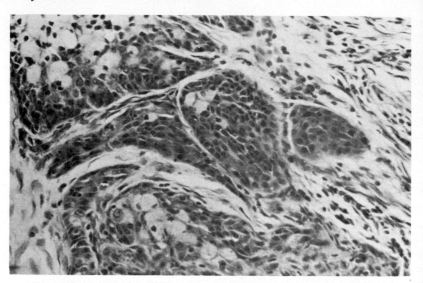

Figure 9.16. Muco-epidermoid tumour. Solid area of tumour showing 'epidermoid' cells and mucus-secreting cells. (× 150.)

comprise 15 to 20 per cent with a predilection for the palatal glands. Complete excision is associated with a very favourable prognosis whilst up to 40 per cent of lesions will recur if removal is incomplete. Muco-epidermoid tumours infiltrate locally and although on rare occasions may metastasise, this potential appears limited (Bhaskar and Bernier, 1962). Although it may

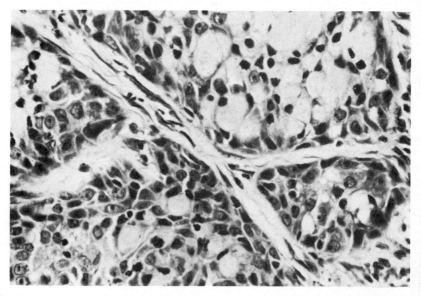

Figure 9.17. Higher magnification showing mucus-secreting cells in a muco-epidermoid tumour. (× 410.)

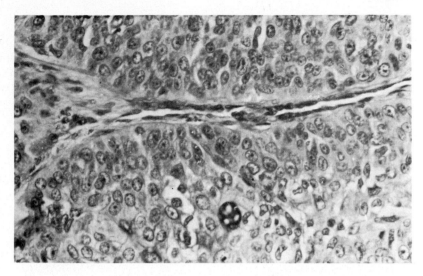

Figure 9.18. Muco-epidermoid tumour of palatal salivary glands. Region of epidermidisation. (× 400.)

be of some value to distinguish between well-differentiated and poorly-differentiated types, the prognostic significance of this is uncertain (Evans and Cruickshank, 1970).

Acinic Cell Tumour

This tumour, which constitutes about one per cent of all salivary gland tumours, arises from cells similar to serous acini of salivary gland tissue (Foote and Frazell, 1954), and the majority arise in the parotid gland. Histologically, the tumour comprises round or polygonal cells, the cytoplasm of which shows a varying degree of basophilia and granularity and are arranged in acinar-like formation or solid sheets. Non-granular cells and clear cells, however, may be present. The so-called clear cell variant may be a morphologically distinct neoplasm (Echevarria, 1967) arising from striated duct cells. Ultrastructurally the tumour cells have many characteristics of normal acinar cells such as abundant endoplasmic reticulum and membrane limited secretory granules (Echevarria, 1967; Kleinsasser, Hübner and Klein, 1967; Hirtzler et al, 1969). Rarely, the tumour may infiltrate locally or metastasise despite a benign histological appearance (Eneroth, Jakobssen and Blank, 1966). It is of interest, in view of the association of neoplasia and auto-immune disease, that a combination of acinic-cell adenocarcinoma and Sjögren's syndrome has been described (Delaney and Balogh, 1966). The marked PAS (Periodic acid Schiff) reaction of granules within neoplastic cells is a most useful histochemical reaction in the diagnosis of acinic-cell tumour.

155

Carcinomas

Malignant disease of the salivary glands is relatively rare. A carcinoma of salivary gland origin may arise ab initio or alternatively originate as a new growth in an antecedent tumour or its recurrence (Evans and Cruickshank, 1970). The clinical signs which herald a malignant neoplasm are rapidity of growth, pain, nerve paralysis and fixation to adjacent tissues.

Adenoid cystic carcinoma

This infiltrative malignant tumour (Figure 9.19) has a characteristic cribriform histological pattern and accounts for approximately six per cent of all salivary gland tumours. The tumour is relatively rare in the parotid gland

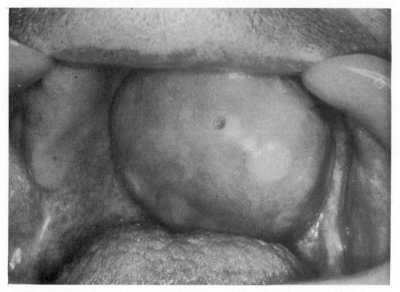

Figure 9.19. Adenoid cystic carcinoma arising in palatal salivary glands.

but is the most common malignant tumour of the submandibular and minor salivary glands (Ranger, Thackray and Lucas, 1956; Eneroth, 1971). The predominant cell type is small and polygonal with a basophilic cytoplasm, although a variable number of myoepithelial-like cells may be present. The tumour cells are arranged either in duct-like masses or in such a fashion as to enclose cyst-like spaces of varying size (Figure 9.20). Rarely, a more solid pattern may be present (Thackray and Lucas, 1960). The cyst-like spaces contain material which has the ultrastructural characteristics of replicated basement-membrane (Figure 9.21). The function of this material in the tumour is unknown, although it may serve some kind of protective role since the cribriform or cylindromatous type, in which this material is abundant, offers a better prognosis than the more solid type (Eneroth et al,

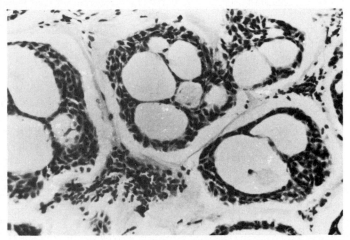

Figure 9.20. Characteristic 'cystic spaces' lined by regular epithelial cells in an adenoid cystic carcinoma. (× 160.)

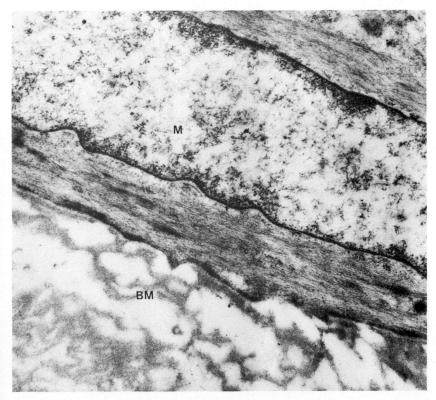

Figure 9.21. Production of basement membrane-like material (BM) in an adenoid cystic carcinoma. A myoepithelial cell (M) is present. (× 8800.)

1968). Ultrastructural features of the adenoid cystic carcinoma are shown in Figures 9.21 to 9.24. It is important to distinguish between adenoid cystic carcinomas and those pleomorphic adenomas containing 'cylindromatous' or cyst-like components. The adenoid cystic carcinoma is isomorphic, lacking the marked and varied stromal changes so characteristic of the pleomorphic adenoma. The adenoid cystic carcinoma grows slowly, has a tendency to grow along nerve sheaths and metastasises late (Quattlebaum, Dockerty and Mayo, 1946; 'Thackray and Lucas, 1960) and should therefore be excised with an adequate margin. With regard to the histogenesis of the adenoid cystic carcinoma, Bauer and Fox (1945), Myluis (1960), Hübner, Kleinsasser and Klein (1969) and Hübner et al (1971) consider the myoepithelial cell to be structurally important. However, Tandler (1971) studying the ultra-structural characteristics of the adenoid cystic carcinoma, has drawn attention to the possibility of myoepithelial-like cells in the tumour, representing remnants of normal salivary parenchyma being replaced by tumour cells. The histogenesis of the tumour for the moment must remain unsettled.

Adenocarcinoma

This is a malignant epithelial tumour, the cells of which show some tubular or papillary glandular formation. No remnants of pleomorphic adenoma are present although occasionally extensive oncocytic change may be present. A

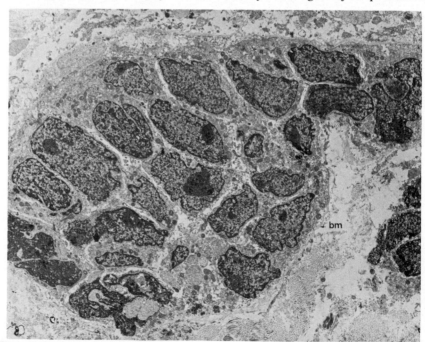

Figure 9.22. Clump of tumour cells in a solid area of an adenoid cystic carcinoma. Basement membrane (BM) is indicated. (× 3375.)

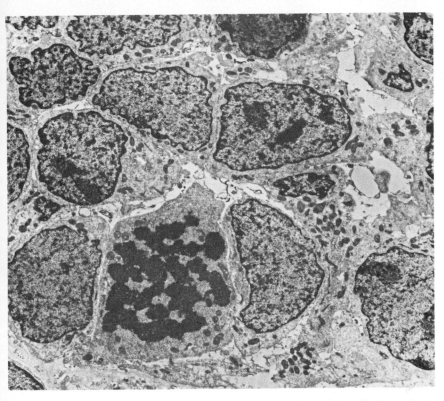

Figure 9.23. Tumour cells in an adenoid cystic carcinoma. Intercellular dilation and the presence of mitosis are shown. ($\times$ 3750.)

subdivision of adenocarcinomas into papillary growths or mucus-secreting growths has little advantage since they are all highly malignant tumours that metastasise widely.

Epidermoid carcinoma

In this malignant epithelial tumour the tumour cells form keratin or exhibit intercellular bridges. Mucus secretion is not a feature. Fortunately the tumour is rare, for the rapid growth with extensive local infiltration and early metastases make the prognosis grave.

Undifferentiated carcinoma

These poorly differentiated malignant tumours of epithelial structure defy inclusion in any other category. However, some workers have felt that even within this group some tumours, although extremely rare, have sufficient

159

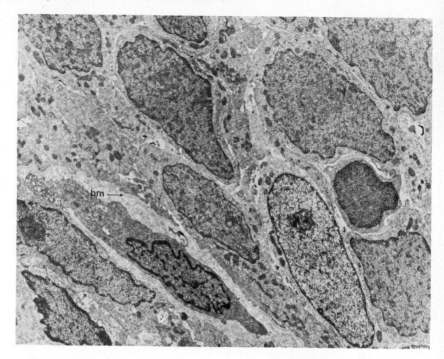

Figure 9.24. Fine structural appearances from a solid area of adenoid cystic carcinoma. Basement membrane region is indicated (BM). ($\times$ 2925.)

characteristics to merit being considered separate entities. These include the solid, undifferentiated carcinoma (Patey, Thackray and Keeling, 1965) trabecular carcinoma and salivary duct carcinoma (Kleinsasser, Klein and Hübner, 1968). This latter lesion shows a marked histological resemblance to duct carcinoma of breast and papillary epithelial proliferation within which tumour duct-like structures are observed. The presence of epithelial and myoepithelial cells in these tumours has been shown by electronmicroscopy (Kleinsasser, Klein and Hübner, 1968; Donath, Seifert and Schmitz, 1972).

Carcinoma in pleomorphic adenoma (Malignant mixed tumour)

This tumour is one in which there is definite evidence of malignancy such as invasive growth and cellular atypia consistent with carcinoma together with histological areas of typical pleomorphic adenoma. It would appear that carcinoma arising in a pleomorphic adenoma is allowed to grow slowly and age over a protracted period (Evans and Cruickshank, 1970). Important clinical features which characterise this tumour are a sudden, painful enlargement of a long-standing, slowly growing lesion and facial nerve paralysis. The tumours carry a poor prognosis and the five-year survival rate is not high (Eneroth, Blanck and Jacobsson, 1968).

NON-EPITHELIAL TUMOURS

The most common stromal tumours of salivary glands are haemangioma, lymphangioma and neurofibroma. These three types of benign tumour represent about 50 per cent of tumours occurring in this site in children, but, interestingly, less than 5 per cent in adults.

UNCLASSIFIED TUMOURS

This category comprises those benign or malignant tumours that cannot be included in the types described above.

SALIVARY GLAND NEOPLASMS IN CHILDREN

Neoplasms of the salivary glands are uncommon in infancy and childhood. Parenchymal neoplasms comprise less than five per cent of those appearing

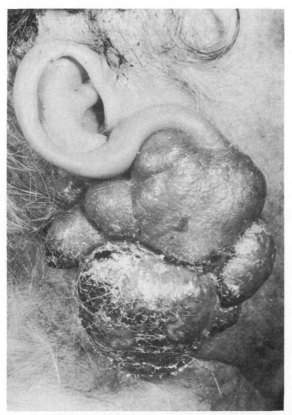

Figure 9.25. Metastatic carcinoma in the extra-parotid lymph nodes. The primary lesion was sited in the scalp.

161

in all age groups (Howard et al, 1950; Byars, Ackerman and Peacock, 1957; Kaufman and Stout, 1963; Reiquam, 1963; Galich, 1969; and Castro et al, 1972). In all reported series in children, haemangioma is the most common salivary gland neoplasm. Pleomorphic adenoma is the most common type of parenchymal neoplasm and appears to favour females; as in adults, recurrences are common. Although the parotid gland is the most common site of origin, the submandibular and minor salivary glands are more frequently involved in children than in adults (Galich, 1969). Children appear more prone to develop malignant lesions, the incidence being around 30 per cent (Byars, Ackerman and Peacock, 1957; Galich, 1969). There appears to be well-documented transformation of the benign tumours into the malignant variant in children. Muco-epidermoid tumours are the most frequently encountered malignant tumour, representing 20 to 25 per cent of all salivary gland tumours in children. Local recurrence or metastases appear in around 30 to 50 per cent of cases. Adenoid cystic carcinoma behaves in similar fashion to the course in adults. The undifferentiated carcinoma is highly malignant with rapid growth and widespread metastases (Kaufman and Stout, 1963).

METASTASIS TO THE SALIVARY GLANDS

Metastatic malignancy in the salivary glands is rare and is usually the result of the involvement of lymph nodes within or around the gland or from direct extension (Figure 9.25) of a neighbouring tumour (Conley and Arena, 1963). Primary growths appear to be lung, kidney, pancreas and stomach (Patey,

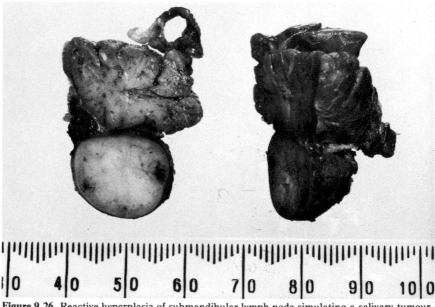

Figure 9.26. Reactive hyperplasia of submandibular lymph node simulating a salivary tumour.

Thackray and Keeling, 1965). Salivary gland involvement in malignant lymphoma of the jaw in African children appears to be quite common (Wright, 1964). Malignant transformation of lymphoid and epithelial structures in Sjögren's syndrome and lympho-epithelial lesions are discussed elsewhere in this book (Chapters 10 and 11). It is worth noting that pathological conditions of the extra-salivary lymph nodes may simulate a localised lesion of salivary gland (Figure 9.26).

REFERENCES

Ackerman, L. V. (1943) Oncocytoma of the parotid gland. *Archives of Pathology,* **36,** 508.
Allegra, S. R. (1971) Warthin's tumour: A hypersensitivity disease? Ultrastructural, light and immunofluorescent study. *Human Pathology,* **2,** 403.
Allen, S. (1974) Elastic Tissue in Pleomorphic Adenomas of Human Minor Salivary Glands. B.Sc. Thesis, University of Glasgow, Glasgow.
Archer, F. L. & Kao, V. C. Y. (1968) Immunohistochemical identification of actomyosin in myoepithelium of human tissues. *Laboratory Investigation,* **18,** 669.
Azzopardi, J. G. & Hou, L. T. (1964) The genesis of adenolymphoma. *Journal of Pathology and Bacteriology,* **88,** 213.
Azzopardi, J. G. & Smith, O. D. (1959) Salivary gland tumours and their mucins. *Journal of Pathology and Bacteriology,* **77,** 131.
Azzopardi, J. G. & Zayid, I. (1972) Elastic tissue in tumours of salivary glands. *Journal of Pathology,* **107,** 149.
Bauer, F. L. & Fox, R. A. (1945) Adenomyo-epithelioma (cylindroma) of palatal mucous glands. *Archives of Pathology,* **39,** 96.
Bauer, W. H. & Byrne, J. J. (1950) Induced tumors of the parotid gland. *Cancer Research,* **10,** 755.
Berg, J. W., Hutter, R. V. P. & Foote, F. W. (1968) The unique association between salivary gland cancer and breast cancer. *Journal of the American Medical Association,* **204,** 771.
Bernier, J. L. & Bhaskar, S. N. (1958) Lymphoepithelial lesions of the salivary gland. Histogenesis and classification based on 186 cases. *Cancer,* **11,** 1156.
Bhaskar, S. N. & Bernier, J. L. (1962) Mucoepidermoid tumors of major and minor salivary glands. *Cancer,* **15,** 801.
Byars, L. T., Ackerman, L. V. & Peacock, E. (1957) Tumours of salivary gland origin in children: A clinical pathologic appraisal of 24 cases. *Annals of Surgery,* **146,** 40.
Castro, E. B., Huvos, A. G., Strong, E. W. & Foote, F. W. (1972) Tumours of the major salivary glands in children. *Cancer,* **29,** 312.
Chaudhry, A. P., Vickers, R. A. & Gorlin, R. J. (1961) Intra-oral minor salivary gland tumors; An analysis of 1,414 cases. *Oral Surgery,* **14,** 1194.
Cherry, C. P. & Glücksman, A. (1965) The histogenesis of carcinomas and sarcomas induced in the salivary glands of rats. *British Journal of Cancer,* **19,** 787.
Chisholm, D. M., Waterhouse, J. P., Kraucunas E. & Sciubba, J. J. (1974) Quantitative ultrastructural study of the pleomorphic adenoma (mixed tumour) of human minor salivary glands. *Cancer,* **34,** 1631.
Christ, T. F. & Crocker, D. (1972) Basal cell adenoma of minor salivary gland origin. *Cancer,* **30,** 214.
Conley, J. & Arena, S. (1963) Parotid gland as a focus of metastasis. *Archives of Surgery,* **87,** 757.
Dawe, C. J., Morgan, W. D. & Slatick, M. S. (1966) Influence of epitheliomesenchymal interactions on tumor induction by polyoma virus. *International Journal of Cancer,* **1,** 419.
Dawe, C. J., Whang-Peng, J., Morgan, W. D., Hearon, E. C. & Knutsen, T. (1971) Epithelial origin of polyoma salivary tumours in mice—evidence based on chromosome marked cells. *Science,* **171,** 394.
Delaney, W. E. & Balogh, Jr. K. (1966) Carcinoma of the parotid gland associated with benign lymphoepithelial lesion (Mikulicz's disease) in Sjögren's syndrome. *Cancer,* **19,** 853.
Deppisch, L. M. & Toker, C. (1969) Mixed tumors of the parotid glands: An ultrastructural study. *Cancer,* **24,** 174.

163

Donath, K., Seifert, G. & Schmitz, R. (1972) Diagnosis and ultrastructure of the tubular carcinoma of the salivary gland ducts. *Virchows Archiv für pathologische Anatomie und Physiologie und für klinische Medizin,* **356,** 16.

Doyle, L. E., Lynn, J. A., Panopio, I. T. & Crass, G. (1968) Ultrastructure of the chondroid regions of benign mixed tumour of salivary gland. *Cancer,* **22,** 225.

Echevarria, R. A. (1967) Ultrastructure of the acinic cell-carcinoma and clear cell carcinoma of the parotid gland. *Cancer,* **50,** 563.

Eneroth, C. M. (1965) Oncocytoma of major salivary glands. *Journal of Laryngology and Otology,* **79,** 1064.

Eneroth, C. M. (1971) Salivary gland tumours in the parotid gland, submandibular gland and the palatal region. *Cancer,* **27,** 1415.

Eneroth, C. M. & Zetterberg, A. (1973) Nuclear DNA content as a criterion of malignancy in salivary gland tumours of the oral cavity. *Acta Otolaryngologica,* **75,** 296.

Eneroth, C. M. & Wersäll, J. (1966) Fine structure of the epithelial cells in mixed tumors of the parotid gland. *Annals of Otology, Rhinology and Laryngology,* **75,** 95.

Eneroth, C. M., Blanck, C. & Jakobsson (1968) Carcinoma in pleomorphic adenoma of the parotid gland. *Acta Oto-Laryngologica,* **66,** 477.

Eneroth, C. M., Jakobsson, P. A. & Blanck, C. (1966) Acinic cell carcinoma of the parotid gland. *Cancer,* **19,** 1761.

Eneroth, C. M., Hjertman, L., Moberger, G. & Wersall, J. (1968) Ultrastructural characteristics of adenoid cystic carcinoma of salivary glands. *Archiv Klinische experimentelle Ohren Nasen Kehlkopfheilkunde,* **192,** 358.

Epker, B. N. & Henry, F. A. (1971) Intra-oral sebaceous gland adenoma. *Cancer,* **27,** 987.

Evans, R. W. & Cruickshank, A. H. (1970) Epithelial tumours of the salivary glands. In *Major Problems in Pathology,* Volume 1. Philadelphia: W. B. Saunders Company.

Eversole, L. R. (1971) Histogenetic classification of salivary tumours. *Archives of Pathology,* **92,** 433.

Foote, F. W. Jr. & Frazell, E. L. (1954) Tumours of the major salivary glands. In *Atlas of Tumour Pathology,* Section 4, Fasicle 11. Washington, D.C.: Armed Forces Institute of Pathology.

Friborsky, V. (1965) Induction of adenoid cystic carcinoma of the submaxillary gland in mice. *Pathologia et Microbiologia,* **28,** 413.

Galich, R. (1969) Salivary gland neoplasms in childhood. *Archives of Otolaryngology,* **89,** 878.

Garrett, J. R. & Harrison, J. D. (1970) Alkaline phosphate and adenosinetriphosphatase histochemical reactions in the salivary glands of cat, dog and man, with particular reference to the myoepithelial cells. *Histochemie,* **24,** 214.

Garrett, J. V., Nicholson, A., Wittaker, J. S., Ridway, J. C. & Bowman, C. M. (1971) Blood groups and secretor status in patients with salivary gland tumours. *Lancet,* **i,** 1177.

Glücksman, A. & Cherry, C. P. (1962) The induction of adenomas by the irradiation of salivary glands of rats. *Radiation Research,* **17,** 186.

Hamperl, H. (1931) Beiträge zur normalen und pathologischen Histologic menschlicher Speicheldrüsen. *Zeitschrift für mikroskopisch-anatomische Forschung,* **27,** 1.

Hamperl, H. (1970) The myothelia (myoepithelial cells). Normal state, regressive changes, hyperplasia; tumours. *Current Topics in Pathology,* **53,** 161.

Hartz, P. H. (1946) Development of sebaceous glands from intralobular ducts of the parotid gland. *Archives of Pathology,* **41,** 651.

Hirtzler, R., Oberman, B., Kulis, M. & Ljubesic, N. (1969) Acinuszelladenocarcinome der Speicheldrüsen. *Archiv klinische experimentelle Ohren Nasen Kehlkopfheilkunde,* **195,** 68.

Howard, J. M., Rawson, J., Koop, C. E., Horn, R. C. & Royster, H. P. (1950) Parotid tumours in children. *Surgery, Gynecology and Obstetrics with International Abstracts of Surgery* **90,** 307.

Hübner, G. & Kleinsasser, O. (1970) Zur Feinstruktur und Genese des Mucoepidermoidtumors der Speicheldrüsen. *Virchows Archiv für pathologische Anatomie und Physiologie und für klinische Medizin,* **349,** 281.

Hübner, G., Kleinsasser, O. & Klein, H. J. (1969) Fine structure and genesis of cylindroma (adenoid cystic carcinoma) of the salivary glands. *Virchows Archiv für pathologische Anatomie und Physiologie und für klinische Medizin,* **347,** 296.

Hübner, G., Kleinsasser, O. & Klein, H. J. (1971) Zur Feinstruktier der Basalzelladenome der Speicheldrüsen. *Virchows Archiv für pathologische Anatomie und Physiologie und für klinische Medizin,* **353,** 333.

Hübner, G., Klein, H. J., Kleinsasser, O. & Schiefer, H. G. (1971) Role of myoepithelial cells in the development of salivary gland tumours. *Cancer,* **27,** 1255.

Kaufman, S. L. & Stout, A. P. (1963) Tumours of the major salivary glands in children. *Cancer,* **16,** 1317.

Kierszenbaum, A. L. (1968) The ultrastructure of human mixed salivary tumour. *Laboratory Investigation,* **18,** 391.

Kierszenbaum, A. L. (1969) Relationship between nucleolus and nuclear bodies in human mixed salivary tumours. *Journal of Ultrastructure Research,* **29,** 459.

Kino, I., Richart, R. M. & Lattes, R. (1973a) Nuclear DNA in salivary gland tumors. I. Warthin tumors, benign mixed tumors and mucoepidermoid carcinomas. *Archives of Pathology,* **95,** 245.

Kino, I., Richart, R. M. & Lattes, R. (1973b) Nuclear DNA in salivary gland tumors. II. Adenocystic carcinomas. *Archives of Pathology,* **95,** 325.

Kleinsasser, O. & Klein, H. J. (1967) Basalzelladenome der Speicheldrüsen. *Archiv klinische experimentelle Ohren Nasen Kehlkopfheilkunde,* **189,** 302.

Kleinsasser, O., Hübner, G. & Klein, H. J. (1967) Acinuszelltumoren der Glandula parotis. *Archiv klinische experimentelle Ohren Nasen Kehlkopfheilkunde,* **192,** 100.

Kleinsasser, O., Klein, H. J. & Hübner, G. (1968) Duct carcinoma of salivary glands. *Archiv klinische experimentelle Ohren Nasen Kehlkopfheilkunde,* **192,** 100.

Kleinsasser, O., Klein, H. J., Steinbach, E. & Hübner, G. (1966) Onkocytäre adenomartige Hyperplasien, Adenolymphone and Oncocytome den Speicheldrusen. *Archiv klinische experimentelle Ohren Nasen Kehlkopfheilkunde,* **186,** 317.

Kondo, T., Muragishi, H. & Imaizumi, M. (1971) A cell from a human salivary gland mixed tumour. *Cancer,* **27,** 403.

Lee, C. M. (1949) Intra parotid sebaceous glands. *Annals of Surgery,* **129,** 152.

Lennox, B., Pearse, A. G. E. & Richards, H. G. H. (1952) Mucin-secreting tumours of the skin: with special reference to the so-called mixed salivary tumour of the skin and its relation to hidradenoma. *Journal of Pathology and Bacteriology,* **64,** 865.

Little, J. W. & Rickles, N. H. (1965) Malignant papillary cystadenoma lymphomatosum. *Cancer,* **18,** 851.

Luna, M. A., Stimson, P. G. & Bardwil, J. M. (1968) Minor salivary gland tumors of the oral cavity. *Oral Surgery, Oral Medicine and Oral Pathology,* **25,** 71.

Meza-Chávez, L. (1949) Sebaceous glands in normal and neoplastic parotid glands—possible significance of sebaceous glands in respect to the origin of tumours of the salivary gland. *American Journal of Pathology,* **25,** 627.

Morgan, M. N. & Mackenzie, D. H. (1968) Tumours of salivary glands; a review of 204 cases with 5-year follow up. *British Journal of Surgery,* **55,** 284.

Murad, T. M. & Haam, E. V. (1968) Ultrastructure of myoepithelial cells in human mammary gland tumours. *Cancer,* **21,** 1137.

Mylius, E. A. (1960) The identification and the role of the myoepithelial cell in salivary gland tumours. *Acta Pathologica et Microbiologica Scandinavica,* Suppl. **139,** 1.

McFarland, J. (1943) The mysterious mixed tumors of the salivary glands. *Surgery, Gynecology and Obstetrics with International Abstracts of Surgery,* **76,** 23.

McGavran, M. H. (1965) The ultrastructure of papillary cystadenoma lymphomatosum of the parotid gland. *Virchows Archiv für pathologische Anatomie und Physiologie und für klinische Medizin,* **338,** 195.

McGavran, M. H., Bauer, W. C. & Ackerman, L. V. (1960) Sebaceous lymphadenoma of the parotid salivary gland. *Cancer,* **13,** 185.

Oota, K. & Takahashi, N. (1958) Electromicroscopic studies on the so-called benign mixed tumor of the salivary gland. *Gann,* **49,** 234.

Ozzello, L. (1971) Ultrastructure of the human mammary gland. *Pathology Annual.* (Ed.) Sommers S. C. pp. 1-59. New York: Appleton-Century-Crofts.

Patey, D. H., Thackray, A. L. & Keeling, D. H. (1965) Malignant disease of the parotid. *British Journal of Cancer,* **19,** 712.

Pava, S., Knutson, G. H., Mukhtar, F. & Pickren, J. W. (1965) Squamous cell carcinoma arising in Warthin's tumor of the parotid gland. *Cancer,* **18,** 790.

Quattlebaum, F. W., Dockerty, M. B. & Mayo, C. W. (1946) Adenocarcinoma, cylindroma type of the parotid gland. *Surgery, Gynecology and Obstetrics with International Abstracts of Surgery,* **82,** 342,

Quintarelli, G. & Robinson, L. (1967) The glycosaminoglycans of salivary gland tumors. *American Journal of Pathology,* **51,** 19.

Ranger, D., Thackray, A. C. & Lucas, R. B. (1956) Mucous gland tumours. *British Journal of Cancer,* **10,** 1.

Rawson, A. J. & Horn, R. C. (1950) Sebaceous gland containing tumours of parotid salivary gland with consideration of histogenesis of papillary cystadenoma lymphomatosum, *Surgery,* **27,** 93.

Reiquam, C. W. (1963) Salivary gland tumours in children. *Archives of Surgery,* **86,** 313.

Rowe, N. H., Grammer, F. C., Watson, F. R. & Nickerson, N. H. (1970) A study of environmental influence upon salivary gland neoplasia in rats. *Cancer,* **26,** 436.

Silver, H. & Goldstein, M. A. (1966) Sebaceous cell carcinoma of the parotid region. *Cancer,* **19,** 1773.

Stebner, F. C., Eyler, W. R., Du Sault, L. A. & Block, M. A. (1968) Identification of Warthin's tumours by scanning of salivary glands. *American Journal of Surgery,* **116,** 513.

Stewart, F. W., Foote, F. W. & Becker, W. F. (1945) Mucoepidermoid tumors of salivary glands. *Annals of Surgery,* **122,** 820.

Stewart, S. E., Eddy, B. E. & Borgese, N. (1958) Neoplasms in mice innoculated with tumor agent carried in tissue culture. *Journal of the National Cancer Institute,* **20,** 1223.

Sykes, J. A, Recher, L., Jernstrom, P. H. & Whitescarver, J. (1968) Morphologic investigation of human breast cancer. *Journal of the National Cancer Institute,* **40,** 195.

Tandler, B. (1965) Ultrastructure of the human submandibular gland. III. Myoepithelium. *Zeitschrift für Zellforschung,* **68,** 852.

Tandler, B. (1971) Ultrastructure of adenoid cystic carcinoma of salivary gland origin. *Laboratory Investigation,* **24,** 504.

Tandler, B. & Shipkey, F. H. (1964a) Ultrastructure of Warthin's tumor. I. Mitochondria. *Journal of Ultrastructure Research,* **11,** 292.

Tandler, B. & Shipkey, F. H. (1964b) Ultrastructure of Warthin's tumor. II. Crystalloids. *Journal of Ultrastructure Research,* **11,** 306.

Thackray, A. C. (1968) Salivary gland tumours. *Proceedings of the Royal Society of Medicine,* **61,** 1089.

Thackray, A. C. (1972) *International Histological Classification of Tumours. Histological Typing of Salivary Gland Tumours.* Geneva: World Health Organisation.

Thackray, A. C. & Lucas, R. B. (1960) The histology of cylindroma of mucous gland origin. *British Journal of Cancer,* **14,** 612.

Thackray, A. C. & Lucas, R. B. (1974) *Tumours of the Major Salivary Glands.* Washington, D.C.: Armed Forces Institute of Pathology.

Veronesi, J. & Corbetta, L. (1960) Adenolymphoma of the lower lip. *Acta Otolaryngologica,* **52,** 1.

Welsh, R. A. & Meyer, Adele, T. (1968) Mixed tumors of human salivary gland. *Archives of Pathology,* **85,** 433.

Willis, R. A. (1967) *Pathology of Tumours,* 4th Edition. London: Butterworth.

Wright, D. H. (1964) Burkitt's tumour: A post-mortem, study of 50 cases. *British Journal of Surgery,* **51,** 245.

Wyatt, A. P., Henry, L. & Curwen, M. P. (1967) Salivary tumours: A clinico-pathological study and follow-up of 156 cases. *British Journal of Surgery,* **54,** 636.

Yates, P. O. & Paget, G. E. (1952) A mixed tumour of salivary gland showing bone formation, with a histochemical study of the tumour mucoids. *Journal of Pathology and Bacteriology,* **64,** 881.

CHAPTER 10

Sjögren's Syndrome

In recent years considerable interest has been shown in Sjögren's syndrome. It appears probable that, if we could understand the basic mechanisms concerned in Sjögren's syndrome, then aetiological factors in rheumatoid arthritis and lymphoid neoplasia, which are associated with the disorder, might be revealed.

Sjögren's syndrome, first described in 1933 (Sjögren, 1933) consists of the triad of xerostomia, keratoconjunctivitis sicca and, in half to two-thirds of patients, rheumatoid arthritis. Salivary gland and/or lacrimal gland enlargement may or may not be present. In some cases, rheumatoid arthritis may be replaced by another connective tissue disease such as polyarteritis nodosa, systemic lupus erythematosus, progressive systemic sclerosis, polymyositis or dermatomyositis. The presence of two of these three main components is generally sufficient for the diagnosis of the syndrome. The term 'sicca syndrome' is used when the connective tissue disorder is absent, i.e. xerostomia and keratoconjunctivitis only are present (Bloch et al, 1965).

GENERAL FEATURES OF SJÖGREN'S SYNDROME

Sjögren's syndrome is primarily a disorder which affects middle-aged females, although occasionally males and younger individuals may be affected (O'Neill, 1965; Duncan, Epker and Sheldon, 1969). The frequency with which Sjögren's syndrome is recognised depends largely upon the awareness of the examiner who first sees the patient (Shearn, 1971).

Several studies suggest that Sjögren's syndrome is a common complication of rheumatoid arthritis alone (Holm, 1949; Bloch and Bunim, 1963; Shearn, 1971). Our experience indicates that approximately one per cent of patients with rheumatoid arthritis develop the salivary gland manifestations of the syndrome (Buchanan, 1973). However, patients with the sicca syndrome accounted for 40 per cent of all cases of Sjögren's syndrome recently reported by Whaley et al (1973).

With regard to the incidence of the syndrome, it is to be noted that among the connective tissue diseases, Sjögren's syndrome ranks second only to rheumatoid arthritis (Shearn, 1971). In Sjögren's syndrome, the association with other connective tissue diseases and the effect of therapeutic measures

167

such as corticosteroids and immunosuppressive drugs make difficult an assessment with regard to the prognosis of the condition. At the present time, however, it appears that Sjögren's syndrome is progressive and may carry an increased risk of early death. From post-mortem studies, infection, malignant lymphoma, renal failure and hepatic failure are the likely causes of death (Cardell and Gurling, 1954; Bloch et al, 1965; Talal, Sokoloff and Barth, 1967; Shearn, 1971).

CLINICAL FEATURES

General manifestations

The symptoms, signs, laboratory findings and radiographic changes of patients with rheumatoid arthritis complicated by Sjögren's syndrome closely resemble those of classic rheumatoid arthritis. It is of interest that arthritic symptoms are the most frequent initial complaint of patients who develop full-blown Sjögren's syndrome (Bloch et al, 1965; Shearn, 1971). Kerato-conjunctivitis sicca manifests as a dryness, together with a gritty burning sensation of the eyes; redness, photophobia and discharge are other symptoms of note. Lacrimal gland enlargement is uncommon (Hughes and Whaley, 1972). In view of the co-existence with various connective tissue diseases it is not surprising that recent investigations have revealed multi-system abnormalities in some patients with Sjögren's syndrome (Bloch and Bunim, 1953; Bloch et al, 1965; Steinberg and Talal, 1971; Whaley et al, 1973a, b). In addition to dryness of the mouth and eyes, hypofunction of exocrine glands may lead to nasal (Figure 10.1), pharyngeal (Doig et al, 1971), vaginal and vulvar dryness. Dryness of the skin with pruritus and

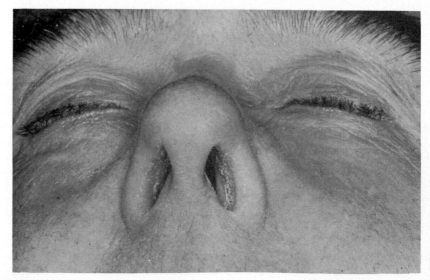

Figure 10.1. Dryness of the nasal mucosa in a patient with Sjögren's syndrome.

Table 10.1. *Clinical features of patients with Sjögren's syndrome.*

	No. of patients	Mean age (years)	Sex	Mean duration of disease (years)	Kerato-conjuncti-vitis sicca	Xerostomia	Lacrimal gland enlarge-ment	Salivary gland enlarge-ment	Skin dryness	Vaginal dryness
Sicca syndrome	71	63.2	7 M 64 F	7.3	71	62	6	24	15	2
Sjögren's syndrome + rheumatoid arthritis	94	59.7	11 M 83 F	15.2	88	52	1	17	21	3
Sjögren's syndrome + systemic lupus erythematosus	4	40.8	4 F	7.3	2	4	..	2	2	..
Sjögren's syndrome + progressive systemic sclerosis	1	40.0	1 F	3.0	1	1	..	..	1	..
Sjögren's syndrome + psoriatic arthritis	1	45.0	1 F	8.5	1	1	..	1	1	..
Total	171	57.2	18 M 153 F		163	118	7	44	40	5

From Whaley et al (1973a).

169

scaling, thrombocytopenic purpura (Steinberg, Green and Talal, 1971) and Raynaud's phenomenon are not infrequently seen. Various gastro-intestinal, pulmonary (Bloch et al, 1965), renal (Shearn and Tu, 1965, 1968; Talal, Zisman and Schur, 1968), neurological (Kaltreider and Talal, 1969), muscle (Denko and Old, 1969), cardiac and endocrine abnormalities (Bloch et al, 1965) in Sjögren's syndrome have been described and are well reviewed by Shearn (1971) and Whaley et al (1973b). The incidence of clinical auto-immune thyroiditis appears not to be increased in patients with Sjögren's syndrome (Williamson et al, 1967; Whaley et al, 1973b) as thought previously (Bloch et al, 1965). Elevation of the erythrocyte sedimentation rate, anaemia, leucopenia and eosinophilia have been reported (Stoltze et al, 1960; Vanselow et al, 1963; Bloch et al, 1965; Whaley et al, 1973b). Finally, the association between Sjögren's syndrome and malignant lymphoreticular disease is now well documented and will be discussed in more detail later in the chapter. Clinical features of patients with Sjögren's syndrome are shown in Tables 10.1 and 10.2.

Table 10.2. *Oral symptoms and signs in Sjögren's syndrome.*

		Sicca syndrome 54 patients		Sjögren's syndrome Rheumatoid arthritis 66 patients	
		Number	per cent	Number	per cent
Xerostomia	Complaining of	54	100	64	97
	On examination	54	100	48	72.7
Mean duration		4.4 years		2.8 years	
Nature	Intermittent	30	55.5	39	60.9
	Persistent	24	43.7	25	39.1
Increased fluid intake		42	77.8	46	69.7
Nature	Related to meals	22	40.7	28	42.4
	Persistent	30	55.5	24	36.4
Oral soreness		32	59.3	49	74.2
Oral ulceration		13	24.1	24	36.4
Abnormality of taste		1	1.9	1	1.5
Lingual changes[a]		38	70.4	46	69.7
	Grade 1	19	35.2	28	42.4
	Grade 2	14	25.9	11	16.7
	Grade 3	5	9.3	7	10.6

[a]Bertram, U., 1967. *Acta Odontologica Scandinavica,* **25** (Suppl. 49).

Oral manifestations

Xerostomia

Decreased salivation, difficulty in swallowing and mastication, increased fluid intake, abnormalities in taste sensation, oral mucosal soreness and ulceration are common symptoms (Table 10.2) (Bloch et al, 1965; Henkin et al, 1972; Chisholm and Mason, 1973; Whaley et al, 1973a). The oral mucous membranes appear dry, smooth and glazed (Figure 10.2) whilst lingual changes varying from slight reddening with mild fissuring to pronounced reddening with sever lobulation (Figures 10.3 to 10.5) and deep fissuring are often present (Bertram, 1967).

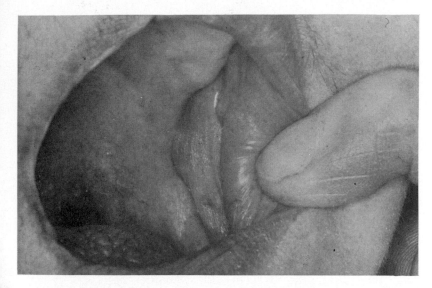

Figure 10.2. Extreme oral dryness, atrophic mucosae and lobulated tongue in patient with long-standing Sjögren's syndrome.

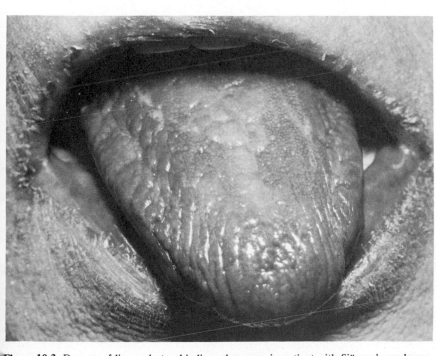

Figure 10.3. Dryness of lips and atrophic lingual mucosa in patient with Sjögren's syndrome.

171

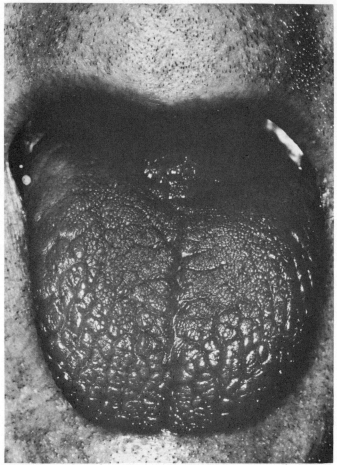

Figure 10.4. Lingual changes in a 66-year-old male patient with Sjögren's syndrome. Mucosal atrophy together with mild fissuring and lobulation is present.

However, these mucosal signs are only suggestive of xerostomia due to Sjögren's syndrome, since they may present in a variety of disorders including pernicious anaemia, folic acid deficiency, sideropenic anaemia and malabsorption (Hjörting-Hansen and Bertram, 1968).

The histopathological appearances of the oral epithelium in Sjögren's syndrome have recently been studied (Adams, 1973). Although basal layer disruption, parakeratinisation, lymphocytic infiltration and atrophy were features of note, they were inconsistent and could not be related to clinical features.

In patients with a natural dentition, a rapidly progressive dental caries may be observed (Figure 10.6). Those patients with dentures have difficulty with retention and suffer angular cheilitis (Figures 10.7, 10.8). Recently, an association between Sjögren's syndrome and oral candidosis (Figure 10.9) has been noted (MacFarlane and Mason, 1974).

172

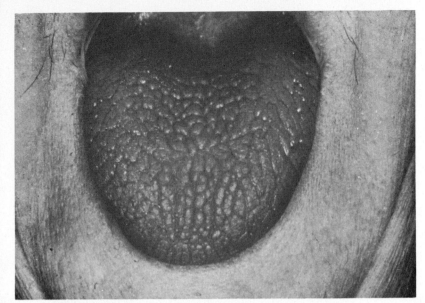

Figure 10.5. Severe lobulation and fissuring of tongue in patient with Sjögren's syndrome and xerostomia of 22 years' duration.

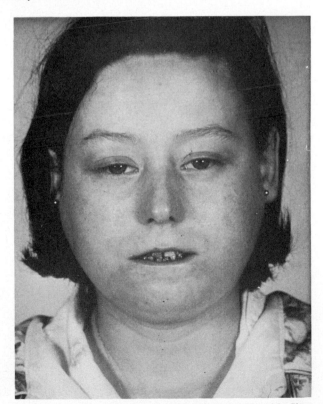

Figure 10.6. Bilateral parotid swelling in a 26-year-old female with Sjögren's syndrome complicated by SLE. Dental decay is present and was of recent onset.

173

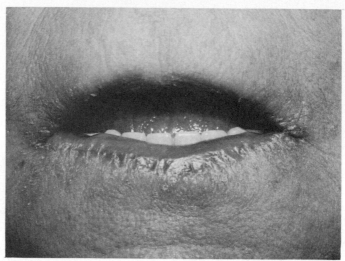

Figure 10.7. Dry lips and angular cheilitis in a patient with Sjögren's syndrome of 8 years duration.

Salivary gland enlargement

Bloch et al (1965) reported salivary gland enlargement to be present in half of 62 patients studied, but our experience over a 10-year period has been that although a history of salivary gland enlargement may be elicited from approximately 30 per cent of patients, its presence is clinically apparent in only half that number (Table 10.1). Most studies agree that salivary swelling in Sjögren's syndrome occurs bilaterally and that the parotid glands are more commonly affected (Figures 10.6 and 10.10 to 10.11). It is of interest that

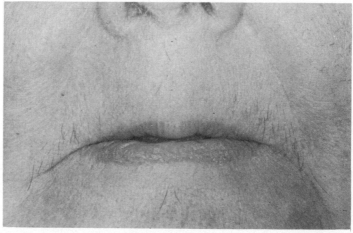

Figure 10.8. Dryness of lips and angular cheilitis in a patient with Sjögren's syndrome.

174

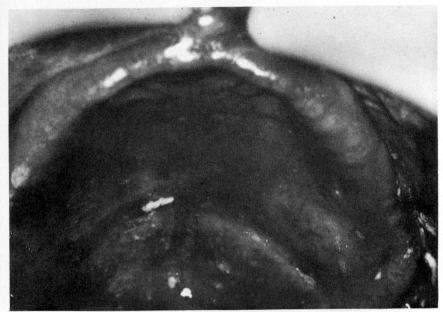

Figure 10.9. Oral candidosis affecting the palatal mucosa of a 66-year-old male with Sjögren's syndrome.

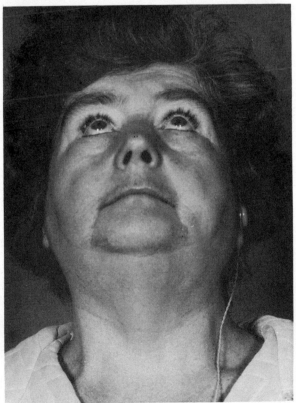

Figure 10.10. Bilateral parotid gland enlargement in a 45-year-old female with sicca syndrome.

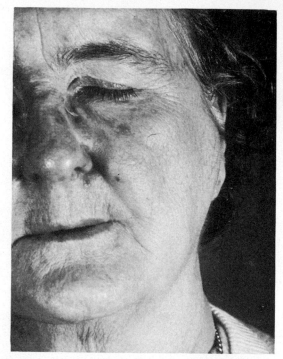

Figure 10.11. Left parotid swelling in a patient with sicca syndrome.

Talal, Sokoloff and Barth (1967) have reported that patients with Sjögren's syndrome who develop lymphoid neoplasia are more likely to show salivary gland enlargement.

DIAGNOSTIC TECHNIQUES

General

Rheumatoid arthritis and keratoconjunctivitis sicca are diagnoses made by well-defined criteria. The American Rheumatism Association criteria (Ropes et al, 1958) have been used in most recent studies. The diagnosis of keratoconjunctivitis sicca is made by demonstrating diminished lacrimation by the use of the Schirmer tear test and the finding of filamentary or punctate keratitis on slip lamp examination of the cornea after the instillation of rose bengal dye into the conjunctival sac (Williamson et al, 1967).

Oral

At the present time, there is no entirely satisfactory diagnostic test for the salivary gland component of Sjögren's syndrome. Xerostomia is a common

Table 10.3. *Citric acid (5% solution) stimulated parotid flow rates (ml/min ± SEM) in 171 control subjects, 32 patients with sicca syndrome and 86 patients with Sjögren's syndrome.*

		Age range (Years)		
		21-40	41-60	61+
Controls	Male	1.73±0.09	1.69±0.11	1.58±0.16
	Female	1.76±0.09	1.36±0.12	1.15±0.08
Sicca syndrome	Male	—	—	0.43±0.08
	Female	—	0.24±0.08	0.27±0.05
Sjögren's syndrome + rheumatoid arthritis	Male	—	0.93±0.17	0.43±0.05
	Female	0.56±0.05	0.47±0.07	0.41±0.05

clinical complaint with a multiplicity of causes and predisposing factors (Bertram, 1967; Mason and Glen, 1967). In recent years, however, much attention has been directed towards the diagnostic value of salivary function tests such as flow rate estimation, labial salivary gland biopsy, hydrostatic sialography and pertechnetate scintiscanning, and these will now be considered in relation to Sjögren's syndrome. Details of these techniques are considered in later chapters of this text.

Table 10.4. *Sialographic appearances and salivary flow results in 64 patients with Sjögren's syndrome.*

	Normal	Sialectasis			Atrophy	Main duct dilatation
		Punctate	Globular	Cavitary		
Total number of parotid glands examined	45	29	15	15	14	6
Number with sicca syndrome	8	10	5	11	4	2
Sex distribution	8 ♀ 0 ♂	10 ♀ 0 ♂	3 ♀ 2 ♂	11 ♀ 0 ♂	4 ♀ 0♂	2 ♀ 0 ♂
Number with Sjögren's syndrome and rheumatoid arthritis	37	19	10	4	10	4
Sex distribution	29 ♀ 9 ♂	17 ♀ 2♂	10 ♀ 0 ♂	4 ♀ 0 ♂	10 ♀ 0 ♂	4 ♀ 0 ♂
Mean parotid flow rate (lemon juice) ml/min	0.85	0.38	0.34	0.13	0.25	0.32
SE	0.07	0.04	0.06	0.04	0.05	0.07
Range	0.26—2.00	0.0—0.8	0.0—1.0	0.0—0.42	0.01—0.5	0.08—0.48

From Chisholm et al (1971).

177

Salivary Glands in Health and Disease

Salivary flow rate estimation

This method is a fairly reliable test of salivary gland function and 90 per cent of patients with Sjögren's syndrome, observed over a 10-year period, had flow rate values below the normal range (Tables 10.3 to 10.4; Figure 10.12a, b) (Chisholm and Mason, 1973). Reduced salivary flow rates in patients with Sjögren's syndrome have been reported by Bloch et al (1965) and Bertram (1967).

Labial salivary gland biopsy

The presence of focal lymphocytic adenitis in the minor salivary glands in a small number of cases of Sjögren's syndrome has been reported (Cifarelli, Bennett and Zaino, 1966; Calman and Reifman, 1966; Mason, 1966; Cahn, 1967; Bertram, 1967). Using the labial salivary glands, Chisholm and Mason (1968) studied the histopathological features of groups of patients with various connective tissue disorders, including Sjögren's syndrome (Table 10.5). In this and subsequent studies (Chisholm, 1969; Talal, Asofsky and Lightbody, 1970; Berry, Bacon and Davis, 1973; Greenspan et al, 1974), focal lymphocytic sialadenitis (Figures 10.13 to 10.18) was demonstrated in approximately 70 per cent of patients with Sjögren's syndrome. In a histo-

Table 10.5. *Grades of lymphocytic infiltration in the labial salivary glands in the clinical groups studied.*

Clinical group	No.	Grade of lymphocytic infiltrate					Per cent with foci
		0	1	2	3	4	
Sicca syndrome	21	1	3	4	5	8	61.9
Rheumatoid arthritis + Sjögren's syndrome	50	1	10	4	15	20	70.0
Rheumatoid arthritis	73	30	20	9	12	2	19.2
Psoriatic arthritis	16	12	2	1	1	0	6.3
Ankylosing spondylitis	12	8	1	1	2	0	16.7
Reiter's syndrome	12	10	2	0	0	0	0
Systemic lupus erythermatosus	5	1	1	1	0	2[a]	40.0
Progressive systemic sclerosis	4	1	2	0	0	1[a]	25.0
Dermatomyositis	1	1	0	0	0	0	0
Gout	2	2	0	0	0	0	0
Osteoarthritis	20	16	1	1	1	0	5.0

[a]These patients also had Sjögren's syndrome.
From Chisholm (1970).

pathological study Greenspan et al (1974) have noted that these accumulations of lymphoid cells are related to blood vessels adjacent to the ducts. They reported that the size of the lymphocytic focus is directly related to the number of foci (focus score) in each specimen and that the focus score correlates well with the stimulated parotid flow rate and the uptake and concentration of ^{99m}Tc pertechnetate as revealed in scintigraphy. The focus

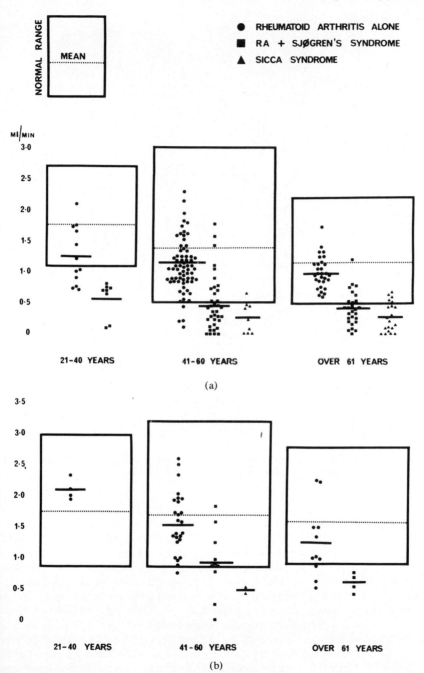

Figure 10.12. Citric acid (5% solution) stimulated parotid flow rates in patients with Sjögren's syndrome with and without rheumatoid arthritis and with rheumatoid arthritis alone, compared with age- and sex-matched control subjects. a. Females. b. Males.

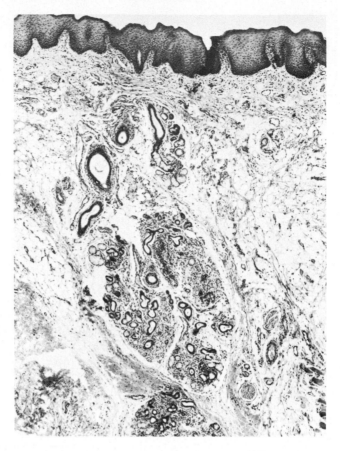

Figure 10.13. Labial mucosa in Sjögren's syndrome. Minor salivary glands lie close to the surface epithelium and show acinar atrophy and lymphocytic adenitis ($\times$ 42).

score is therefore a valuable index for the severity of salivary gland involvement in this disease. The finding of focal lymphocytic adenitis in the labial salivary glands in approximately 20 per cent of patients with rheumatoid arthritis alone is of interest, for this lesion may represent a sub-clinical form of Sjögren's syndrome in these patients (Chisholm and Mason, 1968; Chisholm, 1969). Focal lymphocytic adenitis of major salivary and lacrimal glands occurs commonly in human post-mortem subjects in the absence of evidence of gland infection (Waterhouse, 1963b). A high prevalence of severe focal lymphocytic sialadenitis in 9 per cent of males and 23 per cent of females, especially in the age group 35 to 64 years, has been reported and shown to have a highly significant association with rheumatoid arthritis (Waterhouse and Doniach, 1966). These investigators suggest that such lesions (Figure 10.19) represent a focal manifestation of the lesion in Sjögren's syndrome. Conceptual support for the labial biopsy technique has been provided (Chisholm, Waterhouse and Mason, 1970) by a post-mortem

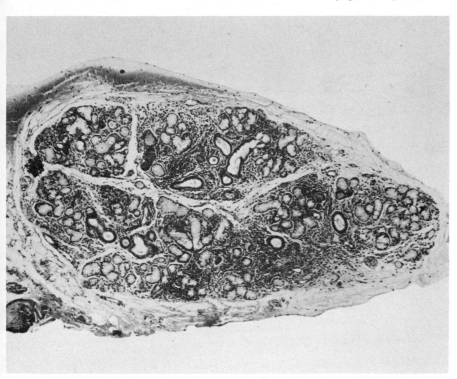

Figure 10.14. Lobule of minor salivary gland tissue in Sjögren's syndrome showing replacement of functional parenchyma by severe lymphocytic infiltration ($\times$ 60).

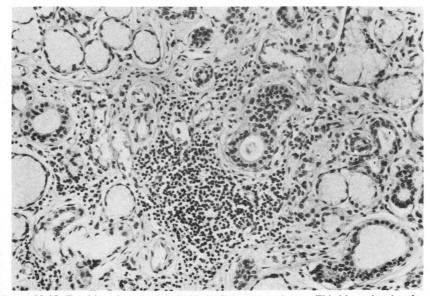

Figure 10.15. Focal lymphocytic sialadenitis in Sjögren's syndrome. This biopsy is taken from the labial glands of the lower lip ($\times$ 21).

181

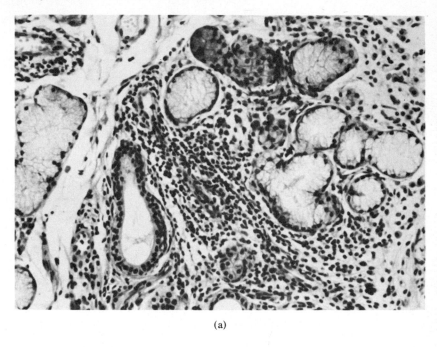

(a)

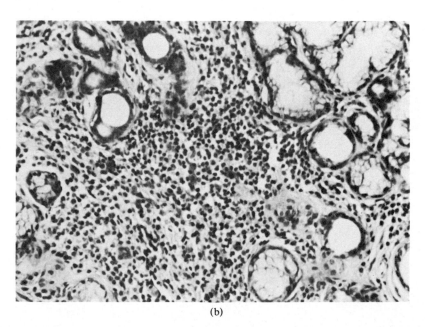

(b)

Figure 10.16. Severe lymphocytic and plasma cell infiltration of minor salivary glands in Sjögren's syndrome. a. Focal aggregate. ($\times$ 36). b. Diffuse aggregate ($\times$ 36).

182

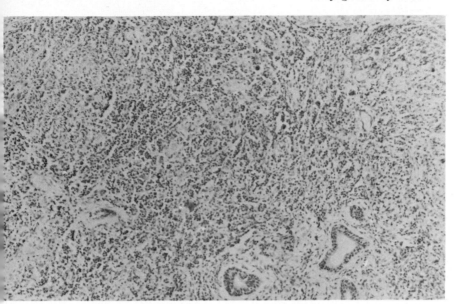

Figure 10.17. Diffuse chronic inflammatory cell infiltrate affecting minor salivary glands in a patient with sicca syndrome. Numerous histiocytes and a pseudo-sarcoid appearance are present (× 20).

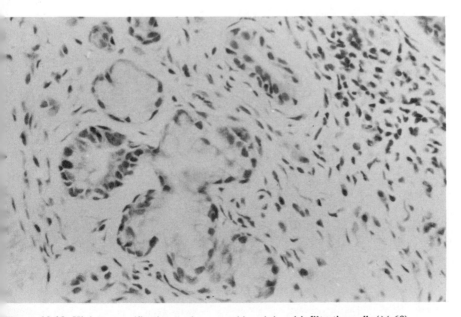

Figure 10.18. Higher magnification to show atrophic acini and infiltrating cells (× 60).

183

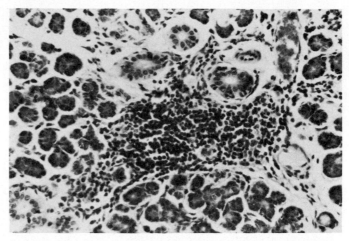

Figure 10.19. A focus of lymphocytes having a periductal distribution in human submandibular salivary gland ($\times$ 30).

study in which focal labial lymphocytic sialadenitis could not be demonstrated in a control series. This study also showed that changes in the minor glands reflected those in their major counterparts. Mucous glands of the nasal cavity (Powell, Larson and Henkin, 1974) and the lacrimal glands (Figure 10.20) show similar changes to those in the labial glands.

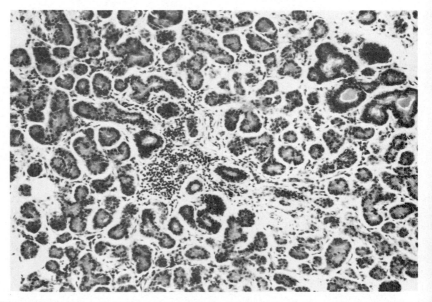

Figure 10.20. Focus of lymphocytes within the lacrimal gland of a patient with Sjögren's syndrome. ($\times$ 7).

184

Hydrostatic sialography

The hydrostatic technique used in our clinic has been described by Park and Mason (1966) and allows a water-soluble contrast medium (Hypaque) to be introduced into the salivary duct system at a constant pressure. Interpretation of sialographic abnormalities is based on criteria laid down by Blatt et al (1956) and modified by Bloch et al (1965). Varying degrees of sialectasis (Figures 10.21 to 10.23) are consistent findings (Table 10.4) in patients with Sjögren's syndrome (Bloch et al, 1965; Mason, 1966; Chisholm et al, 1971; Blair, 1973).

Salivary scintiscanning

Salivary gland scanning appears promising as a method of assessing salivary gland function in man. ^{99m}Tc pertechnetate is an almost ideal scanning agent and, like iodide, is concentrated in the major salivary glands (Harden and Alexander, 1967) and minor salivary glands (Chisholm et al, 1971). Following recent work it appears, both qualitatively (Harden et al, 1967, 1968; Abramson, Goodman and Kolodny, 1968; Grove and Di Chiro, 1968) and quantitatively (Stephen et al, 1971) that ^{99m}Tc pertechnetate uptake by the salivary glands is reduced in patients with Sjögren's syndrome (Figures 18.1d to 18.3). The recent study by Stephen et al (1971) showed that two-thirds of patients with Sjögren's syndrome had uptake values below the lowest value recorded in the control group. Furthermore, investigations with this technique have shown that parotid gland involvement is more common than submandibular; that although the parotid glands may be involved without submandibular glands, the reverse does not hold; and finally that gland involvement is usually bilateral (Stephen et al, 1971). It is of interest that sequential salivary scintigraphy has been shown to closely parallel reduction in flow rates and sialographic abnormalities in the syndrome (Schall et al, 1971). The uptake of ^{99m}Tc pertechnetate by salivary gland tissues in patients with Sjögren's syndrome, rheumatoid arthritis alone and control subjects is shown in Table 10.6.

Evaluation of clinical tests of salivary gland function

The relative value of these salivary gland function tests as diagnostic aids has been assessed by Chisholm and Mason (1973). They found reduced stimulated parotid flow rate to be the most sensitive index of salivary gland dysfunction in Sjögren's syndrome, followed by labial gland biopsy and sialography. Flow rate estimation, however, has the disadvantage of examining the secretions from one group of glands only. Since the parotid glands make the main contribution to whole saliva on stimulation, and are the most commonly involved clinically and as demonstrated by scintiscanning, we feel justified in recommending this technique as an initial screening test. Labial gland biopsy is a simple and safe technique and, in our experience, is well tolerated by patients. It is the only test which gives an indication of the nature of the disease process in the salivary glands. Sialography is time-consuming, since

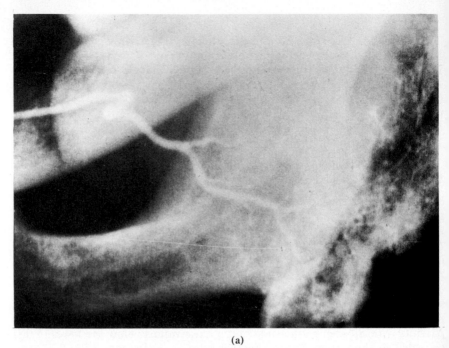

(a)

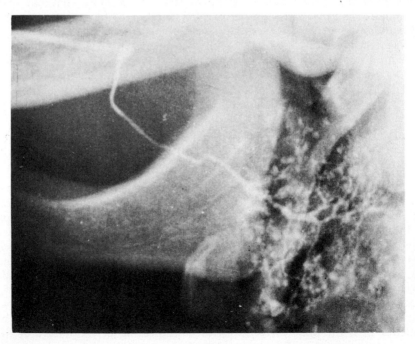

(b)

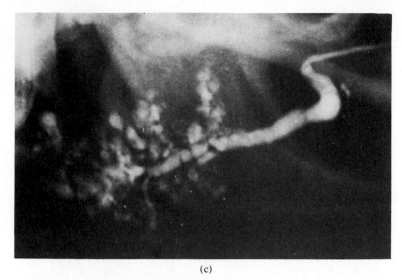

(c)

Figure 10.21. Degrees of sialectasis in Sjögren's syndrome. a. Punctate. b. Globular. c. Cavitary with main duct dilatation. Lateral oblique sialography.

each gland has to be examined individually. The new method of quantitative scintiscanning with ^{99m}Tc pertechnetate is promising, but has not yet been fully evaluated as a test of salivary gland function in disease states. It has the advantage of examining both parotid and submandibular glands at the same time.

Diagnosis

In order to diagnose Sjögren's syndrome with salivary gland involvement, the following steps are undertaken when a patient presents with xerostomia and possible Sjögren's syndrome.
1. A careful clinical examination and history is taken to exclude all other causes of xerostomia or salivary gland enlargement.
2. Swabs and smears are taken from tongue, palate, buccal mucosa and fitting surface of dentures.
3. Stimulated parotid salivary flow rates are measured.
4. A labial salivary gland biopsy is performed to confirm the nature of the disease process if this is in doubt. Major salivary gland biopsy is seldom necessary and only when a salivary or lymphoid neoplasm is suspected.
5. Sialography and/or scintiscanning are undertaken if the flow rate values are equivocal.
6. Ophthalmological and general medical examinations are arranged including haematological and serological work-up. Serological studies should include salivary duct antibody, anti-nuclear factor, rheumatoid factor, anti-thyroid, gastric parietal cell antibody and mitochondrial antibody estimations.

187

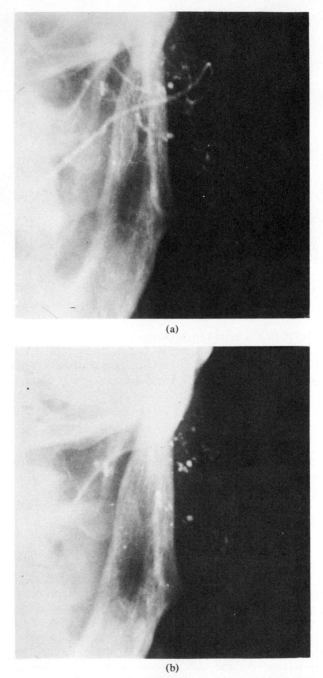

(a)

(b)

Figure 10.22. a. Sjögren's syndrome. Postero-anterior view of the filling phase reveals poor peripheral duct filling and punctate sialectasis. b. Secretory phase showing characteristic retention of contrast immediately in the punctate areas after the main ducts have emptied.

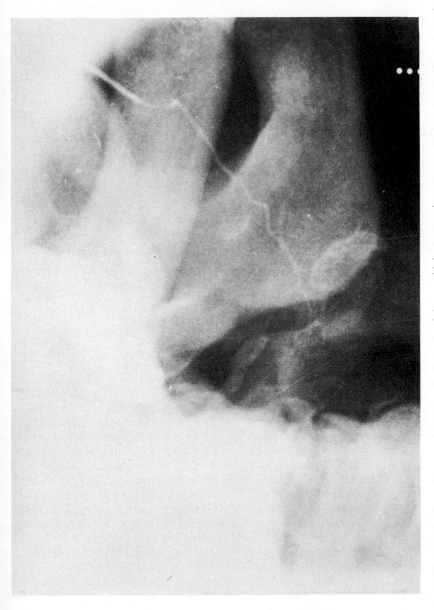

Figure 10.23. Lateral oblique sialogram showing marked atrophy of the parotid duct system in a 31-year-old female with Sjögren's syndrome.

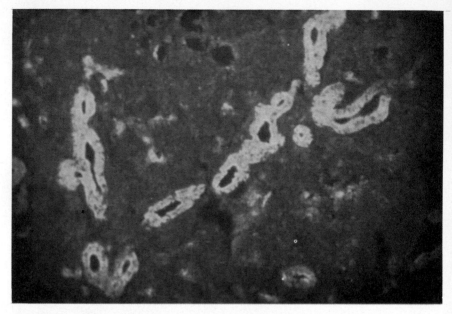

Figure 10.24. Indirect immunal fluorescent staining of salivary duct epithelia in a case of Sjögren's syndrome.

LABORATORY INVESTIGATIONS

General

The remarkable prevalence of abnormal immunological features represent a striking feature of Sjögren's syndrome (Table 10.7). Indeed, the disease ranks second only to systemic lupus erythematosus in its abundance of serum auto-antibodies, both organ specific and non-organ specific. Hypergamma-globulinaemia and circulating auto-antibodies, of both organ-specific and non-organ specific type, are invariably present (Anderson, Buchanan and Goudie, 1967; Whaley et al, 1973b) in Sjögren's syndrome. Although an increased prevalence of organ specific auto-antibodies has been demonstrated, no association has been found between organ specific auto-immune diseases and Sjögren's syndrome. Rheumatoid factor is present in 52 to 100 per cent of patients with Sjögren's syndrome, even in the absence of rheumatoid arthritis (Bloch et al, 1965; Whaley et al, 1973b). Anti-nuclear antibodies are found in approximately two-thirds of patients, speckled or nucleolar patterns being common (Beck, 1961). Tests for lupus erythematosus cells are positive in roughly 10 per cent of patients with Sjögren's syndrome (Bloch et al, 1965). Auto-antibodies to thyroglobulin and thyroid microsomes (Bloch and Bunim, 1963), gastric parietal cell antibody (Buchanan et al, 1966) and mitochondrial antibody (Whaley et al, 1970) have been reported in

190

Table 10.6. *Uptake of ^{99m}Tc pertechnetate by parotid and submandibular salivary glands at mid-scan times of 3, 8 and 13 min.*

Gland	Time (min)	Group A (Normal subjects)		Group B (Rheumatoid arthritis)			Group C (RA and KCS)			Group D (Sjögren's syndrome with salivary involvement)		
		Mean % dose	SE	Mean % dose	SE	P	Mean % dose	SE	P	Mean % dose	SE	P
Parotid	3	0.21	0.02	0.19	0.03	NS	0.18	0.04	NS	0.10	0.01	<0.005
	8	0.30	0.02	0.29	0.04	NS	0.23	0.03	NS	0.15	0.02	<0.005
	13	0.31	0.02	0.36	0.06	NS	0.28	0.05	NS	0.17	0.02	<0.005
Submandibular	3	0.17	0.03	0.15	0.02	NS	0.16	0.03	NS	0.12	0.01	<0.025
	8	0.18	0.01	0.18	0.01	NS	0.14	0.02	NS	0.13	0.02	<0.01
	13	0.18	0.02	0.20	0.02	NS	0.17	0.02	NS	0.13	0.01	<0.025

Groups B, C and D are compared with the normal subjects (Group A) by using Wilcoxon's one-tailed sign-ranked test. RA = Rheumatoid arthritis; KCS = keratoconjunctivitis sicca.
From Stephen et al (1971).

Table 10.7. *Auto-antibodies in Sjögren's syndrome.*

	Rheumatoid factor	Anti-nuclear factor	Salivary duct antibody	Gastric parietal cell antibody	Thyro-globulin antibody	Thyroid microsomal antibody
Sicca syndrome	52% (96%)[a]	37% (88%)[a]	10%	29%	34%	43%
Rheumatoid arthritis + Sjögren's syndrome	99% (100%)[a]	55% (56%)[a]	65%	27%	18%	21%
Total	78%	63%	38%	28%	24%	30%
Lab. controls	9%	9%		15%	10%	16%

[a]The figures in brackets are those of Bloch et al (1965) for comparison.
After Whaley et al, 1973b.

Sjögren's syndrome. Serum IgG, IgM and IgA levels are elevated and serum secretory IgA levels are markedly raised (Gumpel and Hobbs, 1970; Whaley et al, 1973b). However, due to the wide variation of serum immunoglobulin levels in patients with Sjögren's syndrome, their measurement has no specific diagnostic value. In addition to abnormalities of humoral antibody concentrations, cell-mediated immunity has been shown to be impaired in patients with Sjögren's syndrome. In vitro transformation of peripheral blood lymphocytes in response to phytohaemagglutinin and streptolysin O has been studied by Leventhal, Waldorf and Talal (1967). These studies showed significant reduction in response to these mitogenic agents in patients with Sjögren's syndrome, especially those cases complicated by rheumatoid arthritis or lymphoma, compared with controls. Leventhal, Waldorf and Talal (1967) have also shown that the skin of patients with Sjögren's syndrome has a reduced ability to become sensitised to the contact allergen 2,4-dinitrochlorobenzene (DNCB). Hyperviscosity with the presence of intermediate complexes has been reported (Blaylock, Waller and Normansell, 1974).

Oral

An auto-antibody to the cytoplasm of salivary duct cells (Figure 10.24) has been demonstrated by indirect fluorescence (Bertram and Halberg, 1964; Halberg et al 1965; MacSween et al, 1967; Feltkamp and Van Rossum, 1968). However, this antibody is considered to be a reflection of rheumatoid arthritis alone, rather than a manifestation of Sjögren's syndrome per se, since it has a low prevalence in patients with sicca syndrome and shows no correlation with focal lymphocytic sialadenitis (Whaley et al, 1969). Its pathogenic significance appears doubtful (Feltkamp and Van Rossum, 1968). When fluorescence is detected in sera from sicca syndrome patients it is possible that this finding is a reflection of the non-organ-specificity of mitochondrial antibody which appears to occur in association with salivary duct antibody in this condition. The inverse relationship between the presence of antibody and labial gland infiltrates may reflect an imbalance or interplay between humoral and cellular immune responses in Sjögren's syndrome (Anderson et al, 1973). Ductal antigens may elicit a humoral response with salivary duct antibody (SDA) acting as a 'blocking-antibody' or, alternatively, in the absence of sufficient SDA, evoke a cellular response whereby the accumulation of lymphoid cells leads to tissue destruction and gland dysfunction (Anderson et al, 1973). The inhibition of migration of cells by antigen is characteristic of sensitivities of the delayed type. Inhibition of macrophage migration in vitro by salivary gland extracts has been demonstrated in patients with Sjögren's syndrome (Søborg and Bertram, 1968). Recently Berry, Bacon and Davis (1972), using the leucocyte migration test, showed reactivity to parotid gland extract antigen in 93 per cent of patients with Sjögren's syndrome and a good correlation existed between the degree of focal lymphocytic labial sialadenitis and reactivity in this test. From material obtained at labial salivary gland biopsy, Talal et al (1970) have demonstrated a greater synthesis of immunoglobulins, especially IgM and IgG, in Sjögren's syndrome compared with controls, whilst Anderson et al (1972) have demonstrated that the local synthesis of rheumatoid factor in labial salivary gland tissue is distinctive for Sjögren's syndrome.

The renewed interest in the role of infective agents, including mycoplasmas in association with rheumatoid arthritis and other connective tissue disorders (Bartholomew, 1965; Duthie et al, 1967; Brostoff and Roitt, 1970) prompted our group to search for mycoplasmal infection in labial salivary gland tissue and parotid saliva in patients with Sjögren's syndrome. However, mycoplasma (*M. orale* type 1) was recovered from saliva in only one of 26 patients (Gordon, Chisholm and Mason, 1971). Although disappointing, this study does not exclude the possibility of the occurrence of hitherto uncultivatable agents or of 'latent' mycoplasma infection in this and allied conditions. Recent mycological studies from our laboratory have shown that an association exists between Sjögren's syndrome and oral candidosis (MacFarlane and Mason, 1974). This finding is of special interest in view of the occurrence of chronic candidosis in patients with a wide variety of immune defects (*British Medical Journal,* 1972). Other factors which could explain this finding include lack of cleansing action or antibacterial factors in saliva, low pH of saliva, iron deficiency and the use of corticosteroid drugs. There is a paucity of information regarding the constituents of saliva from patients with Sjögren's syndrome. Recently Mandel and Baurmash (1973) reported significant elevations in sodium and chloride and reduction in phosphorus in saliva from patients with Sjögren's syndrome. In 1968, Fischer et al showed that the electrophoretic pattern of parotid saliva was specific for Sjögren's syndrome, anodal proteins migrating more rapidly with advancing severity of the disease. In Sjögren's syndrome, parotid salivary proteins have been separated by the more sensitive tehcnique of isoelectric focusing in polyacrylamide gels (Chisholm, Beeley and Mason, 1973). This study demonstrated additional proteins, with low isoelectric points compared to control samples (Figure 10.25).

HISTOPATHOLOGY; PATHOGENESIS AND LYMPHORETICULAR NEOPLASIA

The most characteristic histopathological feature of affected tissue in Sjögren's syndrome is lymphocytic infiltration. Lymphoid infiltrates may be observed in the lacrimal glands, the mucus-secreting glands of the conjunctivae, the nasal cavity, pharynx, larynx, trachea and bronchi, leading to atrophy of these glands. The sweat glands may be similarly affected. Ultrastructural studies of renal biopsies have shown the presence of viral-like inclusion bodies within renal endothelial cells (Shearn et al, 1970).

The histopathological features of the major salivary glands are well documented (Cardell and Gurling, 1954; Bloch and Bunim, 1963; Ericson, 1968) and include acinar atrophy, focal lymphocytic sialadenitis and ductal

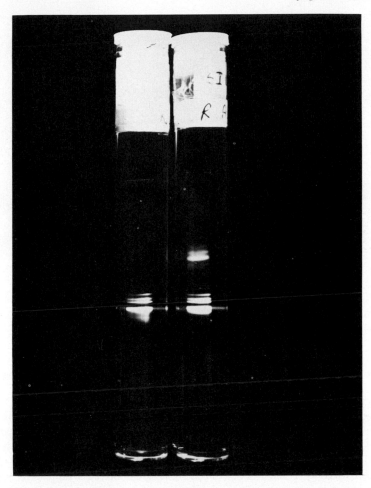

Figure 10.25. Iso-electric focusing of parotid saliva in polyacrylamide gels. Separation of protein bands is shown on the left. Additional protein bands from patient with rheumatoid arthritis and Sjögren's syndrome is shown on right. Photographed in oblique light.

hyperplasia (Figures 10.26 to 10.28) leading to the formation of 'epi-myoepithelial' cell islands (Morgan and Castleman, 1953). It is of interest that ultrastructural studies have failed to reveal the presence of myoepithelial cells in these cell islands (Boquist, Kumlien and Östberg, 1970; Kitamura, Kanda and Ishikawa, 1970). The minor salivary glands show similar features to these described above for their major gland counterparts, with the exception that epi-myoepithelial cell islands do not appear to be a feature (Chisholm and Mason, 1968; Talal, Asofsky and Lightbody, 1970; Eisenbud et al, 1973; Davies et al, 1973). Histopathological features such as interstitial fibrosis, acinar atrophy and ductal changes in the labial glands have been semi-quantitated (Chisholm, 1969; Davies et al, 1973) and shown to be more

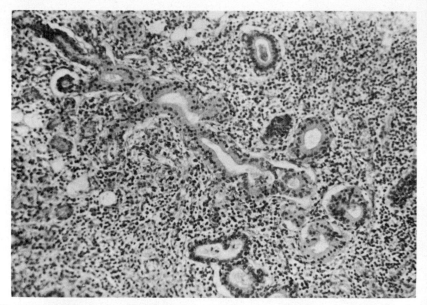

Figure 10.26. Lymphocytic infiltration and duct proliferation within the submandibular salivary glands of a patient with Sjögren's syndrome (× 28).

severe in Sjögren's syndrome than in rheumatoid arthritis or other connective tissue disorders.

Two major sub-populations of lymphocytes, thymus dependent (T) and bursa equivalent (B) are now recognised, and these are separated in distinct anatomical compartments within secondary lymphoid organs. Both T and B lymphocytes are capable of mediating specific cytotoxicity to target cells in vitro. B-cell cytotoxicity is dependent on antibody for this function whilst T-cell cytotoxicity is not. Therefore, determination of which cell type is present in the lesion may help to clarify the mechanism of tissue destruction involved in the salivary glands in Sjögren's syndrome. Sheep erythrocytes coated with 19S antibody and activated third component of complement adhere to human bone marrow-derived (B) cells and monocytes in tissue sections. Erythrocytes coated with 7S antibody adhere only to monocytes. The localisation of these reagents in tissue sections has been used by Chused et al (1974) to demonstrate that the majority of mononuclear cells in labial glands from patients with Sjögren's syndrome are B cells. From their recent histopathological studies on labial salivary gland biopsies, Greenspan et al (1974) have demonstrated that the small lymphocytic foci have a large proportion of plasma cells and perhaps lymphocytes of the B-cell lineage, whereas the larger foci contain a greater proportion of T cells. This is a similar situation to changes observed in the salivary and lacrimal glands of NZB/NZW mice. These workers make the interesting suggestion that the first cells should be concerned with antigen recognition and/or early tissue destruction whilst the later T cells might be involved thereafter as a result of

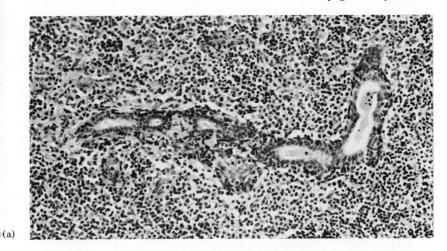

(a)

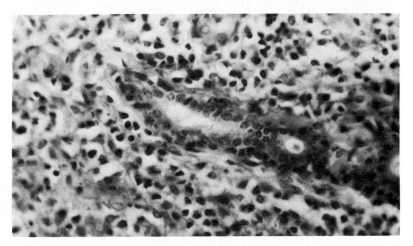

(b)

Figure 10.27. Sjögren's syndrome—submandibular gland. a. Dense lymphocytic infiltrate, acinar atrophy and ductal hyperplasia (× 210). b. Ductal hyperplasia (× 260).

auto-antigen released by B-cell cytotoxicity or as non-specific recruits in this delayed inflammatory reaction.

Amyloid infiltration of lung (Bonner et al, 1973) and labial salivary glands (Chisholm, 1970; Bonner et al, 1973) in Sjögren's syndrome may be associated with immunological disturbance, since immunoglobulin proteins have been shown to be a source of amyloid fibres in human amyloidosis (Glenner, Ein and Terry, 1972). Amyloidosis, however, may mimic other diseases and infiltration of parotid, labial (Figure 10.29) and lacrimal glands may give rise to symptoms similar to sicca syndrome (Kuczynski, Evans and Mitchinson, 1971). It is of interest that virus-like particles, similar to murine C-type oncogenic virus, have been reported within endothelial cells

197

and lymphocytes in the kidney (Shearn et al, 1970), parotid gland (Albegger and Auböck, 1972) and labial glands (Daniels et al, 1973) in recent ultrastructural studies of biopsies from patients with Sjögren's syndrome.

Attempts to produce the salivary gland lesion of Sjögren's syndrome in experimental animals by immunisation with salivary gland homogenates and Freund's adjuvant have met with limited success (Waterhouse, 1963a; Chan, 1964). Perhaps the most exciting development in this field has been the discovery that a series of abnormalities resembling those of Sjögren's syndrome occur spontaneously in NZB/NZW mice. These abnormalities appear about the fourth month, hand in hand with other auto-immune phenomena and increase in severity with age, particularly in females. In these animals, salivary amylase is reduced and the salivary protein concentration is elevated. The incidence of malignant neoplastic disease in elderly

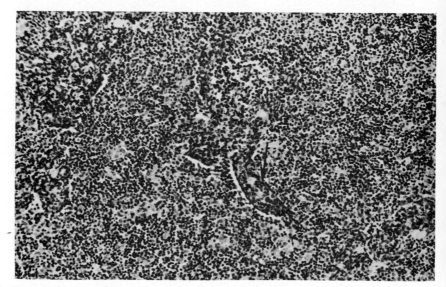

Figure 10.28. Parotid gland. Massive lymphocytic infiltration and ductal hyperplasia (arrowed) in Sjögren's syndrome (× 154).

patients with rheumatoid arthritis appears higher than in age- and sex-matched groups in the general population (Moesmann, 1969) and recently several reports of malignant lymphoma complicating Sjögren's syndrome have appeared (Bloch et al, 1965; Hornbaker, Foster and Williams, 1966; Mellors, 1966; Talal, Sokoloff and Barth, 1967). Generally, such neoplastic change has an extra-salivary distribution, although recent reports have demonstrated that malignant transformation may originate within the salivary glands (Azzopardi and Evans, 1971). Lattes (1962) reported the occurrence of one case each of Sjögren's syndrome, rheumatoid arthritis and scleroderma in a series of 107 cases of thymoma. The interesting observation has been made that lymphoid infiltration or hyperplasia of the thymus,

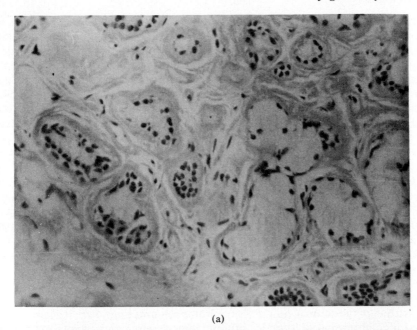

(a)

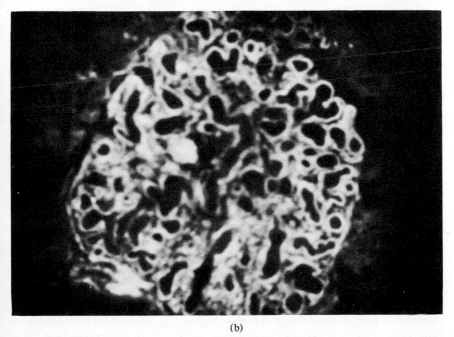

(b)

Figure 10.29. Amyloid infiltration in labial salivary glands in patient with Sjögren's syndrome and severe rheumatoid arthritis. a. Congo Red ($\times$ 75). b. Thioflavine T and ultra-violet light ($\times$ 30).

199

thyroid and salivary glands may give rise to auto-immune disease. Each of these glands are of epithelial derivation from the pharyngeal pouch and have a special affinity for lymphoid tissue (Bunim et al, 1964). The prolonged state of immunological and lymphoid hyperactivity in patients with Sjögren's syndrome, especially those with the sicca syndrome, may be predisposing factors in the development of lymphoid neoplasia (Talal and Bunim, 1964). Such patients are also more likely to show salivary gland enlargement (Talal, Sokoloff and Barth, 1967). Although the selective distribution or bilateral symmetry of parotid gland involvement by malignant lymphoma in an auto-immune disorder such as Sjögren's syndrome may be antigen-dependent, it is possible that the tumour could develop in a clone of circulating lymphocytes which home on a special tissue by a process akin to ecotaxis and there tend to proliferate (Goudie, Macfarlane and Lindsay, 1974). Sjögren's syndrome, therefore, provides a link between disease affecting immunological responses and the development of neoplasia (Fudenberg, 1966). The concept of a virus being the common stimulus for auto-immune disease and lymphoid neoplasia is attractive, and although viral agents have not been isolated nor viral antigens demonstrated in Sjögren's syndrome, further studies in this area are warranted (Anderson and Talal, 1972; Miller, 1967).

Although the cause of Sjögren's syndrome remains unknown, it seems likely that a combination of genetic, immunological, viral and/or environmental factors may play a role in the pathogenesis (Anderson and Talal, 1972). There is strong evidence that Sjögren's syndrome should be considered an auto-immune disorder, since the criteria of such a disease as laid down by MacKay and Burnet (1963) are satisfied (Shearn, 1971). The possibility that Sjögren's syndrome may have a hereditary component is based largely on observations of a familial incidence (Lisch, 1937; Hamilton, 1940; Coverdale, 1948; Bloch et al, 1965). A polygenic hereditary component, the expression of which depends upon certain environmental factors, as yet unknown, may exist in Sjögren's syndrome (Shearn, 1971). Recently, the possible role of an infectious agent in the pathogenesis of Sjögren's syndrome and other connective tissue diseases and arthritides has received much attention (Shearn, 1971). The implication of infectious agents in certain animal models of auto-immune disease, such as Aleutian mink disease, together with the concept of a slow virus disease, have accounted for this interest and are admirably reviewed by Shearn (1971).

TREATMENT AND MANAGEMENT

A broad approach, directed both locally and systemically, is required in the treatment and management of the distressing symptoms of Sjögren's syndrome. The multi-system involvement in Sjögren's syndrome, like other connective tissue diseases, requires attention in the specialties of medicine, rheumatology, immunology, ophthalmology, otolaryngology, oral medicine and pathology and microbiology.

General

Approaches to treatment of rheumatoid arthritis or associated connective tissue disease are identical to those which would be employed if Sjögren's syndrome were absent. The measures aimed at reducing inflammation, pain, joint dysfunction and deformity have been reviewed (Shearn and Englemann, 1968). The use of drugs such as salicylates, gold salts, corticosteroids and anti-malarial drugs all have a place in the treatment of selected cases. Anti-malarial drugs, however, may produce side effects such as nausea, blindness, leucopenia and cutaneous and mucosal pigmentation. Recently, Watson and MacDonald (1974) have reported amodioquine (camoquin)-induced oral pigmentation and confirmed ultrastructurally that melanin was present in the epithelium and in macrophages in the underlying connective tissues. The use of immuno-suppressive drugs and anti-viral agents such as amantadine have not been fully evaluated at the present time. The early recognition and treatment of keratoconjunctivitis sicca with lubricating agents such as 1% methyl cellulose is essential if long-term complications such as corneal ulceration are to be avoided. Electrocoagulation of the lacrimal puncta and canaliculi appears to have limited value. The mucolytic agent acetylcysteine shows promise in the treatment of keratoconjunctivitis sicca but requires further evaluation (Hughes and Whaley, 1972).

Oral

It is important that the oral mucous membranes be kept as moist as possible and, to this end, glycerine lozenges and methylcellulose (2% solution) as a lubricant and the salivary stimulant effect of boiled sweets may be of benefit to edentulous patients. A mouthwash containing citric acid (12.5 g), essence of lemon (20 ml) and glycerine (made up to 1 litre) has been used with success in our clinics. Patients should be encouraged to increase their fluid intake and the importance of meticulous oral and dental hygiene stressed. Local infections such as candidosis should be detected and treated with appropriate anti-fungal agents. Salivary gland swelling usually subsides but painful recalcitrant swellings may be treated with analgesics and antibiotics. In selected cases, especially those where a neoplasm is suspected, surgical removal of enlarged salivary glands has been reported as giving rise to a general symptomatic improvement in Sjögren's syndrome (Berényi, 1974).

Irradiation is contra-indicated for persistent salivary swelling in view of the known association of Sjögren's syndrome and lymphoid neoplasia. The use of corticosteroids does not appear to improve the sicca symptoms (Bloch et al, 1965). Drugs which may cause or increase xerostomia, such as certain tranquillisers and hypotensive agents, should be avoided or changed if possible. Parasympathominetic drugs are contra-indicated in heart cases. Immunosuppressive drugs, such as cyclophosphamide, have been shown to cause an improvement of sicca symptoms in severe cases (Anderson et al, 1972). However, this approach requires further study and cannot be recommended as a routine measure at the present time. In view of the known predisposition to drug allergy in Sjögren's syndrome (Bloch et al, 1965;

Salivary Glands in Health and Disease

Whaley et al, 1973b) it is clear that the response to any drug administered should be carefully monitored. The most frequent offending drug is penicillin whilst other drugs include streptomycin, phenobarbitone, tetracycline and phenylbutazone. Drug allergy is more common in rheumatoid arthritis and Sjögren's syndrome than in sicca syndrome (Whaley et al, 1973b).

REFERENCES

Abramson, A. L., Goodman, M. & Kolodny, H. (1968) Sjögren's syndrome. Additional diagnostic tools. *Archives of Otolaryngology*, **88**, 91.

Adams, D. (1973) *Saliva, the Mucus Barrier and the Health of the Oral Mucosa*. Ph.D. Thesis, University of Wales.

Albegger, K. W. & Auböck, L. (1972) The evidence of 'virus-like' inclusions in myoepithelial sialadenitis of Sjögren's syndrome by electron microscopy. *Archiv klinische experimentelle Ohren Nasen Kehlkopfheilkunde*, **203**, 153.

Anderson, J. R., Buchanan, W. W. & Goudie, R. B. (1967) *Autoimmunity, Clinical and Experimental*. Springfield, Illinois: Charles C. Thomas.

Anderson, L. G. & Talal, N. (1972) The spectrum of benign to malignant lymphoproliferation in Sjögren's syndrome. *Clinical and Experimental Immunology*, **9**, 199.

Anderson, L. G., Cummings, N. A., Asofsky, R., Hylton, Martha B., Tarpley, T. M., Tomasi, T. B., Wolf, R. O., Schall, G. L. & Talal, N. (1972) Salivary gland immunoglobin and rheumatoid factor synthesis in Sjögren's syndrome. *American Journal of Medicine*, **53**, 456.

Anderson, L. G., Tarpley, T. M., Talal, N., Cummings, N. A., Wolf, R. O. & Schall, G. L. (1973) Cellular-versus-humoral autoimmune response to salivary gland in Sjögren's syndrome. *Clinical and Experimental Immunology*, **13**, 335.

Azzopardi, J. G. & Evans, D. J. (1971) Malignant lymphoma of parotid associated with Mikulicz disease (Benign lymphoepithelial lesion). *Journal of Clinical Pathology*, **24**, 744.

Bartholomew, L. E. (1965) Isolation and characterisation of mycoplasmas (PPLO) from patients with rheumatoid arthritis, systemic lupus erythematosus and Reiter's syndrome. *Arthritis and Rheumatism*, **8**, 376.

Beck, J. S. (1961) Variations in the morphological patterns of 'auto-immune' nuclear fluorescence. *Lancet*, **i**, 1203.

Berényi, B. (1974) Oral surgical approach to the treatment of Sjögren's syndrome. *International Journal of Oral Surgery*, **3**, 309.

Berry, H., Bacon, P. A. & Davis, J. D. (1972) Cell-mediated immunity in Sjögren's syndrome. *Annals of the Rheumatic Diseases*, **31**, 298.

Bertram, U. (1967) Xerostomia. Clinical aspects, pathology and pathogenesis. *Acta Odontologica Scandinavica*, **25**, Suppl. 49, 1.

Bertram, U. & Halberg, P. (1964) A specific antibody against the epithelium of the salivary ducts in sera from patients with Sjögren's syndrome. *Acta Allergologica*, **19**, 458.

Blair, G. S. (1973) *Oral and Dental Manifestations of Adult Rheumatoid Arthritis*. M.D.S. Thesis, University of Glasgow.

Blatt, I. M., Rubin, P., French, A. J., Maxwell, J. H. & Holt, J. F. (1965) Secretory sialography in diseases of the major salivary glands. *Annals of Otology, Rhinology and Laryngology*, **65**, 293.

Blaylock, W. M., Waller, M. & Normansell, D. E. (1974) Sjögren's syndrome: Hyperviscosity and intermediate complexes. *Annals of Internal Medicine*, **80**, 27.

Bloch, K. J. & Bunim, J. J. (1963) Sjögren's syndrome and its relation to connective tissue diseases. *Journal of Chronic Diseases*, **16**, 915.

Bloch, K. J., Buchanan, W. W., Wohl, M. J. & Bunim, J. J. (1965) Sjögren's syndrome: A clinical, pathological and serological study of sixty-two cases. *Medicine*, **44**, 187.

Bonner, H., Ennis, R. S., Geelhoed, G. W. & Tarpley, T. M. (1973) Lymphoid infiltration and amyloidosis of lung in Sjögren's syndrome. *Archives of Pathology*, **95**, 42.

Boquist, L., Kumlien, A. & Östberg, Y. (1970) Ultrastructural findings in a case of benign lymphoepithelial lesion (Sjögren's syndrome). *Acta Oto-Laryngologica*, **70**, 216.

British Medical Journal (1972) Editorial—Candida Infection. **iv**, 505.

Buchanan, W. W., Cox, A. G., Harden, R. McG., Glen, A. I. M., Anderson, J. R. & Gray, K. G. (1966) Gastric studies in Sjögren's syndrome. *Gut,* **7,** 351.

Buchanan, W. W. (1973) Personal communication.

Bunim, J. J., Buchanan, W. W., Wertlake, P. T., Sokoloff, L., Bloch, K. J., Beck, J. S. & Alepa, F. P. (1964) Clinical, pathologic and serologic studies in Sjögren's syndrome. *Annals of Internal Medicine,* **61,** 509.

Cahn, L. (1967) A milder type (forme fruste) of Sjögren's syndrome. *Oral Surgery, Oral Medicine and Oral Pathology,* **23,** 8.

Calman, H. I. & Reifman, S. (1966) Sjögren's syndrome—report of a case. *Oral Surgery, Oral Medicine and Oral Pathology,* **21,** 158.

Cardell, B. S. & Gurling, K. J. (1954) Observations on the pathology of Sjögren's syndrome. *Journal of Pathology and Bacteriology,* **68,** 137.

Chan, W. C. (1964) Experimental sialo-adenitis in guinea pigs. *Journal of Pathology and Bacteriology,* **88,** 592.

Chisholm, D. M. (1969) Minor salivary gland pathology in Sjögren's syndrome and rheumatoid arthritis. In *Fourth Proceedings of the International Academy of Oral Pathology.* New York: Gordon and Breach.

Chisholm, D. M. (1970) *The Salivary Glands and their Secretions in Connective Tissue Disease.* Ph.D. Thesis, University of Glasgow.

Chisholm, D. M. & Mason, D. K. (1968) Labial salivary gland biopsy in Sjögren's disease. *Journal of Clinical Pathology,* **21,** 656.

Chisholm, D. M. & Mason, D. K. (1973) Salivary gland function in Sjögren's syndrome—a review. *British Dental Journal,* **135,** 393.

Chisholm, D. M., Waterhouse, J. P. & Mason, D. K. (1970) Lymphocytic sialadenitis in major and minor glands: a correlation in postmortem subjects. *Journal of Clinical Pathology,* **23,** 690.

Chisholm, D. M., Blair, G. S., Low, P. S. & Whaley, K. (1971) Hydrostatic sialography as an index of salivary gland disease in Sjögren's syndrome. *Acta Radiologica,* **11,** 577.

Chisholm, D. M., Beeley, J. A. & Mason, D. K. (1973) Salivary proteins in Sjögren's syndrome: separation by isoelectric focusing in acrylamide gels. *Oral Surgery, Oral Medicine and Oral Pathology,* **35,** 620.

Chused, T. M., Hardin, J. A., Frank, M. M. & Green, I. (1974) Identification of cells infiltrating the minor salivary glands in patients with Sjögren's syndrome. *Journal of Immunology,* **112,** 641.

Cifarelli, P. S., Bennett, M. J. & Zaino, E. C. (1966) Sjögren's syndrome. *Archives of Internal Medicine,* **117,** 429.

Coverdale, H. (1948) Some unusual cases of Sjögren's syndrome. *British Journal of Ophthalmology,* **32,** 669.

Daniels, T., Sylvester, R., Silverman, S. & Talal, N. (1973) Virus-like structure occurring within labial salivary glands in Sjögren's syndrome. *International Association for Dental Research* (North American Division), Abstract No. 428.

Davies, J. D., Berry, H., Bacon, P. A., Issa, M. A. & Schofield, J. J. (1973) Labial sialadenitis in Sjögren's syndrome and in rheumatoid arthritis. *Journal of Pathology,* **109,** 307.

Denko, C. W. & Old, J. W. (1969) Myopathy in the siccas syndrome (Sjögren's syndrome). *American Journal of Clinical Pathology,* **51,** 631.

Doig, J. A., Whaley, K., Dick, W. C., Nuki, G., Williamson, J. & Buchanan, W. W. (1971) Otolaryngological aspects of Sjögren's syndrome. *British Medical Journal,* **iv,** 460.

Duncan, H., Epker, B. N. & Sheldon, G. M. (1969) Sjögren's syndrome in childhood. *Henry Ford Hospital Medical Journal,* **17,** 35.

Duthie, J. J. R., Stewart, S., Alexander, W. R. M. & Dayhoff, R. (1967) Isolation of diptheroid organisms from rheumatoid synovial membrane and fluid. *Lancet,* **i,** 142.

Eisenbud, L., Platt, N., Stern, M., D'Angelo, W. & Sumner, P. (1973) Palatal biopsy as a diagnostic aid in the study of connective tissue diseases. *Oral Surgery, Oral Medicine and Oral Pathology,* **35,** 642.

Ericson, S. (1968) The parotid gland in subjects with and without rheumatoid arthritis. *Acta Radiologica,* Suppl. 275, 1.

Feltkamp, T. E. & Van Rossum, A. L. (1968) Antibodies to salivary duct cells and other autoantibodies in patients with Sjögren's syndrome and other idiopathic autoimmune diseases. *Clinical and Experimental Immunology,* **3,** 1.

Salivary Glands in Health and Disease

Fischer, C. J., Wyshak, G. H. & Weisberger (1968) Sjögren's syndrome. Electrophoretic and immunological observations on serum and salivary proteins of man. *Archives of Oral Biology*, **13**, 257.

Fudenberg, H. H. (1966) Immunological deficiency, autoimmune disease and lymphoma: Observations, implications and speculations. *Arthritis and Rheumatism*, **9**, 464.

Glenner, G. G., Ein, D. & Terry, W. D. (1972) The immunoglobulin origin of amyloid. *American Journal of Medicine*, **52**, 141.

Gordon, A. M., Chisholm, D. M. & Mason, D. K. (1971) Oral mycoplasmas in Sjögren's syndrome. *Journal of Clinical Pathology*, **24**, 810.

Goudie, R. B., Macfarlane, P. S. & Lindsay, M. K. (1974) Homing of lymphocytes to non-lymphoid tissues. *Lancet*, **i**, 292.

Greenspan, J. S., Daniels, T. E., Talal, N. & Sylvester, R. A. (1974) The histopathology of Sjögren's syndrome in labial salivary gland biopsies. *Oral Surgery, Oral Medicine and Oral Pathology*, **37**, 217.

Grove, A. S. Jr. & Di Chiro, G. (1968) Salivary gland scanning with technetium ^{99m}Tc pertechnetate. *American Journal of Roentgenology, Radium Therapy and Nuclear Medicine*, **102**, 109.

Gumpel, J. M. & Hobbs, J. R. (1970) Serum immune globulins in Sjögren's syndrome. *Annals of the Rheumatic Diseases*, **29**, 681.

Halberg, P., Bertram, U., Söberg, M. & Nerup, J. (1965) Organ antibodies in disseminated lupus erythematosus. *Acta Medica Scandinavica*, **178**, 291.

Hamilton, J. B. (1940) Keratitis sicca, including Sjögren's syndrome. *Transactions of the Ophthalmological Society of Australia*, **2**, 63.

Harden, R. McG. & Alexander, W. D. (1967) The relation between the clearance of iodide and pertechnetate in human parotid saliva and salivary flow rate. *Clinical Science*, **33**, 425.

Harden, R. McG., Hilditch, T. E., Kennedy, I., Mason, D. K., Papadopoulos, S. & Alexander, W. D. (1967) Uptake and scanning of the salivary glands in man using pertechnetate ^{99m}Tc. *Clinical Science*, **32**, 49.

Harden, R. McG., Alexander, W. D., Shimmins, J. & Russell, R. J. (1968) Quantitative uptake measurements of ^{99m}Tc in salivary glands and stomach and concentration of ^{99m}Tc, ^{132}I and ^{82}Br in gastric juice and saliva. In *Radioaktive Isotope in Klinik und Forschung*, **8**, 76. Fellinger, K. & Hofer, R. (Eds.)

Henkin, R. I., Talal, N., Larson, A. L. & Mattern, C. T. F. (1972) Abnormalities of taste and smell in Sjögren's syndrome. *Annals of Internal Medicine*, **76**, 375.

Hjörting-Hansen, E. & Bertram, U. (1968) Oral aspects of pernicious anaemia. *British Dental Journal*, **125**, 266.

Holm, S. (1949) Keratoconjunctivitis sicca and the sicca syndrome. *Acta Opthalmologica*. Suppl. 33, 1.

Hornbaker, J. H., Foster, E. A. & Williams, G. S. (1966) Sjögren's syndrome and nodular reticulum cell sarcoma. *Archives of Internal Medicine*, **118**, 449.

Hughes, G. R. V. & Whaley, K. (1972) Sjögren's syndrome. *British Medical Journal*, **iv**, 533.

Kaltreider, H. B. & Talal, N. (1969) The neuropathy of Sjögren's syndrome—trigeminal nerve involvement. *Annals of Internal Medicine*, **70**, 751.

Kitamura, T., Kanda, T. & Ishikawa, T. (1970) Parotid gland of Sjögren's syndrome. *Archives of Otolaryngology*, **91**, 64.

Kuczynski, A., Evans, R. J. C. & Mitchinson, M. J. (1971) Sicca syndrome due to primary amyloidosis. *Lancet*, **i**, 506.

Lattes, R. (1962) Thymoma and other tumors of the thymus: an analysis of 107 cases. *Cancer*, **15**, 1224.

Leventhal, B. G., Waldorf, D. S. & Talal, N. (1967) Impaired lymphocyte transformation and delayed hypersensitivity in Sjögren's syndrome. *Journal of Clinical Investigation*, **46**, 1338.

Lisch, K. (1937) Über hereditäres Vorkomen des mit keratoconjuncitivitis sicca verbundenen Sjögrensched Symptomenkomplexes. *Archiv für Augenheilkunde*, **110**, 357.

MacFarlane, T. W. & Mason, D. K. (1974) Changes in the oral flora in Sjögren's syndrome. *Journal of Clinical Pathology*, **27**, 416.

MacSween, R. N. M., Goudie, R. B., Anderson, J. R., Armstrong, E. M., Murray, M. A., Mason, D. K., Jasani, M. K., Boyle, J. A., Buchanan, W. W. & Williamson, J. (1967) Occurrence of antibody to salivary duct epithelium in Sjögren's diseases, rheumatoid arthritis and other arthritides. A clinical and laboratory study. *Annals of the Rheumatic Diseases*, **26**, 402.

Mackay, I. R. & Burnet, F. M. (1963) *Autoimmune Diseases*. Springfield, Illinois: Charles C. Thomas.

Mandel, I. D. & Baurmash, H. (1973) Biochemical profile in salivary gland disease. *International Association for Dental Research* (North American Division), Abstract No. 672.

Mason, D. K. & Glen, A. I. M. (1967) The aetiology of xerostomia. *Dental Magazine and Oral Topics*, **84**, 235.

Mason, D. K., Harden, R. McG., Boyle, J. A., Jasani, M. K., Williamson, J. & Buchanan, W. W. (1967) Salivary flow rates and iodide trapping capacity in patients with Sjögren's syndrome. *Annals of the Rheumatic Diseases*, **26**, 311.

Mellors, R. C. (1966) Autoimmune disease in NZBL/BL mice II. *Blood*, **27**, 435.

Miller, D. G. (1967) The association of immune disease and malignant lymphoma. *Annals of Internal Medicine*, **66**, 507.

Moesmann, G. (1969) Malignancy and mortality in subacute rheumatoid arthritis in old age. *Acta Rheumatologica Scandinavica*, **15**, 193.

Morgan, W. S. & Castleman, B. (1953) A clinicopathologic study of Mikulicz's disease. *American Journal of Pathology*, **29**, 471.

O'Neill, E. M. (1965) Sjögren's syndrome with onset at 10 years of age. *Proceedings of the Royal Society of Medicine*, **58**, 689.

Park, W. M. & Mason, D. K. (1966) Hydrostatic sialography. *Radiology*, **86**, 116.

Powell, R. D., Larson, A. L. & Henkin, R. I. (1974) Nasal mucous membrane biopsy in Sjögren's syndrome: A new diagnostic technique. *Annals of Internal Medicine*, **81**, 25.

Ropes, M. W., Bennett, G. A., Cobb, S., Jacox, R, & Jessar, R. A. (1958) Diagnostic criteria for rheumatoid arthritis. *Bulletin on Rheumatic Diseases*, **9**, 175.

Schall, G. L., Anderson, L. G., Wolf, R. O., Herdt, Jean R., Tarpley, T. M., Cummings, N. A., Zeiger, L. S. & Talal, T. (1971) Xerostomia in Sjögren's syndrome. *Journal of the American Medical Association*, **216**, 2109.

Shearn, M. A. & Engleman, E. P. (1968) *The Rheumatic Diseases, Cyclopedia of Medicine, Surgery Specialties*. Philadelphia: F. A. Davis & Co.

Shearn, M. A. & Tu, W. H. (1965) Nephrogenic diabetes insipidus and other defects of renal tubular function in Sjögren's syndrome. *American Journal of Medicine*, **39**, 312.

Shearn, M. A. & Tu, W. H. (1968) Latent renal tubular acidosis in Sjögren's syndrome. *Annals of the Rheumatic Diseases*, **27**, 27.

Shearn, M. A., Tu, W. H., Stephens, B. G. & Lee, J. C. (1970) Virus-like structures in Sjögren's syndrome. *Lancet*, **i**, 568.

Shearn, M. A. (1971) Sjögren's syndrome. In *Major Problems in Internal Medicine*, Vol. 2. Philadelphia: W. B. Saunders Company.

Sjögren, H. (1933) Zur Kenntnis der Keratoconjunctivitis sicca (Keratitis filiformis bei Hypofunktion der Träsendrüsen). *Acta Opthalmologica*. (Suppl. 2), **11**, 1.

Söborg, M. & Bertram, U. (1968) Cellular hypersensitivity in Sjögren's syndrome. *Acta Medica Scandinavica*, **184**, 319.

Steinberg, A. D. & Talal, N. (1971) The co-existence of Sjögren's syndrome and systemic lupus erythematosus. *Annals of Internal Medicine*, **74**, 55.

Steinberg, A. D., Green, W. T. & Talal, N. (1971) Thrombotic thrombocytopenic purpura complicating Sjögren's syndrome. *Journal of the American Medical Association*, **215**, 757.

Stephen, K. W., Chisholm, D. M., Harden, R. McG., Robertson, J. W. K., Whaley, K. & Stuart, Agnes (1971) Diagnostic value of quantitative scintiscanning of the salivary glands in Sjögren's syndrome and rheumatoid arthritis. *Clinical Science*, **41**, 555.

Stoltze, C. A., Hanlon, D. G., Pease, G. L. & Henderson, J. W. (1960) Keratoconjunctivitis sicca and Sjögren's syndrome. Systemic manifestations and hematologic and protein abnormalities. *Archives of Internal Medicine*, **106**, 513.

Talal, N. & Bunim, J. J. (1964) The development of malignant lymphoma in the course of Sjögren's syndrome. *American Journal of Medicine*, **36**, 259.

Talal, N., Sokoloff, L. & Barth, W. F. (1967) Extrasalivary lymphoid abnormalities in Sjögren's syndrome (reticulum cell sarcoma 'Pseudolymphoma', macroglobulinemia). *American Journal of Medicine*, **43**, 50.

Talal, N., Zisman, E. & Schur, P. H. (1968) Renal tubular acidosis, glomerulonephritis and immunologic factors in Sjögren's syndrome. *Arthritis and Rheumatism*, **11**, 774.

Talal, N., Asofsky, R. & Lightbody, P. (1970) Immunoglobulin synthesis by salivary gland lymphoid cells in Sjögren's syndrome. *Journal of Clinical Investigation*, **49**, 49.

205

Salivary Glands in Health and Disease

Vanselow, N. A., Dodson, V. N., Angell, D. C. & Duff, I. F. (1963) A clinical study of Sjögren's syndrome. *Annals of Internal Medicine,* **58,** 124.
Waterhouse, J. P. (1963a) *Focal Adenitis of Salivary and Lacrimal Glands.* M.D. Thesis, University of London.
Waterhouse, J. P. (1963b) Focal adenitis in salivary and lacrimal glands. *Proceedings of the Royal Society of Medicine,* **56,** 911.
Waterhouse, J. P. & Doniach, I. (1966) Post-mortem prevalence of focal lymphocytic adenitis of the submandibular salivary gland. *Journal of Pathology and Bacteriology,* **91,** 53.
Watson, I. B. & MacDonald, D. G. (1974) Amodioquine induced oral pigmentation—a light and electronmicroscopic study. *Journal of Oral Pathology,* **3,** 16.
Whaley, K., Chisholm, D. M., Goudie, R. B., Downie, W. W., Dick, W. C., Boyle, J. A. & Williamson, J. (1969) Salivary duct autoantibody in Sjögren's syndrome: Correlation with focal sialadenitis in the labial mucosa. *Clinical and Experimental Immunology,* **4,** 273.
Whaley, K., Goudie, R. B., Willamson, J., Nuki, G., Dick, W. C., & Buchanan, W. W. (1970) Liver disease in Sjögren's syndrome and rheumatoid arthritis. *Lancet,* **i,** 861.
Whaley, K., Williamson, J., Chisholm, D. M., Webb, J., Mason, D. K. & Buchanan, W. W. (1973a) Sjögren's syndrome 1. Sicca components. *Quarterly Journal of Medicine,* **166,** 279.
Whaley, K., Webb, J., McAvoy, B. A., Hughes, G. R. V., Lee, P., MacSween, R. N. M. & Buchanan, W. W. (1973b) Sjögren's syndrome. 2. Clinical and immunological phenomena. *Quarterly Journal of Medicine,* **167,** 513.
Williams, M. H., Brostoff, J. & Roitt, I. M. (1970) Possible role of *Mycoplasma fermentans* in pathogenesis of rheumatoid arthritis. *Lancet,* **ii,** 277.
Williamson, J., Cant, J. S., Mason, D. K., Greig, W. R. & Boyle, J. A. (1967) Sjögren's syndrome and thyroid disease. *British Journal of Ophthalmology,* **51,** 721.

CHAPTER 11

Lymphoepithelial Lesions

In this chapter the term lymphoepithelial lesion is used to denote a condition of bilateral salivary gland enlargement (Figure 11.1), the histopathological features of which show epimyoepithelial cell islands and marked lymphocytic infiltration (Figure 11.2). In a number of cases, however, unilateral gland involvement only is present (Morgan and Castleman, 1953; Bhaskar and Bernier, 1960). The lacrimal glands and palatal salivary glands (Lancaster and Hughes, 1963) may also be affected. The condition may also be referred to as Mikulicz's disease or benign lymphoepithelial lesion of Godwin. However, in recent years, it has been shown that this condition has a malignant potential so that the term benign now appears inappropriate. The presence of salivary gland enlargement together with the characteristic histopathological appearance are features shared with Sjögren's syndrome (Chapter 10). However, at the present time, the authors feel that the absence of other systemic abnormalities in patients with lymphoepithelial lesions justify a separation of the two entities. The historical background, clinical features and histopathological appearances are now described.

HISTORICAL AND HISTOPATHOLOGICAL CONSIDERATIONS

In 1888, Johann von Mikulicz, at a meeting of the Society for Scientific Medicine in Königsberg, described a case of benign, asymptomatic symmetrical enlargement of the lacrimal and salivary glands. Histologically, excised lacrimal tissue showed lymphoid infiltration and acinar atrophy. The enlargement recurred and was again excised but the patient died two months later from peritonitis. Mikulicz's paper describing this original case was published in 1892, and on the basis of the benign course manifested by the patient without evident generalised lymphatic involvement and regression of the swellings, Mikulicz concluded that the condition was one of a chronic low-grade infection.

Following this original report, much confusion was caused by the fact that all types of cases with similar glandular enlargements were labelled as Mikulicz's disease Howard, (1909). The first attempt to classify the syndrome on an aetiological basis was made by Thursfield (1914). This grouping was modified by Schaffer and Jacobsen (1927) into two main categories, Mikulicz's disease proper of unknown aetiology, and Mikulicz's syndrome

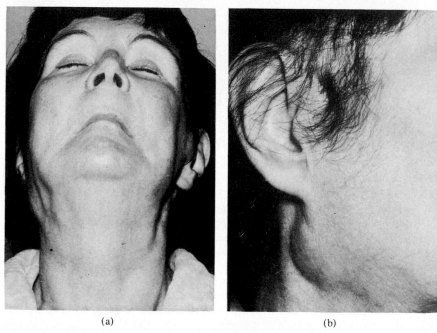

(a)   (b)

Figure 11.1. a. Bilateral parotid and submandibular salivary gland swelling in a 62-year-old female patient with lymphoepithelial lesion (Mikulicz's disease). A partial parotidectomy has been performed on the L side. b. Parotid swelling on R side of this patient.

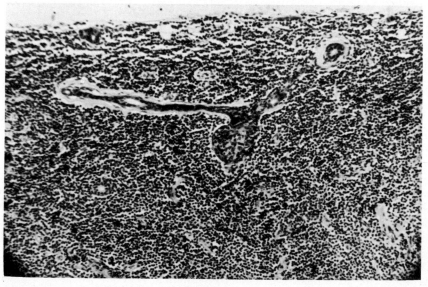

Figure 11.2. Epimyoepithelial cell island and massive lymphoid infiltrate in parotid gland in patient with lymphoepithelial lesion. ($\times$ 75.)

caused by leukaemia, lymphosarcoma, tuberculosis, syphilis or sarcoidosis. The diagnosis of Mikulicz's disease should then be reserved for those benign cases without any known cause (Schaffer and Jacobsen, 1927; Du Plessis, 1958). Where the lesion is confined to one gland the possibility of neoplasia must be considered. In a series of 81 tumours reported by Swinton and Warren (1938), seven such lesions were present, but these workers suggested that the lesion represented a localised form of Mikulicz's disease rather than neoplasia. However, the 'lymphoepithelioma' reported by Fein (1940) was probably a neoplasm. The first well-documented clinicopathological study of Mikulicz's disease was published in 1953 by Morgan and Castleman. In considering the clinical and pathological aspects of 18 cases, they concluded that the disease was benign, chronic, occurred predominately in women in the fifth and sixth decades and might involve one or more salivary or lacrimal glands. Frequently, the disease was confined to one salivary gland. The lacrimal glands were less often involved than the salivary glands. Histologically, the disease was characterised by replacement of acinar parenchyma by lymphoid tissue together with a characteristic proliferation of ductal epithelium in the form of 'epimyoepithelial cell islands'. Morgan and Castleman suggested the appearance of the epithelial and myoepithelial component offered the most reliable means by which Mikulicz's disease could be distinguished from malignant lymphoma. They further suggested that on the basis of certain clinical and pathological similarities, Mikulicz's disease could be considered as a manifestation of the more generalised symptom complex of Sjögren's syndrome.

The following year, Morgan (1954) published a comparative histological study of the 18 previously reported cases of Mikulicz's disease and microscopic material from the original series of Sjögren's syndrome. The pathological appearances were found to be identical and a re-examination of the clinical records of cases of Mikulicz's disease showed that a number had other components of Sjögren's syndrome, such as keratoconjunctivitis sicca, xerostomia and rheumatoid arthritis. Morgan concluded that Mikulicz's disease may be a less highly developed variant of Sjögren's syndrome.

Earlier, Godwin (1952) had reviewed 11 cases of parotid gland lesions which had been reported previously either lymphoepithelioma, lymphocytic tumour, chronic inflammation, Mikulicz's disease or adenolymphoma. Histologically, the lesions consisted of masses of lymphoid tissue containing scattered foci of epithelial cells, traceable to a ductal origin. Grossly, two types of lesions were noted, a well-circumscribed and a diffuse variety. Discomfort, occasional pain, xerostomia and parotid enlargement either unilateral or bilateral were the presenting symptoms. The lesion was more common in middle-aged females and responded well to radio-therapy. In none of the cases were the lacrimal glands involved and the condition pursued a benign course. Godwin stated that the condition may arise either in the parotid lymph nodes which contain glandular tissue or may be a hyperplastic reactive manifestation unique to the parotid gland, and culled the term 'benign lymphoepithelial lesion'. This term rapidly gained acceptance since it was aetiologically non-committal and included the term benign. However, as Azzopardi and Evans (1971) have demonstrated, malignant lymphoma may develop at the same site as the so-called 'benign' lymphoepithelial lesion. These workers draw attention to the fact that epimyoepithelial islands do not necessarily indicate a benign pathological process.

In a study of 186 cases of lymphoepithelial lesions of the salivary glands, Bernier and Bhaskar (1958) showed Mikulicz's disease or benign lymphoepithelial lesion of Godwin to be primarily a lesion of lymphoid tissue which because of its site, involved the salivary gland incidentally. It represented a reactive hyperplasia of lymphatic tissue and a nodular and diffuse type was recognised. The reactive nature of the lesion was based on the fact that the parotid nodes drain a wide area of the face, some nodes are not encapsulated, that in some instances a history of regional infection was reported, that the lesion showed regression in some instances following removal of suspected local factor and finally that the infiltrating element was lymphocytic rather than epithelial.

In an excellent review of the literature and a report of three cases Du Plessis (1958) takes the view that Mikulicz's disease is the result of chronic irritation and not a variant of Sjögren's syndrome. He pointed out that too often the diagnosis of Mikulicz's disease is made on histological grounds alone. He suggested that the application of the strict criteria of clinical picture, sialography and histology in considering the diagnosis will prevent confusion with Sjögren's syndrome. Du Plessis suggests the term idiopathic chronic parotitis. In 1964, Grage and Lober published the results of a retrospective study of ten patients who had been diagnosed as having benign lymphoepithelial lesion on histopathological evidence. Six patients had experienced symptoms of xerostomia, dryness of the eyes and polyarthritis, and these workers considered the lesion to be a manifestation of Sjögren's syndrome.

In a collection of 11 cases Cruickshank (1965) showed the benign lymphoepithelial lesion to be an isolated one. Although the histopathological features were identical to those of Sjögren's syndrome the sicca component was absent in each case. Furthermore, from long-term follow-up studies there appeared to be no evidence for an eventual onset of symptoms of Sjögren's syndrome.

It is of interest that the ultrastructural studies of Yarington and Zagibe (1969) and Boquist, Kamlien and Östberg (1970) failed to demonstrate the presence of myoepithelial cells in the epimyoepithelial cell islands. The former investigators believed that the epithelial component of the lesion arises from embryonic rests in the salivary glands. However, Boquist, Kamlien and Östberg (1970) provided strong evidence that the islands of epithelial tissue are derived from ducts by a process of proliferation together with the occurrence of squamous metaplasia of duct epithelium.

It is important to note that Pincus and Dekker (1970) and Azzopardi and Evans (1971) have drawn attention to the malignant potential of this condition. Azzopardi and Evans (1971) reported five cases which developed malignant lymphoma and suggested that the presence of tracts of immature lymphocytes, foci of necrosis and histiocystic infiltration were features associated with the transition from a benign to malignant nature. The epithelial component of the lesion has also been reported (Hilderman et al, 1962; Gravanis and Giansanti, 1970; Arthaud, 1972) as developing malignant change.

NATURE OF THE LESION AND ITS MANAGEMENT

It is clear that lymphoepithelial lesion is characterised by persistent bilateral salivary gland enlargement though localised lesions may occur. The condition is generally painless and there is no firm evidence to suggest widespread systemic involvement or immunological derangement. The histopathological features are characteristic and have been described in the preceding section.

The nature of the condition remains obscure and our understanding of it is far from complete. Evans and Cruickshank (1970) consider the lesion to be essentially reactive in nature though the stimulus which evokes the change remains unknown. Although the lesion may represent a variant of Sjögren's syndrome definite evidence is lacking. However, the malignant transformation which may occur in some cases may be viewed as a good example of an auto-immune disease followed by the development of malignant disease (Azzopardi and Evans, 1971).

Many cases are referred to surgeons since the salivary gland swelling is the predominant clinical feature. Accordingly partial parotidectomy or irradiation therapy have been employed or recommended in the treatment of the condition. However, the majority of cases remain benign and the authors recommend a conservative approach to treatment until the nature of the condition is more fully understood. In view of the malignant potential, patients should be reviewed at regular intervals. Irradiation would appear to be contra-indicated. A biopsy, especially in the localised form, may be necessary to exclude neoplasia.

The authors feel that there is justification for considering lymphoepithelial lesion separately from Sjögren's syndrome at the present time. In the past there has been a failure to establish exact criteria for these conditions when studies have been reported in the literature. It is only in recent years indeed, that diagnostic tests of salivary dysfunction in Sjögren's syndrome have been developed. Lymphoepithelial lesion appears rare but it is clear that in the light of recent studies an interdisciplinary approach to diagnosis must be taken and an effort made to compare and contrast all the features of the condition, especially salivary gland dysfunction and immunological abnormalities. The aim of future investigations must be the establishment of firm criteria. Detailed longitudinal clinical studies and broad-based laboratory studies are necessary before conclusions with regard to the exact nature of this condition can be established.

REFERENCES

Arthaud, J. B., (1972) Anaplastic parotid carcinoma ("malignant lymphoepithelial lesion") in seven Alaskan natives. *American Journal of Clinical Pathology*, **57**, 275.

Azzopardi, J. G. & Evans, D. J. (1971) Malignant lymphoma of parotid associated with Mikulicz disease (benign lymphoepithelial lesion). *Journal of Clinical Pathology*, **24**, 744.

Bernier, J. L. & Bhaskar, S. N. (1958) Lymphoepithelial lesions of the salivary glands. *Cancer*, **11**, 1156.

Bhaskar, S. N. & Bernier, J. L. (1960) Mikulicz's disease: Clinical features, histology and histogenesis; Report of seventy-three cases. *Oral Surgery, Oral Medicine and Oral Pathology*, **13**, 1387.

Boquist, L., Kumlien, A. & Ostberg, Y. (1970) Ultrastructural findings in a case of benign lymphoepithelial lesion (Sjögren's syndrome). *Acta Oto-Laryngologica*, **70**, 216.

Cruickshank, A. H. (1965) Benign lymphoepithelial salivary lesion to be distinguished from adenolymphoma. *Journal of Clinical Pathology*, **18**, 391.

Du Plessis, D. J. (1958) The problem of Mikulicz's disease. *South African Medical Journal*, **32**, 264.

Evans, R. W. & Cruickshank, A. H. (1970) *Epithelial Tumours of the Salivary Glands*. Philadelphia: W. B. Saunders Company.

Fein, M. J. (1940) Lymphoepithelioma of the parotid gland. *American Journal of Cancer*, **40**, 434.

Godwin, J. T. (1952) Benign lymphoepithelial lesion of the parotid gland. *Cancer*, **5**, 1089.

Grage, T. B. & Lober, P. H. (1964) Benign lymphoepithelial lesion of the salivary glands. *American Journal of Surgery*, **108**, 495.

Gravanis, M. B. & Giansanti, J. S. (1970) Malignant histopathologic counterpart of the benign lymphoepithelial lesion. *Cancer*, **26**, 1332.

Hilderman, W. C., Gordon, J. S., Large, H. L. & Carroll, C. F. (1962) Malignant lymphoepithelial lesion with carcinomatous component apparently arising in parotid gland. *Cancer*, **15**, 606.

Howard, C. P. (1909) Mikulicz's disease and allied conditions. *International Clinics*, **1**, 30.

Lancaster, J. E. & Hughes, K. W. (1963) Mikulicz's disease involving multiple salivary glands. *Oral Surgery, Oral Medicine and Oral Pathology*, **16**, 1266.

Morgan, W. S. (1954) The probable systemic nature of Mikulicz's disease and its relation to Sjögren's syndrome. *New England Journal of Medicine*, **251**, 5.

Morgan, W. S. & Castleman, B. (1953) A clinicopathologic study of "Mikulicz's disease". *American Journal of Pathology*, **29**, 471.

Pincus, G. S. & Dekker, A. (1970) Benign lymphoepithelial lesion of the parotid glands associated with reticulum cell sarcoma. *Cancer*, **25**, 121.

Schaffer, A. J. & Jacobsen, A. W. (1927) Mikulicz's syndrome; report of 10 cases. *American Journal of Diseases of Children*, **34**, 327.

Sprinkle, P. M. & Yarington, C. T. (1968) Disease of the salivary glands and benign lymphoepithelial lesion. *Southern Medical Journal*, **61**, 971.

Swinton, N. W. & Warren, S. (1938) Salivary gland tumours. *Surgery, Gynecology and Obstetrics with International Abstracts of Surgery*, **67**, 424.

Thursfield, H. (1914) Bilateral salivary swellings (Mikulicz's disease). A clinical review. *Quarterly Journal of Medicine*, **7**, 237.

Von Mikulicz, J. (1892) Über eine eigenartige symmetrische Erkrankung der Thränenund Mundspeicheldrüsen. In *Beiträge zur Chir., Festschrift.* pp. 610-630. Stuttgart: Theodor Billroth.

Yarington, C. T. & Zagibe, F. T. (1969) The ultrastructure of benign lymphoepithelial lesion. *Journal of Laryngology and Otology*, **83**, 361.

CHAPTER 12

Sialosis

Sialosis is the term which is used to describe a non-inflammatory non-neo-plastic recurrent bilateral swelling of the salivary glands (Thackray, 1972). The parotid glands are much more commonly affected than the submandi-bular, sublingual or minor salivary glands. The cause is not known but the condition is associated with numerous other conditions, such as endocrine abnormalities, nutritional deficiencies and those following the ingestion of various drugs. Regardless of the numerous associated conditions in sialosis there is a striking uniformity in the clinical appearances, histopathological changes and salivary enzyme constituents in affected individuals. The onset of salivary gland enlargement is slow, generally painless and unaccompanied by the signs or symptoms of inflammation. Multiglandular involvement, usually symmetrical, is a characteristic feature. Women are more commonly affected. It is of interest that in the majority of cases the enlargement involves principally the pre-auricular portion of the parotid gland. Rauch (1959) has reported the elevation of potassium in saliva of affected individuals from 25 meq/litre to 35 to 59 meq/litre and this may be an important diagnostic aid. Sialography reveals a duct structure of normal architecture and there appears to be little alteration in stimulated salivary flow rate values. The histology of sialosis is characterised by serous acinar cell hypertrophy, oedema of the interstitial supporting tissue and atrophy of the striated ducts. The cytoplasm of the hypertrophic serous cells is more mucoid and less granular than normal. The lesion may progress to a lipo-matosis of the affected glands.

These general features, then, characterise sialosis. The majority of cases reported have been related to hormonal disturbances, chiefly ovarian, thyroid and pancreatic dysfunction, and to malnutrition, liver cirrhosis and chronic alcoholism (Rauch, 1959). Drug-induced sialosis in experimental animals following the administration of various adrenergic and cholinergic drugs is well known (Selye, Veilleux and Cantin, 1961), whilst in humans, parotid enlargement has been noted in patients taking various medications such as phenylbutazone (Banks, 1968).

Rauch (1959) has classified the various sialoses according to their clinical association or aetiology as hormonal, neurohumoral, dysenzymatic, malnu-tritional and drug induced. These are now discussed.

213

HORMONAL SIALOSIS

Sialosis may occur as a result of dysfunction of the sex hormones. It has been described following ovariectomy (Korp, 1953), in gynaecomastia (Trautmann and Kanther, 1947), during pregnancy (Udsen and Thomsen, 1970) and at the time of menopause (Rauch, 1959). Raised potassium levels in resting saliva appear to be a constant feature.

Recently, the presence of salivary gland enlargement in three patients with active acromegaly has been reported (Thomson, McCrossan and Mason, 1974). Detailed studies of salivary flow rate, biochemistry of saliva from individual glands, sialography and isotope scanning showed no abnormality in function. These authors conclude that the salivary gland enlargement found represented part of the general organomegaly found in acromegaly. In keeping with other reports (Franke and Seige, 1950; del Castillo and Andrada, 1964) selective involvement of the submandibular glands was noted (Thomson, McCrossan and Mason, 1974). Examples of salivary gland enlargement in acromegaly are illustrated in Figures 12.1 and 12.2.

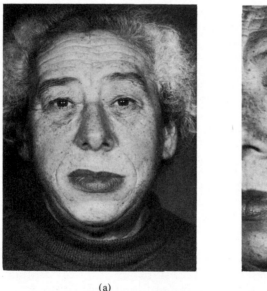 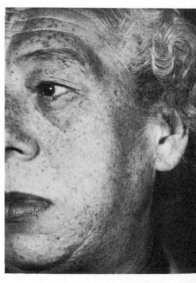

(a)   (b)

Figure 12.1. a and b. Parotid sialosis in a patient with acromegaly.

Bilateral parotid enlargement has been described in diabetes mellitus (Kenawy, 1937; Rauch, 1959; Davidson, Leibel and Berris, 1969). The reduced flow rate values which have been reported in diabetes (Takaoka et al, 1955; Conner, Iranpour and Mills, 1970) together with the increased susceptibility to infection, make sialadenitis a common complication. Sialosis in a patient with diabetes mellitus is shown in Figure 12.3.

214

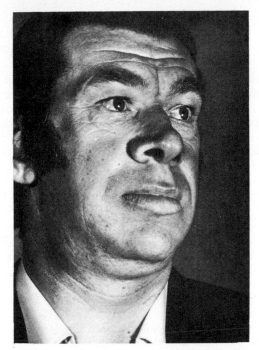

Figure 12.2. Submandibular salivary gland swelling in a patient with acromegaly.

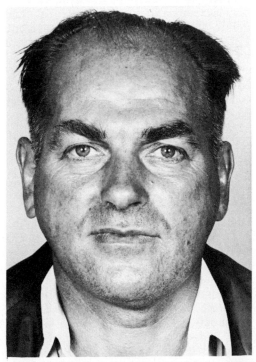

Figure 12.3. Bilateral parotid enlargement in a patient with diabetes mellitus.

215

NEUROHUMORAL SIALOSIS

Sialosis may follow disease or irritation of the autonomic nervous system either peripherally or centrally. Bilateral parotid enlargement has been described with cardiospasm (Nash and Morrison, 1949), with gastric spasm (Pearson, 1935) and in bronchial asthma (Campanacci, 1960). Rauch (1957) has described a small group of patients with severe psychic disturbances who displayed adiposity, oligomenorrhoea and parotid enlargement.

DYSENZYMATIC SIALOSIS

Hepatogenic sialosis affecting the parotid glands is commonly observed in patients with alcoholic cirrhosis (Kenawy, 1937; Rauch, 1959). Sialosis, however, may occur in alcoholics in the absence of cirrhosis (Wolfe, Summerskill and Davidson, 1957) or in cirrhosis due to other causes (Sandstead, Koehn and Sessions, 1955). Biopsy of affected glands has shown marked acinar oedema to be a feature of note. Chronic secondary infection is present in nearly one half of patients (Rauch and Gorlin, 1970). A case of sialosis in a patient with liver damage following malarial infection is shown in Figure 12.4. Nephrogenic sialosis appears to be exceedingly rare (Rauch, 1959). Parotid enlargement and increased parotid flow rates have been reported in patients with chronic relapsing pancreatitis (Alappatt and Aranthachari, 1967). Biopsies from these patients revealed hypertrophy of the acinar cells and no apparent change in the duct elements. An association between recurrent parotid swelling, arterial hypertension and pancreatitis has been reported by Isenberg and Boyle (1968). Salivary gland enlargement, together with stomatitis, may be present in cases of uraemia, though resolution follows renal dialysis (Rothstein et al, 1969).

MALNUTRITIONAL SIALOSIS

Soft, painless enlargement of the salivary glands may occur in nutritional deficiency states (Kenawy, 1937; Gillman, Gilbert and Gillman, 1947; Du Plessis, 1956) especially where there is a qualitative and quantitative lack of protein. Children appear to be more commonly affected in those regions where malnutrition is a problem.

Bilateral, asymptomatic parotid gland enlargement associated with prolonged starch ingestion has also been reported (Merkatz, 1961; Silverman and Perkins, 1966). Iron deficiency was noted in Merkatz's case, but otherwise the reported cases had an adequate nutritional intake. Silverman and Perkins (1966) suggested that parotid gland work hypertrophy due to chronic ingestion might be an aetiological factor in their case.

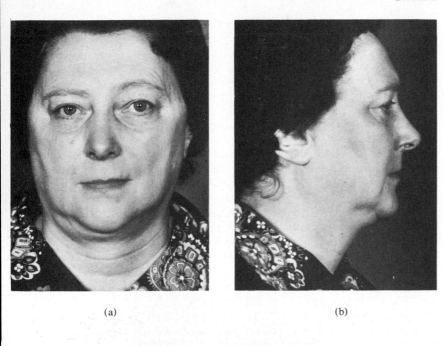

(a)   (b)

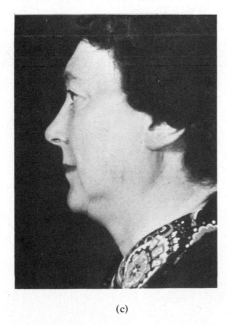

(c)

Figure 12.4. a, b, c. Bilateral parotid gland swelling in a 45-year-old female. The patient had lived in North Africa and suffered liver damage following malaria.

DRUG-INDUCED SIALOSIS

Parotid enlargement has been noted in patients taking medications such as phenylbutazone. The anti-inflammatory effects of phenylbutazone drugs has led to their use in rheumatoid arthritis and allied conditions. The pharmacology is poorly understood although the drug probably acts by decreasing capillary permeability (Goodman and Gilman, 1970). Adverse reactions and allergic responses to phenylbutazone drugs have been reported (Savin, 1970) and it is possible that salivary gland enlargement may reflect this phenomenon. Xerostomia and signs and symptoms of acute sialadenitis may be accompanying features (Rogers, 1966; Simpson, 1966; Murray, 1966; Banks, 1968; Chienes, 1971; Garfunkel et al, 1974). These reactions respond to cessation of drug administration. Antibiotics and/or corticosteroid therapy (Gross, 1969) may be of value in the treatment. Iodide-containing compounds, thiouracil and catecholamines and sulphonamides have also been reported as inducing sialosis (Nash and Morrison, 1949; Nidus, Field and Rammelkamp, 1965; Banks, 1968).

In man iodide is concentrated in saliva to many times the plasma level (Harden, Mason and Alexander, 1966) and there is evidence to suggest that the site of concentration is the salivary ducts (Mason, Harden and Alexander, 1966). Iodine is extensively used in expectorants and asthma preparations, in the pre-operative treatment of hyperthyroidism and as a radio-opaque substance for diagnostic radiography. Toxic reactions including enlargement of the salivary glands (Figure 12.5) may be a complication of iodide administration (Williams and Bakke, 1962; Meyler, 1963;

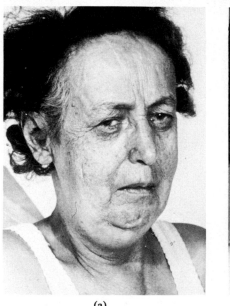 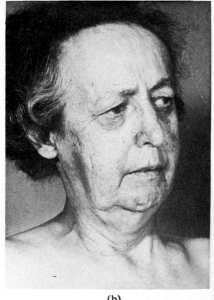

(a) (b)

Figure 12.5. a. Submandibular enlargement in a patient following ingestion of an iodide containing expectorant. b. Reduction in iodide sialosis when medication discontinued.

Harden, 1968). Usually salivary enlargement is associated with long-term administration of iodide although the condition may develop acutely (Sussman and Miller, 1966). Harden (1968) has related the onset of symptoms to the plasma inorganic iodine level and demonstrated that gland enlargement does not occur until the plasma iodide concentration exceeds 11 000 $\mu g/100$ ml. Follis (1961) has studied iodide-induced submandibular adenitis in the hamster and concludes that the inflammation was a direct toxic effect of iodide on the cells of the distal duct system. It must be noted that genetic factors are capable of causing much variability in the response to iodide administration (Bock and Wright, 1964). Kanda and Ghidoni (1970) have studied light and electronmicroscopic changes in iodide-induced sub-mandibular adenitis in hamsters. A predominantly plasma cell infiltrate progressively accumulated throughout the connective tissue stroma. Duct changes included degranulation, degeneration and squamous metaplasia. Acinar cells also showed degranulation.

EXPERIMENTAL STUDIES IN DRUG-INDUCED SIALOSIS

Drug-induced sialosis in experimental animals may follow the administration of various adrenergic and cholinergic drugs. Administration of isoproterenol, a β-adrenergic drug, produced a marked enlargement of the salivary glands of the rat and mouse (Selye, Veilleux and Cantin, 1961; Brown-Grant, 1961). The enlargement of the glands, defined as experimental sialadenosis (Seifert, 1967), occurs by the processes of hypertrophy and hyperplasia of the acinar cells (Schneyer, 1962; Barka, 1965; Baserga and Heffler, 1967; Novi and Baserga, 1971). The drug stimulates DNA and RNA synthesis which is followed by an increase in mitotic activity, formation of polyploid cells, an activation of protein synthesis and accelerated cellular differentiation (Schneyer and Shackleford, 1963; Chan, 1964; Barka, 1965, 1966; Baserga and Heffler, 1967; Radley, 1967; Schneyer, Finley and Finley, 1967; Malamud and Baserga, 1968). The time sequences of changes occurring in acinar cells following administration of the drug have been reported at an ultrastructural level by Takahama and Barka (1967) and Radley (1969). The relative role of each of the processes, hypertrophy and hyperplasia, has been reported for rat parotid salivary glands by Schneyer, Finley and Finley (1967) and for mouse parotid and submandibular glands by Novi and Baserga (1971).

Radley (1969) studied the ultrastructural changes in rat salivary glands following isoprenaline and suggested that a process of adaptation takes place with regard to the level of depletion of secreting granules; i.e., the magnitude of response with regard to the depletion of secretory granules decreased with chronic drug treatment. Since hyperplasia progressively diminishes with time, Radley suggests that virtually total depletion of secretory material may be a necessary condition for the stimulus of cell division. Failure of the mucous cells of the sublingual to show hyperplasia may be explained by the failure of the drug to exhaust these cells of secretory material. However, pilocarpine will exhaust secretory granules in the acinar cells of rat parotid

219

and submaxillary glands without a trophic effect (Scott and Pease, 1964). It is to be noted, however, that replenishment of secretory granules occurs more rapidly following pilocarpine administration (Takahama and Barka, 1967).

Byrt and Glanvill (1967) have studied the effect of isoprenaline on the secretion of sialo-proteins from rat salivary glands. The period of synthesis of amylase in the parotid gland and sialic acid within the submandibular gland were very similar. In contrast the rate of synthesis differed markedly—amylase synthesised at an exponentially increasing rate for 16 hours while the rate of sialic acid synthesis increased slowly between 4 and 12 hours and is approximately linear for the remaining period. Also, isoprenaline appeared to be a less effective stimulant of the submandibular gland secretion.

It is of interest that isoprenaline causes an acceleration of development of salivary glands in early post-natal rats—the effect being especially pronounced in the parotid gland. The effects on differentiation were separate from the influences of the drug on cell size (Schneyer and Shackleford, 1963). In the late phase of isoprenaline treatment, the increased size of parotid gland, without cell proliferation, indicated that hypertrophy is the dominant cytological event at this stage. However, the observation of continued synthesis of DNA prompted Novi and Baserga (1971) to question the classic definition of hypertrophy, especially in view of recent findings that increased cell size may be associated with polyploidy (Eisenstein and Wied, 1970). These workers have shown that for heart muscle the ability to mitose is rapidly lost, but that the ability to replicate DNA is not. DNA is replicated in response to functional demand in adult heart. DNA/protein ratio is not altered in cardiac hypertrophy, and this stability appears to be due to a concomitant increase in DNA and protein in the muscle cells.

Evidence for a reutilisation of DNA by salivary glands has been presented (Barka, 1965). In view of the role of lymphocytes in the transfer of DNA or its catabolites Barka (1965) has discussed the possibility of degenerating lymphocytes being a source of DNA incorporated into the salivary glands. No evidence, however, was obtained for such a role.

Although the increase in cell size following isoproterenol is often considered to be a work-hypertrophy (Seifert, 1962) this seems unlikely since extirpation of the upper cervical ganglion (Wells, 1962) did not affect the enlargement induced by the drug. A direct cellular effect is assumed, therefore (Barka, 1965). However, it must be noted that Pohto (1968) has shown that the increase in salivary flow and amylase secretion, following isoprenaline administration, can be reduced by β-receptor blocking drugs such as propranolol strongly indicating direct action of isoprenaline on β-receptors. Also, the blocking agent dichlorisoprenaline will prevent isoprenaline enlargement of the glands (Pohto, 1966).

Intrinsic differences in secretory mechanisms may play an important role. The effects of isoproterenol on the sublingual mucous salivary gland are minimal. It is to be noted that a possible apocrine secretion has been suggested for the mucous human labial glands (Tandler et al, 1969). In humans, asymptomatic enlargement of the parotid glands has been reported (Borsanyi and Blanchard, 1961) in patients receiving isoproterenol hydrochloride in the treatment of chronic bronchial asthma. In this report a biopsy of the parotid gland from one patient showed hypertrophic changes with increased granularity of the acinar cells.

In summary, it may be said that the pathological conditions which have in common the asymptomatic enlargement of the salivary glands may at first appear as a heterogeneous group of diseases. Further consideration, however, allows a broad classification into those associated with endocrine disease, nutritional states and following drug therapy. Nutritional deficiency, for example, appears to be the aetiological factor in gland enlargement in alcoholic cirrhosis. There appears also to be uniformity with regard to clinical presentation, histopathological appearance and a general lack of salivary functional change. It is clear that further study is required to elucidate the mechanisms involved. It is possible that a final common pathway may operate in all cases although the initial stimulus may vary.

REFERENCES

Alappatt, J. L. & Aranthachari, M. D. (1967) A preliminary study of the structure and function of enlarged parotid glands in chronic relapsing pancreatitis by sialography and biopsy methods. *Gut,* **8,** 42.

Banks, P. (1968) Non neoplastic parotid swellings: A review. *Oral Surgery, Oral Medicine and Oral Pathology,* **25,** 732.

Barka, T. (1965) Stimulation of DNA synthesis by isoproterenol in the salivary gland. *Experimental Cell Research,* **39,** 355.

Barka, T. (1966) Stimulation of RNA synthesis in the salivary gland by isoproterenol. *Experimental Cell Research,* **41,** 573.

Baserga, R. & Heffler, S. (1967) Stimulation of DNA synthesis by isoproterenol and its inhibition by actinomycin D. *Experimental Cell Research,* **46,** 571.

Bock, F. G. & Wright, J. J. (1964) Variations of acute iodide toxicity among inbred strains of mice. *Proceedings of the Society for Experimental Biology and Medicine (N.Y.),* **115,** 551.

Borsanyi, S. J. & Blanchard, C. L. (1961) Asymptomatic enlargement of the parotid glands due to the use of isoproterenol. *Maryland State Medical Journal,* **10,** 572.

Brown-Grant, K. (1961) Enlargement of salivary gland in mice treated with isopropylnoradrenaline. *Nature (London),* **191,** 1076.

Byrt, P. & Glanvill, S. (1967) Effect of isoprenaline on the secretion of sialoproteins from rat salivary glands. *Biochimica et Biophysica Acta* (Amsterdam), **148,** 215.

Campanacci, D. (1960) Das chronische Lungenemphsem durch bronchitisch-asthmatische Obstruktion. *Scientia Medica Italica,* **8,** 303.

Chan, W. C. (1964) Enlargement of the rat's salivary glands and salivary calculus formation induced with isoprenaline. *Journal of Pathology and Bacteriology,* **88,** 563.

Chienes, H. (1971) Phenylbutazone derivatives and pathology of the salivary glands. *Presse Medicale,* **79,** 54.

Conner, S., Iranpour, B. & Mills, J. (1970) Alteration in parotid salivary flow in diabetes mellitus. *Oral Surgery, Oral Medicine and Oral Pathology,* **30,** 55.

Davidson, D., Leibel, B. S. & Berris, B. (1969) Asymptomatic parotid gland enlargement in diabetes mellitus. *Annals of Internal Medicine,* **70,** 31.

Del Castillo, E. B. & Andrada, J. A. (1964) Aumento de Tamano de las glandulas submaxilares en acromegalicos. *Medicina* (Buenos Aires), **24,** 332.

Du Plessis, D. J. (1956) Parotid enlargement in malnutrition. *South African Medical Journal,* **30,** 700.

Eisenstein, R. & Wied, G. L. (1970) Myocardial DNA and protein in maturing and hypertrophied human hearts. *Proceedings of the Society for Experimental Biology and Medicine,* **134,** 176.

Franke, H. & Seige, K. (1950) Über Speicheldrusenvergrösserungen bei Störungen der inneren Sekretion. *Deutsche Zeitschrift für Verdauungs- und Stoffwechselkrankheiten,* **10,** 51.

Follis, R. H. Jr. (1961) Iodine-induced submandibular sialadenitis in the hamster. *Proceedings of the Society for Experimental Biology and Medicine,* **108,** 1332.

Garfunkel, A. A., Roller, N. W., Nichols, C. & Ship, I. L. (1974) Phenylbutazone-induced sialadenitis. *Oral Surgery, Oral Medicine and Oral Pathology,* **38,** 223.

Gillman, J., Gilbert, C. & Gillman, T. (1947) The Bantu salivary glands in chronic malnutrition. *South African Journal of Medical Sciences,* **12,** 99.

Goodman, L. S. & Gilman, A. (1970) *The Pharmacological Basis of Therapeutics,* 4th edition, p. 336. New York: Macmillan.

Gross, L. (1969) Oxyphenbutazone-induced parotitis. *Annals of Internal Medicine,* **70,** 1229.

Harden, R. McG. (1968) Submandibular adenitis due to iodide administration. *British Medical Journal,* **1,** 160.

Harden, R. McG., Mason, D. K. & Alexander, W. D. (1966) The relation between salivary iodine excretion and the plasma inorganic iodine concentration. *Quarterly Journal of Experimental Physiology,* **51,** 130.

Isenberg, J. & Boyle, J. D. (1968) Recurrent parotid swelling, arterial hypertension and pancreatitis. *Gastroenterology,* **55,** 277.

Kanda, T. & Ghidoni, J. J. (1970) Light and electron microscopic observations on iodide-induced sialoadenitis of hamster submaxillary glands. *Laryngoscope,* **80,** 455.

Kenawy, M. R. (1937) Endemic enlargement of parotid gland in Egypt. *Transactions of the Royal Society of Tropical Medicine and Hygiene,* **31,** 339.

Korp, W. (1953) Über die sogenannte Parotishypertrophie. *Medizinische Klinik,* **48,** 1325.

Malamud, D. & Baserga, R. (1968) Glycogen concentration and DNA synthesis in isoproterenol-stimulated salivary glands. *Experimental Cell Research,* **50,** 581.

Mason, D. K., Harden, R. McG. & Alexander, W. D. (1966) The influence of flow rate on the salivary iodide concentration in man. *Archives of Oral Biology,* **11,** 235.

Merkatz, I. R. (1961) Parotid enlargement resulting from excessive ingestion of starch. *New England Journal of Medicine,* **265,** 1304.

Meyler, L. (1963) *Side Effects of Drugs,* 4th edition p. 119. Amsterdam: Excerpta Medica.

Murray, B. (1966) Salivary gland enlargement and phenylbutazone. *British Medical Journal,* **i,** 1599.

Nash, L. & Morrison, L. F. (1949) Asymptomatic chronic enlargement of parotid glands: review and report of case. *Annals of Otology, Rhinology and Laryngology,* **58,** 646.

Nidus, B. D., Field, M. & Rammelkamp, C. J. Jr (1965) Salivary gland enlargement caused by sulfisoxazole. *Annals of Internal Medicine,* **63,** 663.

Novi, A. M. & Baserga, R. (1971) Association of hypertrophy and DNA synthesis in mouse salivary glands after chronic administration of isoproterenol. *American Journal of Pathology,* **62,** 295.

Pearson, R. S. B. (1935) Recurrent swelling of parotid glands. *Archives of Disease in Childhood,* **10,** 363.

Pohto, P. (1966) Catecholamine-induced salivary gland enlargement in rats. *Acta Odontologica Scandinavica,* **24,** No. 45 (Supplement).

Pohto, P. (1968) Effect of isoprenaline, pilocarpine and prenylamine on amylase secretion in rat parotid saliva. *Journal of Oral Therapeutics and Pharmacology,* **4,** 467.

Radley, J. M. (1967) Changes in ploidy in the rat submaxillary gland induced by isoprenaline. *Experimental Cell Research,* **48,** 679.

Radley, J. M. (1969) Ultrastructural changes in the rat submaxillary gland following isoprenaline. *Zeitschrift für Zellforschung und mikroskopische Anatomie,* **97,** 196.

Rauch, S. (1957) Die rezidivierende abakterielle Parotitis bilateralis dienzephaler Genese AOP Syndrom. *Practica Otorhino-laryngologica* (Basel), **19,** 59.

Rauch, S. (1959) *Die Speicheldrusen des Menschen.* Stuttgart: Georg Thieme.

Rauch, S. & Gorlin, R. J. (1970) Diseases of the salivary glands. In *Thoma's Oral Pathology,* Vol. 2. St. Louis: C. V. Mosby Co.

Rogers, R. D. (1966) Salivary gland enlargement and phenylbutazone. *British Medical Journal,* **ii,** 113.

Rothstein, D., Yudis, M., Shaw, A. S. & Onesti, G. (1969) Massive neck swelling secondary to uremic submaxillary gland involvement. *Oral Surgery, Oral Medicine and Oral Pathology,* **27,** 333.

Sandstead, H. R., Koehn, C. J. & Sessions, S. M. (1955) Enlargement of the parotid gland in malnutrition. *American Journal of Clinical Nutrition,* **3,** 198.

Savin, Y. A. (1970) Current causes of fixed drug eruptions. *British Journal of Dermatology,* **83,** 546.

Schneyer, C. A. (1962) Salivary gland changes after isoproterenol-induced enlargement. *American Journal of Physiology,* **203,** 232.

Schneyer, C. A. & Shackleford, J. M. (1962) Accelerated development of salivary glands of early postnatal rats following isoproterenol. *Proceedings of the Society for Experimental Biology and Medicine,* **112,** 320.

Schneyer, C. A., Finley, W. H. & Finley, S. C. (1967) Increased chromosome number of rat parotid cells after isoproterenol. *Proceedings of the Society for Experimental Biology and Medicine,* **125,** 722.

Scott, B. L. & Pease, D. C. (1964) Electron microscopy of induced changes in the salivary gland of the rat. In *International Series of Monographs on Oral Biology,* Ed. Sreebny, L. M. & Meyer, J. Vol. 3, p. 13. Oxford: Pergamon Press.

Seifert, G. (1962) Experimentelle Speicheldrüsenvergrossungen nach Einwirkung von Noradrenalin. *Beiträge zur pathologischen Anatomie und zur allgemeinen Pathologie,* **126,** 321.

Seifert, G. (1967) Experimental sialadenosis by isoproterenol and other agents: Histochemistry and electron microscopy. In *Secretory Mechanism of Salivary Glands,* p. 191. New York: Academic Press.

Selye, H., Veilleux, R. & Cantin, M. (1961) Excessive stimulation of salivary gland growth by isoproterenol. *Science,* **133,** 44.

Silverman, M. & Perkins, R. L. (1966) Bilateral parotid enlargement and starch ingestion. *Annals of Internal Medicine,* **64,** 843.

Simpson, R. W. (1966) Salivary gland enlargement and phenylbutazone. *British Medical Journal,* **ii,** 113.

Sussman, R. M. & Miller, J. (1966) Iodide "mumps" after intravenous urography. *New England Journal of Medicine,* **255,** 433.

Takahama, M. & Barka, T. (1967) Electron microscopic alterations of submaxillary gland produced by isoproterenol. *Journal of Ultrastructure Research,* **17,** 452.

Takaoka, Y., Uono, M., Ninomiya, H., Yoshikawa, M., Yamada, N. & Ishikawa, T. (1955) Der hormonale Einfluss der Parotisdrüsen auf den Eiweiss-Stoffwechsel. *Klinische Wochenschrift,* **33,** 156.

Tandler, B., Denning, C. R., Mandel, I. D. & Kutscher, A. H. (1969) Ultrastructure of human labial salivary glands. I. Acinar secretory cells. *Journal of Morphology,* In press.

Thackray, A. C. (1972) *Histological Typing of Salivary Gland Tumours.* W.H.O., Geneva.

Thomson, J. A., McCrossan, J. & Mason, D. K. (1974) Salivary gland enlargement in acromegaly. *Clinical Endocrinology,* **3,** 1.

Trautmann, F. & Kanther, R. (1947) Über Parotidenschwellung, Pankreatitis, Gynakomastie. *Zeitschrift für die gesamte innere Medizin und ihre Grenzgebiete,* **2,** 582.

Udsen, J. & Thomsen, K. A. (1970) Hormonal sialosis during two consecutive pregnancies. *Acta Oto-Laryngologica,* **263,** 195.

Wells, H. (1962) Submandibular salivary gland weight increase by administration of isoproterenol to rats. *American Journal of Physiology,* **202,** 425.

Williams, R. H. & Bakke, J. L. (1962) In *Textbook of Endocrinology* (Ed.) Williams, R. H., 3rd edition p. 134. Philadelphia: W. B. Saunders Company.

Wolfe, S. J., Summerskill, W. H. & Davidson, C. S. (1957) Parotid swelling, alcoholism and cirrhosis. *New England Journal of Medicine,* **256,** 491.

CHAPTER 13

Age Changes and Oncocytosis

Among the known age-related changes in salivary glands are an increase in fat cells and oncocytes; salivary functional changes may also occur. These are now discussed.

ADIPOSE TISSUE AND AGE

The majority of reports of an age-related accumulation of adipose tissue in human salivary glands (Yamaguchi, 1925; Stormont, 1928; Bauer, 1950; Rauch, 1959; Garrett, 1962) have been of a descriptive nature only. Recently, however, Waterhouse et al (1973) have shown the replacement of functional parenchymal cells by fat and connective tissue in human sub-mandibular glands to be an age-related change.

An increase in fat cells with age in rat salivary glands (Andrew, 1949a), and a semi-quantitative comparison of age changes in human and rat salivary glands (Andrew, 1952) have also been reported. Among other age-related changes which have been described in rat salivary gland tissue are an increase in oncocytes (Hamperl, 1931; Andrew, 1949b), alterations in mitochondria and Golgi substance (Kurtz, 1954), a reduction in total concentration of RNA with an increase in gland acid phosphatase activity (Bogart, 1967) and an intracellular accumulation of lipid droplets (Bogart, 1970).

Andrew (1952) believed the fatty change he observed in human and rat salivary glands to be a destructive one, involving degeneration of parenchymal elements through the accumulation of fat. Garrett (1962) noted a tendency for fat to increase with age in human submandibular glands but suggested that the change is due to replacement, since fusion of fat-droplets indicated true degeneration was not observed in his study. Ultrastructurally, lipid droplets and lipofuscin granules have been observed in salivary acinar cells in humans (Garrett, 1963) and rats (Bogart, 1970), and an age-related increase in membrane-bound pigment granules which consisted of lipid has been reported in rats by Bogart (1970). Lipofuscin granules are considered to be an age-related pigment and may represent an end-product of metabolism that accumulates in lysosomes (Novikoff, 1961).

Wassermann (1965) related the fat associated with the parotid gland to the general body fat comprising the 'fat organ'. However, Waterhouse et al

(1973) found no tendency for submandibular gland fat to be related to the adiposity of the subject, and suggested that the fat cells of the submandibular gland do not behave as a functional part of the bodily 'fat organ'.

Furthermore, Waterhouse et al (1973) have shown from autopsy studies that between childhood and old age a loss occurs on average of a quarter of the morphologically active parenchymal cell volume present in childhood (Figure 13.1). Fat and connective tissue replace the functional parenchymal

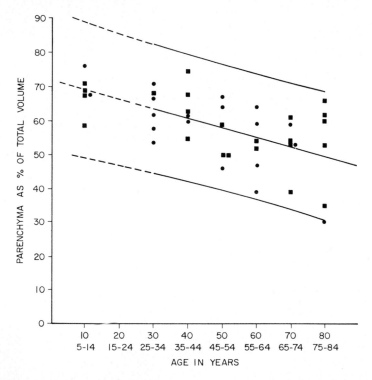

Figure 13.1. Scatter diagram showing percentage of gland volume occupied by parenchyma in a submandibular salivary gland in individuals of a randomly selected sample of 36 autopsy subjects aged 25 to 84, and also six subjects aged 5 to 14, arranged by decade of age. The regression line and upper and lower 95 per cent confidence limits on points on the regression line for values from subjects aged 25 to 84 years are plotted. The regression line and the tolerance limits have been extrapolated (— — — — —) towards the *y*-axis, and these encompass values for six children aged 5 to 14 years. ● = male; ■ = female.

cell loss (Figure 13.2). The loss of perhaps one-half may occur in more extremely affected human submandibular glands. This loss would reduce the functional reserve normally present and might be associated with the reported reduction of salivary flow rate (Meyer and Necheles, 1940; Becks and Wainwright, 1943; Korting and Kleinschmidt, 1953; Bertram, 1967; Ericson, 1968) and also of amylase activity with senescence (Meyer et al, 1937; Meyer and Necheles, 1940). It is important to note that flow rate per se does not appear to influence salivary amylase concentration (Dawes and

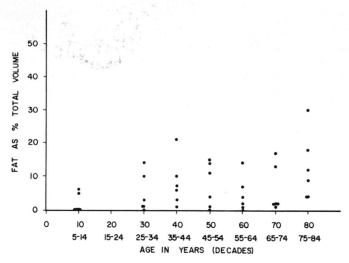

Figure 13.2. Scatter diagram showing individual values for fat as a percentage of total gland volume and age in decades, for same subjects as in Figure 13.1.

Jenkins, 1964). Fat cells in human submandibular salivary gland tissues are shown in Figure 13.3.

It is of interest that salivary gland enlargement has been noted to occur with great frequency in older individuals (Keleman, 1954; Kelemen and Montgomery, 1958; Scott, 1960; Diamant, 1966; and Hall, 1966) although

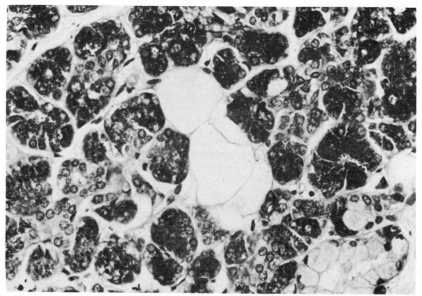

Figure 13.3. Submandibular salivary gland tissue from a 45-year-old female subject. Fat cells are noted centrally (H and E × 325).

whether or not this is due to fat accumulation remains speculative. Waterhouse et al (1973) did not find a relationship between gland wet weight and age. A marginal connection between post-menopausal women and large parotid salivary glands has been observed (Ericson, 1970).

The accumulation of fat cells in the salivary glands has been reported in a number of pathological states. Fatty infiltration was considered to be the only apparent cause of salivary gland enlargement in ten cases of malnutrition (Sandstead, Koehn and Sessions, 1955). An apparent increase in adipose tissue in salivary glands has been reported in isolated cases, following irradiation (Kasbourn, 1953; Garrett, 1962), in pyogenic adenitis (Garrett, 1962), Sjögren's syndrome (Holm, 1949; Cardell and Gurling, 1954; Garrett, 1962; Bloch et al, 1965) and Mikulicz's disease (Morgan and Castleman, 1954). Cases of local lipomatosis of the parotid gland have been described (Johansen and Berdal, 1970).

ONCOCYTOSIS

With increasing age individual cells or groups of cells in various glands undergo a striking change, becoming larger with an eosinophilic, granular cytoplasm. These cells have been called oncocytes and, as we have seen, may give rise to neoplasms. However, a non-neoplastic increase in number of oncocytes in the salivary glands may be termed oncocytosis. Oncocytosis would appear to be an age-related phenomenon (Hamperl, 1931; Andrew, 1949b) although in some instances inflammation or duct obstruction may provide the stimulus for oncocytic hyperplasia (Eversole and Sabes, 1971). An example of oncocytic hyperplasia at the edge of a salivary tumour is shown in Figure 13.4.

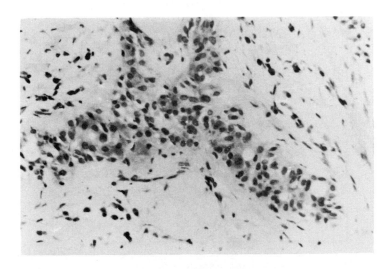

Figure 13.4. Focus of oncocytic hyperplasia at the edge of a pleomorphic adenoma.

HUMAN SALIVARY SECRETION AND AGE

Age of the subject is an important factor with regard to salivary flow rate. In 1940, Meyer and Necheles demonstrated a decrease in salivary secretion in old age in man. Becks and Wainwright (1943) found a lower mean value for salivary secretions in persons 50 to 95 years of age than in the group 5 to 49 years although the difference was not statistically significant. Östlund (1953) and Korting and Kleinschmidt (1953) showed that resting secretions diminished with age. However, Brun and Dominé (1958) could find no difference in salivary flow with increasing age. Differences in division of the

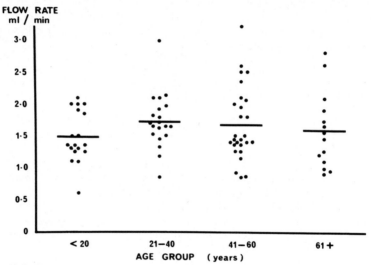

Figure 13.5. Citric acid (5%) stimulated parotid flow rate values in normal male subjects.

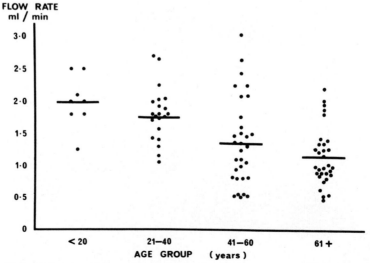

Figure 13.6. Citric acid (5%) stimulated parotid flow rate values in normal female subjects.

228

Table 13.1. *Mean parotid salivary flow rates in normal subjects (ml/min).*

Age range (years)	Resting		Fruit gum		Citric acid (5%)	
	Male	Female	Male	Female	Male	Female
<20 18M 8 F	0.061±0.007 (0.02 —0.12)	0.083±0.02 (0.04 —0.16)	0.66±0.06 (0.36—1.07)	0.46±0.07 (0.27—0.80)	1.49±0.09 (0.60—2.10)	1.99±0.14 (1.25—2.50)
21-40 20M 20 F	0.104±0.008 (0.06 —0.20)	0.09 ±0.01 (0.01 —0.19)	0.47±0.03 (0.32—0.85)	0.50±0.05 (0.09—1.04)	1.73±0.09 (0.85—2.99)	1.76±0.09 (1.03—2.70)
41-60 27 M 31 F	0.078±0.02 (0.01 —0.31)	0.064±0.01 (0.01 —0.34)	0.59±0.08 (0.15—1.76)	0.52±0.05 (0.13—1.15)	1.68±0.11 (0.85—3.20)	1.36±0.12 (0.50—3.02)
>61 14 M 31 F	0.084±0.02 (0.03 —0.20)	0.06 ±0.02 (0.01 —0.5)	0.050±0.08 (0.15—1.26)	0.43±0.03 (0.14—0.83)	1.58±0.16 (0.90—2.76)	1.15±0.08 (0.47—2.20)

Mean ± Standard error of the mean (S.E.M.).
Ranges indicated in parenthesis.

groups, however, may be of importance. Brun and Dominé (1958) divided their subjects into two groups at 50 years, whilst Korting and Kleinschmidt (1953) divided their groups at 65 years of age. Bertram (1967) also divided his subjects at 65 years of age and concluded from his material that men had higher salivary secretion than women, that secretion diminished in senility and that persons in poor health produced less saliva but that xerostomia was not likely to arise as a result of the ageing process. Ericson (1967) showed that parotid secretion at relative rest diminished with increasing age. Chisholm (1970) has shown that five per cent citric acid stimulated parotid flow rates decrease with age in both males and females, although the difference was significant only for the female group (Table 13.1 and Figures 13.5 and 13.6).

With regard to parotid gland size, Ericson (1970), using sialographic and planimetric techniques, has shown that the parotid glands diminish in size with age. Interestingly, this study demonstrated a great variation in parotid gland size in healthy individuals from the age of 26 to 64 years. This variation in size of the parotid gland may be a contributory factor to the differences in salivary secretion in normal individuals. Atrophy of the salivary glands with advancing age has been observed by Janczuk and Jedrzejwska (1966).

Direct comparison between the results obtained by different investigators requires care since even the various methods used in the recording of salivary flow have a considerable influence on flow rate (Kerr, 1961). Some investigations have not taken into account other factors such as time of collection, mental stress, infection, drug therapy and fatigue. Furthermore, some studies have been concerned with total saliva secretion whilst others have reported secretion from individual glands.

REFERENCES

Andrew, W. (1949a) Age changes in the salivary glands of Wistar Institute rats with particular reference to the submandibular glands. *Journal of Gerontology,* **4,** 95.

Andrew, W. (1949b) Age changes in the parotid glands of Wistar Institute rats with special reference to the occurrence of oncocytes in senility. *American Journal of Anatomy,* **85,** 157.

Andrew, W. (1952) A comparison of age changes in salivary glands of man and of the rat. *Journal of Gerontology,* **7,** 178.

Bauer, W. H. (1950) Old age changes in human parotid glands with special reference to peculiar cells in uncommon salivary gland tumors. *Journal of Dental Research,* **29,** 686.

Becks, H. & Wainwright, W. W. (1943) Human Saliva. XIII. Rate of flow of resting saliva of healthy individuals. *Journal of Dental Research,* **22,** 391.

Bertram, U. (1967) Xerostomia. *Acta Odontologica Scandinavica,* **25,** Supplement 49.

Bloch, K. J., Buchanan, W. W., Wohl, M. J. & Bunim, J. J. (1965) Sjögren's syndrome; A clinical, pathological and serological study of sixty two cases. *Medicine* (Baltimore), **44,** 187.

Bogart, B. I. (1967) The effect of ageing on the histochemistry of the rat submandibular gland. *Journal of Gerontology,* **22,** 372.

Bogart, B. I. (1970) The effect of ageing on the rat submandibular gland: an ultrastructural, cytochemical and biochemical study. *Journal of Morphology,* **130,** 337.

Brun, R. & Domine, E. (1958) Etude sur la transpiration. *Acta Dermato-Venereologica,* **38,** 91.

Cardell, B. S. & Gurling, K. J. (1954) Observations in the pathology of Sjögren's syndrome. *Journal of Pathology and Bacteriology,* **68,** 137.

Chisholm, D. M. (1970) Ph.D Thesis, University of Glasgow.

Dawes, C. & Jenkins, G. N. (1964) The effects of different stimuli on the composition of saliva in man. *Journal of Physiology,* **170,** 86.

Diamant, H. (1966) Spottkortelaffektioner. *Svensk Läkartidn,* **63,** 4192.

Ericson, S. (1967) Sialographic study of the parotid glands in rheumatoid arthritis. *Odontologisk Revy,* **18,** 163.

Ericson, S. (1968) The parotid gland in subjects with and without rheumatoid arthritis. *Acta Radiologica,* Supplement **275.**

Ericson, S. (1970) The normal variation of the parotid size. *Acta Oto-Laryngologica,* **70,** 294.

Eversole, L. R. & Sabes, W. R. (1971) Minor salivary gland duct changes due to obstruction. *Archives of Otolaryngology,* **94,** 19.

Garrett, J. R. (1962) Some observations on human submandibular salivary glands. *Proceedings of the Royal Society of Medicine,* **55,** 488.

Garrett, J. R. (1963) The ultrastructure of intracellular fat in the parenchyma of human submandibular salivary glands. *Archives of Oral Biology,* **8,** 729.

Hall, M. D. (1966) Diagnosis of diseases of the salivary glands. *Journal of Oral Surgery,* **27,** 15.

Hamperl, H. (1931) Beiträge zur normalen und pathologischen Histologie menschlicher Speicheldrüsen. *Zeitschrift für Zellforschung und mikroskopische Anatomie,* **27,** 1.

Holm, S. (1949) Keratoconjunctivitis and the Sicca syndrome. *Acta Ophthalmologica,* Supplement **33.**

Jańczuk, Z. & Jedrzejwska, T. (1966) Radiological investigation on parotid glands in patients with atrophic stomatitis. *Polish Medical Journal,* **5,** 1215.

Johansen, J. & Berdal, (1970) Lipomatosis of the parotid gland. *Acta Oto-laryngologica,* **263,** 167.

Kasbourn, W. J. (1953) Histopathology of irradiated salivary glands. *Journal of Dental Research,* **32,** 658.

Keleman, G. (1954) Symmetrical enlargement of submaxillary salivary glands in the aged. *Geriatrics,* **9,** 70.

Keleman, G. & Montgomery, W. W. (1958) Symmetrical asymptomatic submaxillary gland enlargement in older age groups. *New England Journal of Medicine,* **258,** 188.

Kerr, A. C. (1961) *The Physiological Regulation of Salivary Secretions in Man. A Study of the Response of Human Salivary Glands to Reflex Stimulation.* Oxford: Pergamon Press.

Korting, G. W. & Kleinschmidt, W. (1953) Veranderungen der Speichelsekretion bei Hautkrankheiten. *Dermatologische Wochenschrift,* **28,** 772.

Kurtz, S. M. (1954) Cytologic studies of the salivary glands of the rat with reference to the ageing process. *Journal of Gerontology,* **9,** 421.

Meyer, J. & Necheles, H. (1940) Studies in old age. IV. The clinical significance of salivary, gastric and pancreatic secretion in the aged. *Journal of the American Medical Association,* **115,** 2050.

Meyer, J., Golden, J. S., Steiner, N. & Necheles, H. (1937) The ptyalin content of human saliva in old age. *American Journal of Physiology,* **119,** 600.

Morgan, W. S. & Castleman, B. (1954) A clinico-pathologic study of "Mikulicz's disease". *American Journal of Pathology,* **29,** 471.

Novikoff, A. B. (1961) Lysosomes and related particles. In *The Cell* (Eds.) Brachet, J. & Mirsky, A. E. Vol. II, pp. 423-488. New York: Academic Press.

Östlund, S. G. (1953) Palatine glands and mucin. Disp. MALMO.

Rauch, S. (1959) *Die Speicheldrusen des Menschen.* Stuttgart: Georg Thieme.

Sandstead, H. R., Koehn, C. J. & Sessions, S. M. (1955) Enlargement of the parotid gland in malnutrition. *American Journal of Clinical Nutrition,* **3,** 198.

Scott, J. (1960) Prominence of the submaxillary glands in the aged. *Journal of the American Geriatrics Society,* **8,** 53.

Stormont, D. L. (1928) In *Special Cytology* (Ed.) Cowdry, E. V. Vol. I, p. 125. New York: Paul B. Hoeber Inc.

Wassermann, F. (1965) The development of adipose tissue. In *Handbook of Physiology,* Section 5. Adipose Tissue (Eds.) Renold, A. E. & Cahill, G. F. Jr., p. 95-96. Washington, D.C.: American Physiological Society.

Waterhouse, J. P., Chisholm, D. M., Winter, R. B., Patel, M. & Yale, R. S. (1973) Replacement of functional parenchymal cells by fat and connective tissue in human submandibular salivary glands: An age-related change. *Journal of Oral Pathology,* **2,** 16.

Yamaguchi, S. (1925) Studien über die Hundspeicheldrüsen. *Beitraege zur Pathologischen Anatomie und zur Allgemeinen Pathologie,* **73,** 113.

CHAPTER 14

Surgical Treatment of Salivary Gland Disease

It is only in the last twenty years that satisfactory methods of salivary gland excision have been outlined. Special attention has been paid to parotid excision by the French school (Redon, 1955). In the past, the approach to parotid surgery has been cautious due to the fear of damage to the facial nerve and the fact that biopsy of the gland carried the risk of implantation recurrence of malignant tumours. Equally, removal of the submandibular gland was complicated by possible damage to important neuro-vascular structures at that site.

In the surgical treatment of salivary gland neoplasia, as well as of some chronic inflammatory disease, it is essential to recognise the importance of designing an operation that will meet the requirements of total and safe resection of the affected gland with preservation of the important nerve involved.

In the approach to salivary gland surgery, the general principles include sufficient incision with the development of adequate flaps which should be reflected from the surface of the gland. The entire anatomical area should be exposed and the lesion outlined to delineate an adequate margin. Immediate control of the important blood supply to the area is established and the lesion approached from the uninvolved area.

SALIVARY GLAND SURGERY

Indications

In arriving at the decision to operate upon the salivary glands it is of course important to consider the differential diagnosis of salivary gland swellings. Intrinsic lesions of the salivary glands are discussed elsewhere in this book, but the possibility of an extra salivary cause such as masseteric enlargement disease of regional lymph nodes must also be considered. With such entities salivary gland functional tests are within normal limits. It should be noted that teeth clenching will increase the swelling at the angle of jaw in cases of masseteric enlargement and that plain antero-posterior radiographs often reveal a lateral spur at the angle. In these cases, surgical treatment is essentially cosmetic (Lash, 1963). Swellings due to infections of the glands may be modified by the tight fascia which encloses the gland, especially the parotid. Pain and rapid swelling are characteristic of acute infections, whilst with chronic infections their temporary nature helps to distinguish them. Predisposing factors such as low flow rate with secondary retrograde infection of gland are common (Maynard, 1965). Parotid secretion rate is particularly sensitive to obstruction and infection (Patey, 1965) so that a vicious circle is created which ultimately destroys the gland both functionally and anatomically, whilst histological changes reflect this conception (Patey and Thackray, 1955).

It should be noted that parotid calculi tend to arise at the junction of the duct with its main branches and ultimately lead to gland destruction (Maynard, 1967). Response to conservative therapy together with presence or absence of gland dysfunction are important factors when surgery is contemplated. Where flow rate and sialography are normal then spontaneous remission may be expected. This may be hastened by measures aimed at increasing flow rate such as chewing and use of sialogogues. Where salivary function tests reveal marked changes and severe symptoms continue despite conservative measures, surgical intervention must be considered. In some conditions intra-oral parotid duct ligation which results in acinar atrophy and parotid ablation (Laage-Hellman, 1955; Diamant and Enfors, 1965; Maynard, 1965) may be of value and still leaves open the option to perform a total parotidectomy.

With regard to tumour surgery, a single lump in the parotid is nearly always a neoplasm and mostly non-malignant (*British Medical Journal,* 1970). Exceptions are tumours of the sublingual gland which, although rare, have a 70 per cent incidence of malignancy. Only about three-quarters of slow-growing masses in the parotid prove to be neoplasms; the rest are other tumours arising without the gland (Hobsley, 1970). Recently the W.H.O. (Thackray, 1972) have classified tumours according to their histological type and fortunately the frankly malignant tumours of salivary tissue are rare. The ratio of malignant to other tumours is 1:5.8 (Patey, 1965). Benign tumours are slow growing and located superficially in the parotid towards the lower pole. Rapid growth, local pain, early lymph node involvement and facial nerve involvement are characteristic of malignant tumours. Enucleation should be abandoned as a method of treatment and radiotherapy must be considered unsatisfactory in itself, although it may usefully be combined with surgery. Cysts (Pratt, 1965), secondary tumours, intra-parotid lymph nodes and connective tissue neoplasms are other causes of salivary swelling which may warrant a surgical approach to treatment.

It may be concluded that the modern technique of superficial and total conservative parotidectomy and preservation of the facial nerve allows most tumours to be treated by wide excision.

Biopsy

Pre-operative biopsy of parotid tumours is generally undesirable since it may encourage spread of tumour (Patey and Thackray, 1958). However, in special cases, if a tissue diagnosis is required pre-operatively, then surgical biopsy under direct vision is the method of choice (Chapter 19). The procedure is best carried out under endotracheal general anaesthesia and the incision is placed in such a way that, if necessary, it can be removed with the entire biopsy at a subsequent operative procedure. Flaps are not elevated and in most instances the incision is placed near the posterior edge of the gland so as to give as much room as possible between the proposed biopsy area and the relatively deep facial nerve trunk. If definitive surgical treatment is to be carried out at the same time then the biopsy wound is closed and dressed. The entire biopsy incision and its tract are then excised in continuity with the tumour (Anderson and Byars, 1965).

PAROTID GLAND EXCISION

Anatomical considerations

The following anatomical points may usefully be made in relation to parotid gland surgery. Developmentally, the relationship of the parotid gland to the facial nerve is a secondary one, since the gland migrates backwards from its original site of pharyngeal outpouching. A majority view suggests that the parotid gland is H-shaped (McWhorter, 1917; McCormack, Cauldwell and Anson, 1945). The facial nerve lying between two lobes of the parotid partially separates the gland into a large superficial and a small deep portion, the two parts being connected by a slender isthmus which passes between the two diverging portions of the nerve.

The facial nerve divides into two main divisions, the temporofacial and cervicofacial portions. This point of bifurcation occurs 5 to 7 mm dorsal to the ramus of the mandible and 4.1 to 4.7 cm above the external angle of the mandible (McCormack, Cauldwell and Anson, 1945).

As an approximate measurement of surgical value, the point of bifurcation lies posterior and slightly medial to the ramus of the mandible and superiorly two-thirds of the distance between the external angle of the mandible and the palpable condyoid process (Figure 14.1). The temporofacial branch is the larger by far. The pattern of branching from these two main trunks varies but eight general types of configuration may be distinguished (McCormack, Cauldwell and Anson, 1945). These are illustrated in Figure 14.2, and it is of interest that patterns of anastomoses appear to be governed by the shape and position of the deep lobe of the gland and the presence of the isthmus. Further, where anastomoses between branches of the two main trunks occur, then the isthmus is the common site (McCormack, Cauldwell and Ånson, 1945). In terms of the surgical exposure of the parotid gland these authors suggest that the parotid fascia should be opened posteriorly and reflected forward from a preauricular incision. The upper border of the superficial lobe, which coincides with the line of the zygomatic arch, is thus exposed. At the apex of this lobe the parotid duct and buccal branches of the facial nerve may be identified. Using the isthmus as a guiding landmark the branches and main trunks of the facial nerve may be traced back to the point of bifurcation of the nerve.

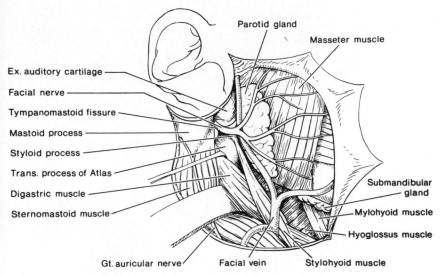

Ex. auditory cartilage

Facial nerve

Tympanomastoid fissure

Mastoid process

Styloid process

Trans. process of Atlas

Digastric muscle

Sternomastoid muscle

Parotid gland

Masseter muscle

Submandibular gland

Mylohyoid muscle

Hyoglossus muscle

Gt. auricular nerve   Facial vein   Stylohyoid muscle

Figure 14.1. Diagram showing bony landmarks around main trunk of the facial nerve.

Parotidectomy

The approach to the facial nerve is selected by the surgeon depending on the location of the lesion within the gland. However, the distribution of the peripheral branches is variable, whereas the exit of the trunk from the stylomastoid foramen is constant. The tip of the mastoid process, the transverse process of the second cervical vertebra, the tympano-mastoid fissure and the styloid process are encircling bony landmarks which help in locating the trunk (Figure 14.1). In addition the facial nerve usually divides into an upper temporofacial division and a lower cervicofacial division and then into five peripheral branches superficial to the posterior facial vein. This neurovenous plane is a valuable soft tissue guide when bony landmarks are obliterated. With regard to parotid tumours the vast majority occur in the superficial portion of the gland lateral to the facial nerve. In these cases, the surgical specimen can be the entire superficial portion of the gland, obtained by lateral parotidectomy. If the tumour is located within the deeper medial portion of the gland, lateral parotidectomy is first completed and the facial nerve carefully elevated to allow the medial portion to be delivered as the surgical specimen. The use of an electrical stimulator or pinching with forceps is a useful technique to avoid section of an unsuspected branch of the nerve.

Parotidectomy should be considered as a dissection of the gland away from the facial nerve. A typical incision for a tumour of the lower pole of the gland is shown in Figure 14.3. The flap is raised over the surface of the upward extension of the investing layer of the deep cervical fascia. The dissection is begun posteriorly and inferiorly where the facial nerve or its branches are least likely to be encountered. The upper and anterior borders of the gland are approached and retrograde dissection begun. Once the tumour is

235

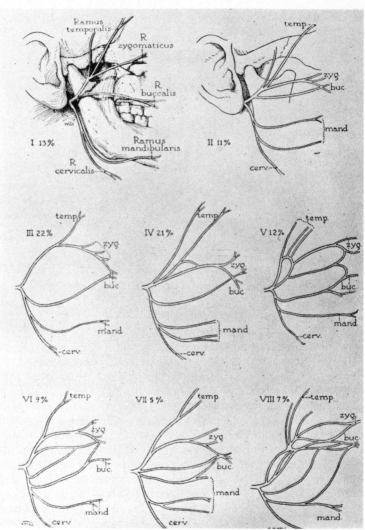

Figure 14.2. Major types of facial nerve branching and anastomosis; I: Major divisions (Temporal and facial) independent; II: anastomosis between rami of the temporal division; III: connection between adjacent rami from the major divisions; IV: anastomoses representing a composite of those in II and III; V: proximal anastomosis within the temporal component, distal interconnection between the latter and the cervical component; VI: two anastomotic rami sent from the buccal division of the cervical to the zygomatic part of the temporal; VII: transverse ramus, from the trunk of the nerve, contributing to the buccal ramus formed by anastomosis between the two major divisions; VIII: richly plexiform communications, especially within the temporal portion of the nerve.

reached, dissection is begun around it with a layer of normal tissue left around the capsule. The isthmus may be divided to permit elevation of the superficial lobe which is swung back so that resection takes place with the facial nerve and its branches in view. For malignant tumours and lesions in the deep portion of the gland a total parotidectomy is advisable. The operation must be carefully planned and preparations made for radical neck dissection and facial nerve repair should they be necessary. A total parotidectomy is begun posteriorly by dissecting along the anterior border of the mastoid process. Dissection follows the anatomic border of the parotid. Nerve stimulation, identification and marking should be undertaken as already described. Following closure a drain should be inserted and a pressure dressing applied. An approach to parotidectomy is illustrated in Figures 14.4a to 14.4e. It is worth noting that the intra-ductal instillation of a dye, such as methylene blue, may facilitate parotid gland surgery (Forrest and Robinson, 1957). It has been shown that this technical adjunct to operations for removal of parotid tumours stains normal tissue but not tumour (Figure 14.5). Spillage of dye is negligible and the facial nerve does not stain (Robinson, Masters and Forrest, 1960; Shedd and Robinson, 1966). Limitations of the method include the presence of ductal change due to previous surgery, duct involvement or occlusion by tumour.

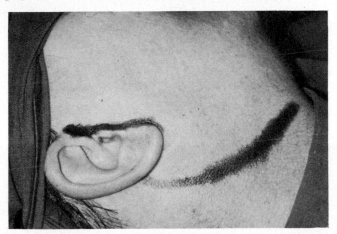

Figure 14.3. Pre-operative field showing the line of incision for the removal of a parotid gland tumour.

COMPLICATIONS AND THEIR MANAGEMENT

Facial nerve damage

The accidental division of the nerve or the intentional division of the nerve in a difficult parotidectomy will result in the distressing condition of postoperative facial paralysis. Although late repairs may be achieved by crossover anastomoses from convenient cranial nerves such as the accessory or hypoglossal: an immediate repair, where feasible, is to be preferred (Rankow, 1973). This is achieved either by direct anastomoses of the severed nerve or by the interposition of a free nerve graft. Conley (1955) first reported the effective use of free grafts from the great auricular nerve or branches of the anterior cervical plexus (C3 and C4), immediately following parotidectomy. The graft must rest within a well-vascularised soft tissue bed. There may be

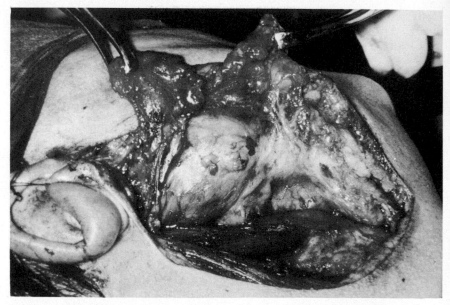

Figure 14.4a. Removal of recurrent pleomorphic adenoma of R parotid gland. The inferior part of the tumour, which involves the deep lobe, is mobilised.

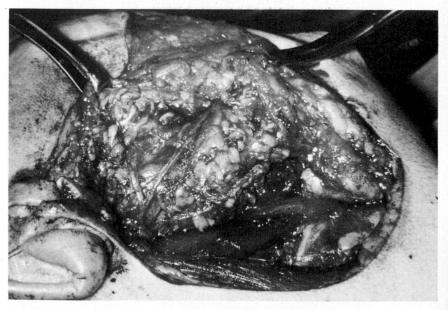

Figure 14.4b. The superficial part of the gland is removed with the branches of the facial nerve in situ.

238

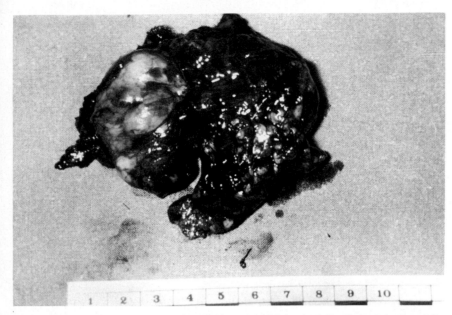

Figure 14.4c. Surgical specimen showing the tumour which involved the whole of the deep lobe of the parotid gland.

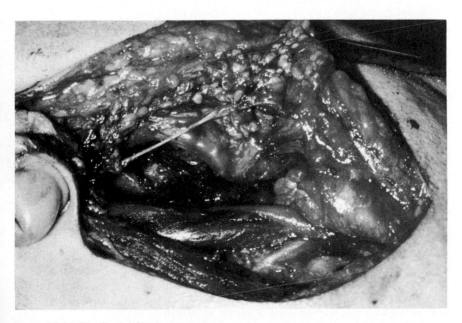

Figure 14.4d. The final defect is shown.

239

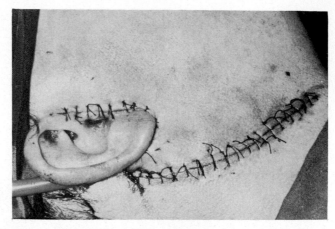

Figure 14.4e. Closure of wound with drain in place.

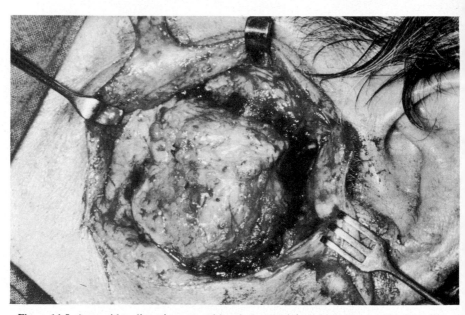

Figure 14.5. As an aid to dissection patent blue dye can be injected into the parotid duct. This stains the whole of the gland but not the tumour or facial nerve. This illustration shows the tumour surrounded by the dye stained gland.

an advantage in protecting the anastomoses with small silicone tubes or milli-pore tapes (Rankow, 1973). The final results of the anastomoses may not be refined muscle movement but rather a mass muscle action. Material for nerve suture must be of minimal diameter—No. 7.0 silk—and the sutures are placed in nerve sheath only. Prior to insertion of suture, the nerve ends are cleanly excised to provide surfaces which will appose neatly. The use of a drain and a pressure pack to prevent post-operative swelling are essential. The time of return of function is probably never less than two months.

Permanent facial nerve paralysis produces serious cosmetic deformity and functional impairment. Static support of the resting face makes a major contribution to reducing the overall deformity. A satisfactory surgical method is the insertion of multiple strips of fascia lata, attached at one end to the soft tissues around the mouth and at the other end to the temporal muscle and pre-auricular fascia. In elderly patients it may be combined with the face-lift type of operation. The average face requires four fascial implants to obtain satisfactory support. The first two go to the mid-line of the upper and lower lips; a third forms a wide loop supporting the naso-labial fold whilst the fourth supports the lower lip just medial to the angle of the mouth.

The auriculotemporal syndrome (Frey's syndrome; gustatory sweating)

This is an uncommon complication of parotid surgery. It consists of sweating in the region of the skin of the forehead and cheek supplied by the auriculo-temporal nerve following a stimulus to salivary secretion. Gardner and McCubbin (1956) have suggested that parasympathetic impulses, intended for the salivary gland and misdirected to supply sweat glands, take place due to a short circuiting within the auriculotemporal nerve. Injury to this nerve, either direct or following compression by scar tissue, may give rise to the syndrome. Although curable by division of the intra-cranial portion of the glosso-pharyngeal nerve the condition rarely warrants this approach; the syndrome is explained to the patient and usually left untreated.

Salivary fistula

The formation of a fistula most probably follows division of the duct without the limits of the gland. Following injury, the application of a pressure dressing is the best way to prevent salivary fistula formation. Persistent salivary drainage from a site of injury is best treated surgically by repair of the duct. In some instances it may be necessary to ligate the proximal portion of the duct as it leaves the gland, so producing atrophy of the gland proximal to this point. Parotid fistulas may be treated by freeing the proximal portion and transferring it to the buccal mucosa. The external scar may be removed by an elliptical excision around the lesion, the skin undermined and the wound closed. Extra-oral fistulas of the submandibular and sublingual glands usually require excision of these glands.

ACUTE SUPPURATIVE PAROTITIS

Antibiotic therapy alone is satisfactory in treating some cases of staphylococcal parotitis (Speirs and Mason, 1972). Petersdorf, Forsyth and Bernanke (1958) treated a number of cases with antibiotics and avoided surgery but most other workers have stressed the need for early incision of the parotid gland in some cases (Spratt, 1961; Krippaehne, Hunt and Dunphy, 1962; Carlson and Glas, 1963; Goldberg and Harrigan, 1965).

Rapid progression of pain and swelling with associated general manifestations of acute bacterial infection despite conservative treatment requires surgical incision and drainage. The procedure is carried out under general anaesthesia and an incision following the anterior border of the ear and extending into a skin fold of the neck is made. The entire gland should be exposed and drainage is achieved by the use of a pointed haemostat, although prior incision of the parotid capsule may be necessary. Drains may be inserted, and the wound packed but not closed.

PAROTID CALCULI

If the calculus is small and readily palpated in Stensen's duct it may on occasion be 'milked' towards the papilla. If the calculus lies right at the papilla then a simple incision under local anaesthesia is sufficient to liberate the mass and the papilla left unsutured. Calculi lying further back in the duct are removed under general anaesthesia, a longitudinal incision being made in the duct in the region of the lesion. A calculus not palpable in the mouth is best approached by an external incision, parallel to the course of the duct. The duct is opened longitudinally and sutured once the calculus has been delivered. As a precaution the duct may be ligated on either side of the calculus prior to the duct incision being made. Soft tissue and skin are carefully sutured and a pressure dressing applied.

RECONSTRUCTION OF PAROTID DUCT

Reconstruction of the parotid duct involves the formation of a tubed mucosal pedicle from buccal mucosa. This is transferred to the lateral cheek. The diameter of severed duct and pedicle are different and must be adjusted to match by selective bevelling. It should be noted that no sphincteric action is present and that air pressure in the mouth may inflate the duct also.

In recent years a surgical method has been developed for the treatment of excessive salivation or drooling. As mentioned in Chapter 8, this most distressing condition may affect patients with cerebral palsy. Essentially the surgical procedure (Wilkie, 1967, 1970) is a parotid duct transplantation. A vertical incision is made, just behind the papilla of the parotid duct, and a submucosal tunnel is made to the tonsillar fossa. With the parotid papilla at its base, a flap is raised, folded backwards and drawn as a strip through the tunnel. It is then sutured to the anterior pillar of the fauces. Finally the mucosal defect is closed (Wilkie, 1967). Thus, parotid saliva is diverted to the tonsillar fossa and directed down the throat away from an uncontrollable oral cavity.

SUBMANDIBULAR GLAND EXCISION

The broad general principles of surgery to the submandibular gland will be discussed in relation to the treatment of salivary calculi (Seward, 1968a-g). The removal of anterior submandibular calculi may be performed under local anaesthesia. To prevent the calculus moving distally, a suture is passed around the duct behind the calculus and tied gently. The duct is identified following initial incision in the floor of the mouth followed by blunt dissection. The duct is mobilised and clamped to provide a firm base while it is being incised with a longitudinal incision over the calculus. The calculus is removed, the duct irrigated and sutures removed. The mucosal wound only is sutured, since attempts to suture the duct usually lead to stricture formation.

Posterior submandibular calculi are best approached under general anaesthesia. The duct is identified and traced backwards. It is important at this stage to identify the lingual nerve, pass a tape around it and have it drawn laterally. The calculus in the posterior portion of the duct or just within the upper pole of the gland may now be identified and removed by incision. It is important to avoid involving the posterior portion of the upper pole since division of the facial artery is a real risk.

Excision of the submandibular gland is necessary for calculi positioned below the junction with Wharton's duct of the most distal intra-lobular duct and also for tumour surgery. Although the gland may be removed through an intra-oral incision (Downton and Quist, 1960), this is an approach which requires special experience (Seward, 1968d).

An extra-oral approach uses a 5-cm long incision parallel to a skin crease at the junction of the upper two-thirds and lower one-third of the palpable part of the gland. Blunt dissection through platysma and deep fascia is undertaken whilst branches of the facial nerve are identified and retracted. The lower pole of the gland is isolated by retraction upwards and forwards. The posterior belly of the digastric and the stylo-hyoid muscles are retracted downwards to expose the facial artery which should be carefully ligated at this stage. The gland is separated from the lower border of the mandible, and turned backwards to expose the border of mylo-hyoid which is separated from the gland. The lingual nerve should now be displayed and freed from the gland. The deep part of the gland may now be enucleated and the duct ligated and divided. The wound is closed in layers and a drain inserted. The most common serious complication of the procedure is surgical trauma to the mandibular branch of the facial nerve. Deviation of the tongue from surgical section of the hypoglossal nerve is a less frequent complication (Frabble, 1970).

RECURRENT AND MALIGNANT TUMOURS

Recurrent lesions from benign tumours are generally the result of inadequate initial surgery. It is clear that the surgical removal of these is complicated by the presence of scar and fibrous tissue. Total excision of the affected gland should be considered.

Frankly malignant tumours require a definite surgical plan which may include total gland excision, facial nerve sacrifice and radical neck dissection in continuity with the primary tumour.

SUBLINGUAL AND MINOR GLAND SURGERY

Ranula

Marsupialisation is the treatment of choice for this lesion. Simple incision and drainage inevitably results in recurrence. Due to the thin cystic wall, attempts to enucleate the ranula without rupturing the lining prove extremely difficult. Marsupialisation consists in excision of the anterior-superior wall of the cyst and suturing the cystic lining to the mucous membrane in the floor of the oral cavity. As an initial step the submandibular duct and lingual nerve are identified and isolated. The opening incision allows drainage of the cyst cavity. Robinson (1966) recommends that ¼-inch sterile selvage-edge gauze be introduced to the cyst cavity at this stage. This allows the full extent of the cavity to be outlined. Using No. 9 Dean's scissors, overlying mucosa and lining are cut from the top of the cavity around the greatest perimeter of the cyst. Generally only a few sutures are required around the periphery to join the cystic wall to the mucosa of the floor of the oral cavity.

Excision of the sublingual gland

Tumours of the sublingual gland occur infrequently. The surgical management of tumours at this site is adequate excision of the gland.

An important point to note with regard to sublingual neoplasms is the high proportion of malignant lesions (Rankow and Mignogna, 1969). Surgical removal of the sublingual gland may also be the treatment of choice for sialolithiasis and deep-seated ranulas and a technique has been described (Catone, Merrill and Henry, 1969).

Essentially, a linear incision is made in the superior aspect of the lesion and the submandibular duct identified and retracted. Blunt dissection is undertaken to identify the lingual nerve. The sublingual gland is gently elevated and removed, taking special care to avoid severance of lingual nerve or submandibular duct. The antero-lateral aspect of the gland may be attached to the periosteum of the mandible by fibrous tissue, and this portion of the gland should be freed carefully. Following gland removal the wound is closed in the usual manner.

Mucocele

Mucoceles are simply excised together with the few mucous gland lobules in the vicinity of the lesion.

Surgical Treatment of Salivary Gland Disease

Minor gland tumours

The points made earlier with regard to major gland tumours apply equally to intra-oral salivary tumours. Excision should be wide and enucleation is condemned. Frankly, malignant tumours require careful surgical planning including a consideration of plastic and prosthetic post-operative treatments.

SUMMARY

It is clear that surgical decisions in the treatment of disease of the major salivary glands evolve from certain fundamental procedures. Diagnostic tests described in Part III may be used to establish the nature and extent of disease as an initial step. The selection of a definitive surgical procedure based on the clinical and investigative evidence at hand should be made. An awareness of possible damage to important neuro-vascular structures should always be considered and preparation made beforehand to enable repair to be carried out.

REFERENCES

Anderson, R. & Byars, L. T. (1965) *Surgery of the Parotid Gland,* St. Louis: C. V. Mosby Co.
British Medical Journal (1970) Parotid swellings, **iii,** 662.
Carlson, R. G. & Glas, W. W. (1963) Acute suppurative parotitis. *Archives of Surgery,* **86,** 659.
Catone, G. A., Merrill, R. G. & Henny, F. A. (1969) Sublingual gland mucus-escape phenomenon—treatment by excision of the sublingual gland. *Journal of Oral Surgery,* **27,** 774.
Conley, J. J. (1955) Facial nerve grafting in treatment of parotid gland tumors. *Archives of Surgery,* **70,** 359.
Diamant, H. & Enfors, B. (1965) Treatment of chronic recurrent parotitis. *Laryngoscope,* **75,** 153.
Downton, D. & Quist, G. (1960) Intra-oral excision of the submandibular gland. *Proceedings of the Royal Society of Medicine,* **53,** 543.
Forrest, H. J. & Robinson, D. W. (1957) Delineation of the parotid by in vivo staining. *Plastic and Reconstructive Surgery and The Transplantation Bulletin,* **20,** 311.
Frable, M. A. S. (1970) Submaxillary gland excision. *Surgery, Gynecology and Obstetrics with International Abstracts of Surgery,* **131,** 1155.
Gardner, W. J. & McCubbin, J. W. (1956) Auriculotemporal syndrome; gustatory sweating due to misdirection of regenerating nerve fibres. *Journal of the American Medical Association,* **160,** 272.
Goldberg, M. H. & Harrigan, W. G. (1965) Acute suppurative parotitis. *Oral Surgery, Oral Medicine and Oral Pathology,* **20,** 281.
Hobsley, M. (1970) Affections of the salivary glands and their management. *Annals of the Royal College of Surgeons of England,* **46,** 224.
Krippaehne, W. W., Hunt, T. K. & Dunphy, J. E. (1962) Acute suppurative parotitis. *Annals of Surgery,* **156,** 251.
Laage-Hellman, J. E. (1955) Ligatur av ductus Stenoni som terpeutisk atgard. *Svenska Läkartidningen,* **52,** 3150.
Lash, H. (1963) Benign masseteric hypertrophy. *Surgical Clinics of North America,* **43,** 1357.
Maynard, J. D. (1965) Recurrent parotid enlargement. *British Journal of Surgery,* **52,** 784.
Maynard, J. (1967) Parotid enlargement. *Hospital Medicine,* **1,** 620.
McCormack, L. J., Cauldwell, E. W. & Anson, B. J. (1945) The surgical anatomy of the facial nerve. *Surgery, Gynecology and Obstetrics with International Abstracts of Surgery,* **80,** 620.

McWhorter, G. L. (1917) The relations of the superficial and deep lobes of the parotid gland to the ducts and to the facial nerve. *Anatomical Record*, **12**, 149.

Patey, D. H. (1965) Inflammation of the salivary glands with particular reference to chronic and recurrent parotitis. *Annals of the Royal College of Surgeons of England*, **36**, 26.

Patey, D. H. & Thackray, A. C. (1955) Chronic "sialectatic" parotitis in light of pathological studies on parotidectomy material. *British Journal of Surgery*, **43**, 43.

Patey, D. H. & Thackray, A. C. (1958) The treatment of parotid tumours in the light of a pathological study of parotidectomy material. *British Journal of Surgery*, **45**, 477.

Petersdorf, R. G., Forsyth, B. R. & Bernanke, D. (1958) Staphylococcal parotitis. *New England Journal of Medicine*, **259**, 1250.

Pratt, L. W. (1965) Cystic lesions of the parotid region. *Journal of the Maine Medical Association*, **56**, 21.

Rankow, R. M. (1973) Surgical decisions in the treatment of major salivary gland tumors. *Plastic and Reconstructive Surgery*, **51**, 514.

Rankow, R. M. & Mignogna, F. (1969) Cancer of the sublingual salivary gland. *American Journal of Surgery*, **118**, 790.

Redon, H. (1955) *Chirurgie des Glandes Salivaires*. Paris: Masson.

Robinson, D. W., Masters, F. W. & Forrest, H. J. (1960) Clinical experience with supravital staining in surgery of parotid gland. *Surgery, Gynecology and Obstetrics with International Abstracts of Surgery*, **110**, 121.

Robinson, H. B. G. (1966) Cysts of the oral cavity. In *Oral Surgery: A Step by Step Atlas of Operative Techniques*, 4th edition. (Ed.) Archer, W. H. Philadelphia: W. B. Saunders Co.

Seward, G. R. (1968a) Anatomic surgery for salivary calculi. I. Symptoms, signs and differential diagnosis. *Oral Surgery, Oral Medicine and Oral Pathology*, **25**, 150.

Seward, G. R. (1968b(Anatomic surgery for salivary calculi. II. Calculi in the anterior part of the submandibular duct. *Oral Surgery, Oral Medicine and Oral Pathology*, **25**, 287.

Seward, G. R. (1968c) Anatomic surgery for salivary calculi. III. Calculi in the posterior part of the submandibular duct. *Oral Surgery, Oral Medicine and Oral Pathology*, **25**, 525.

Seward, G. R. (1968d) Anatomic surgery for salivary calculi. IV. Calculi in the intraglandular part of the submandibular duct. *Oral Surgery, Oral Medicine and Oral Pathology*, **25**, 670.

Seward, G. R. (1968e) Anatomic surgery for salivary calculi. V. Calculi in the extraglandular part of the parotid duct. *Oral Surgery, Oral Medicine and Oral Pathology*, **25**, 810.

Seward, G. R. (1968f) Anatomic surgery for salivary calculi. VI. Calculi in the intraglandular part of the parotid duct. *Oral Surgery, Oral Medicine and Oral Pathology*, **26**, 1.

Seward, G. R. (1968g) Anatomic surgery for salivary calculi. VII. Complications of salivary calculi. *Oral Surgery, Oral Medicine and Oral Pathology*, **26**, 137.

Shedd, D. P. & Robinson, R. M. (1964) Facilitation of parotid gland surgery by intraductal instillation of dye. *Archives of Surgery*, **93**, 958.

Speirs, C. F. & Mason, D. K. (1972) Acute septic parotitis; Incidence, aetiology and management. *Scottish Medical Journal*, **17**, 62.

Spratt, J. S. (1961) The etiology and therapy of acute pyogenic parotitis. *Surgery, Gynecology and Obstetrics*, **112**, 391.

Thackray, A. C. (1972) *Histological Typing of Salivary Gland Tumours*. Geneva: World Health Organisation.

Wilkie, T. F. (1967) The problem of drooling in cerebral palsy—a surgical approach. *Canadian Journal of Surgery*, **10**, 60.

Wilkie, T. F. (1970) The surgical treatment of drooling: A follow up report of five years experience. *Plastic and Reconstructive Surgery*, **45**, 549.

PART III

Special Investigations: Basis, Methodology and Application

CHAPTER 15

The Collection of Saliva

Salivary studies may be conducted on samples of mixed or total saliva or on separated secretions of the major salivary glands. The choice depends on the nature of the problem being investigated. For example, separate secretion is necessary if the function of a diseased gland is being assessed but if saliva as part of the dental environment is being considered, mixed saliva is usually collected. Where a particular salivary constituent is being measured, accurate reproducible measurements can only be obtained on separated parotid, submandibular or sublingual secretions as the individual gland contribution to mixed saliva varies in volume and composition under various conditions. Although Tiedemann and Gmelin (1826) first described the collection of separated secretions in animal experiments as long ago as 1826, it is only in the past 20 years that the value of obtaining such samples has been widely appreciated and applied in man.

The following methods have been described for the collection of separated parotid, submandibular, mixed and minor gland saliva:

Parotid:	1. Polyethylene catheter
	2. Suction cup
	3. Combined catheter and suction cup
Submandibular:	1. Polyethylene catheter
	2. Segregator appliance
	3. Suction cup
Sublingual:	1. Segregator appliance
Mixed:	1. Spitting
	2. Drainage
	3. Suction
	4. Cotton wool rolls
Minor:	1. Capillary tubes

Each collection method will now be described in detail.

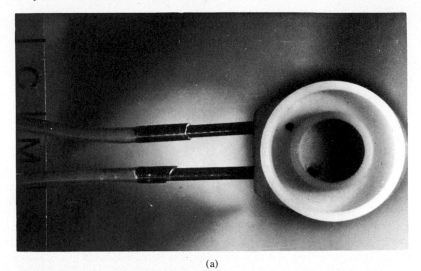

(a)

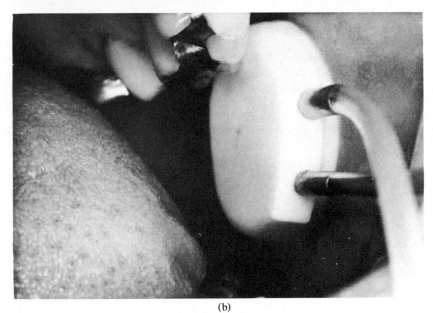

(b)

PAROTID

Polyethylene catheter

Small samples of parotid saliva may be collected using polyethylene tubing of a suitable diameter (0.5 to 1.5 mm). The catheter is introduced through the duct orifice and into the duct for 1 to 2 cm. The ductal end of the catheter may be tapered by heating and pulling out over a bunsen flame. A further requirement is to smooth the edges of the tapered end, on rough cloth (Kerr,

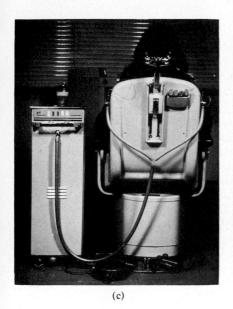

(c)

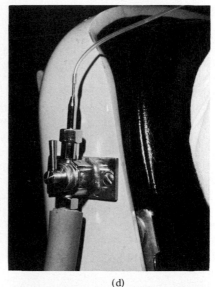

(d)

Figure 15.1. Collection of parotid saliva. a. Modified Carlson-Crittenden cup. The inner chamber is placed over the parotid duct orifice. b. Cup in position over left parotid duct orifice. c. Method of providing air suction at dental chair from conventional aspirator. d. Locking key attached to dental chair. e. Patient having parotid saliva collected.

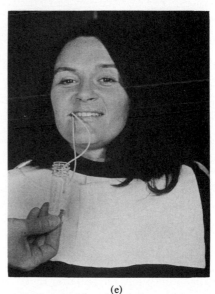

(e)

1961). A major disadvantage with this method is that the catheter is unstable and requires to be held in position whilst in use. It may also be uncomfortable for the patient. This method of parotid saliva collection is indicated only where a small sample is required, e.g. for bacteriological examination. More recently, pre-sterilised disposable catheters tapered for this purpose can be obtained commercially (Portex Plastics, Hythe, England).

251

Suction cup

This basic two-chambered device is often referred to as a 'Lashley Cup' (Lashley, 1916) but, as pointed out by Terry and Shannon (1965) it was first described by Carlson and Crittenden in 1910. The inner chamber is placed over the parotid duct orifice and the cup maintained by air suction applied through the outer chamber (Figure 15.1 a, b).

Since the details of the original Carlson-Crittenden cup were published in 1910, various modifications on the same two-chamber principle have been described (Lashley, 1916; Richter and Wada, 1924; Krasnogorski, 1931; Finesinger and Finesinger, 1937; Gore, 1938; Curby, 1953; Kerr, 1955; Tsaturov, 1957; Miller, 1960; Suhara and Asakawa, 1959; Shannon, Prigmore and Chauncey, 1962). Metals and plastics have been used to construct the basic cup portion of the collecting device.

A simple, reliable two-chambered nylon cup used by the authors in their own clinic is shown in Figure 15.2. The inner chamber diameter is 10 mm with a depth of 4 mm. This cup is well tolerated by the tissues, gives adequate retention and is satisfactory for routine collection of parotid saliva.

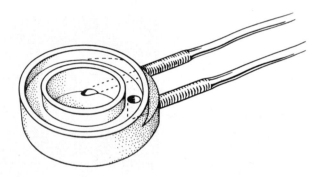

Figure 15.2. Diagram showing internal structure of the modified Carson-Crittenden cup used to collect parotid saliva. Air suction is applied through the outer chamber. The saliva flows from the inner chamber to the outlet tube. The inner and outer chambers are 10 and 20 mm diameter respectively with a depth of 4 mm.

The source of air suction may be a rubber ball syringe if for a portable saliva collection kit (Figure 15.3). However, if the saliva is usually being collected in the same room or laboratory, and a water tap is available, a conventional water pump can be attached. The negative pressure applied to maintain the cup is approximately 200 to 250 mm Hg. If the saliva is being collected in a dental surgery the system illustrated in Figures 15.1c, d, and e is a convenient method using the air suction of the dental unit.

There are two disadvantages of suction cup methods which are occasionally encountered. Firstly, in some patients when intra-oral stimuli are being chewed or sucked, movements of the cup can occur. Secondly, if the air-suction pressure is too great, the buccal mucosa is sucked into the suction

252

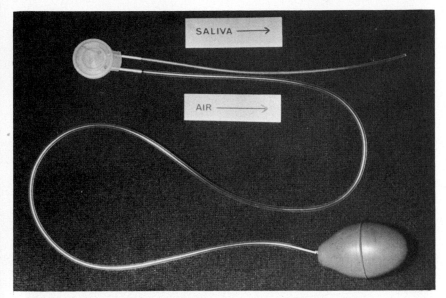

Figure 15.3. Portable saliva collection device—suction cup with rubber ball syringe. In this device a catheter has been inserted through the centre of the cup (combined catheter and suction cup).

tube and occludes it, allowing movement of the cup away from the mucosa elsewhere. Fincsinger and Finesinger (1937) attempted to overcome the latter by introducing a perforated plate over the outer chamber. If this modification is used, it is important to ensure that no sharp edges occur around the perforated areas as tearing of the oral mucosa will result. As a result of both of these above-mentioned complications, air may pass into the inner chamber resulting in air bubbles being included with the saliva as it passes down the saliva collecting tube.

Combined catheter and suction cup

This method was described by Kerr (1961). A suitable polyethylene catheter is selected to fit the parotid duct orifice. The catheter is inserted along the tube to the centre of the modified suction cup and through until it projects ½ to 1 cm beyond the fitting surface of the cup (Figure 15.4). The catheter, with the cup attached, is then inserted into the parotid duct and, when satisfactorily positioned, air suction is applied through an outer chamber which maintains the appliance in position.

The advantages of this method are that the retention is excellent and air inclusion bubbles never occur. However, it is time-consuming for the operator and can cause discomfort to the patient.

This method is therefore not suitable for routine clinical use but may have a place where special investigations requiring great accuracy in a few subjects are being undertaken or where air inclusion must be avoided.

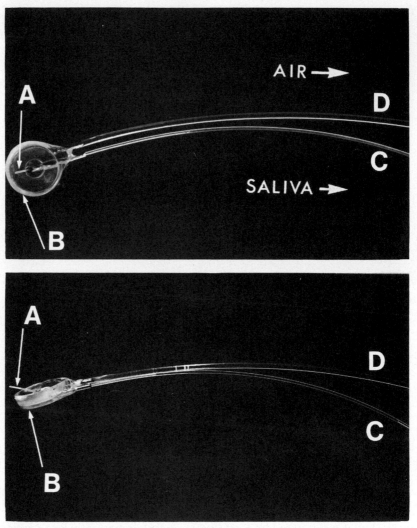

Figure 15.4. Kerr method for parotid saliva collection. A: Polyethylene catheter; B: Suction cup; C: Tube—saliva; D: Air suction.

SUBMANDIBULAR

Polyethylene catheter

Until recently, this was regarded as the only suitable method of collecting submandibular saliva in an edentulous subject. A tapered polyethylene catheter, as described for the parotid, is prepared and inserted through the submandibular duct orifice for 2 to 3 cm along the duct. Usually, the submandibular duct orifice requires dilation and the best instrument for this purpose is the lacrimal probe dilator as demonstrated in Chapter 4 (Figure 4.7). All the disadvantages detailed for the use of catheters in the collection of the parotid saliva can be repeated for the submandibular. In addition, submandibular duct catheterisation is more difficult because the surrounding tissues are looser and more mobile. The area is also less accessible, especially if the lower anterior teeth are inclined lingually. The main disadvantage is, however, lack of retention; tongue movements tend to displace the catheter from the duct after a few minutes. However, it remains the only method by which separated submandibular saliva may be obtained from one gland only. With the other methods (Segregator and Suction Cup) secretions from right and left submandibular duct orifices are collected together.

Segregator appliances

This method of collecting submandibular saliva was first described by Schneyer in 1955. It can only be used where the subject has a sufficient number of lower anterior teeth to provide retention. The appliance, like a partial denture, is made in some form of plastic such as clear acrylic and there is a lingual extension in the form of a hollow chamber which is placed over and around the submandibular duct orifices (Figure 15.5). This method is only as good as the peripheral seal around the chamber in the floor of the mouth. This can be enhanced by adding Kerr's green impression compound to the edges of the lingual chamber. But, on the other hand, too great a downward pressure by the edges of the chamber will occlude the submandibular ducts as they lie in the floor of the mouth. A balance has, therefore, to be obtained and this requires careful adjustment. The efficiency of the peripheral seal can be tested by the use of a simple dye, e.g. Evans Blue.

A modification of the Schneyer method has been described by Block Brottman (1962). They describe a preformed plastic cup as the lingual chamber which is placed over the submandibular duct orifices. This is maintained in position by denture rubber base impression material which is placed over, around and between it and the lingual surfaces of the lower teeth. The complete appliance is quickly constructed at the chairside whereas the Schneyer method requires laboratory preparation. Similar care is required to obtain and prove that there is adequate peripheral seal.

Both of these appliances, once made, can be used for repeated saliva collections. Their only disadvantage is the time required to construct and fit accurately. The segregator method can also be used to collect sublingual saliva at the same time as described by Schneyer (1955).

Suction cup

A two-chambered device, similar in principle to that used for the collection of parotid saliva, was first described by Truelove, Bixler and Merritt (1967) for submandibular saliva. A recent modification of this method (Stephen and Speirs, 1974) is illustrated (Figures 15.6a, b; 15.7). Once in position the subject is required to protrude the tongue slightly so that the undersurface of the tongue rests on the lingual and upper surface of the appliance, thus aiding retention. In the authors' experience this is the most reliable and efficient technique and is used in their own clinic. Unfortunately it does not permit collection of saliva from one gland only, both right and left submandibular secretions being collected together.

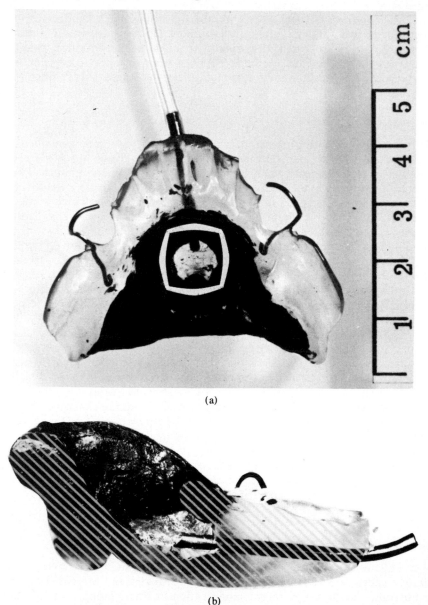

(a)

(b)

Figure 15.5. Schneyer segregator for collection of submandibular saliva. The chamber (circled) is placed over the submandibular duct orifices. a. Seen from below. b. Vertical cross section.

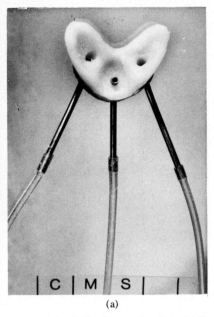 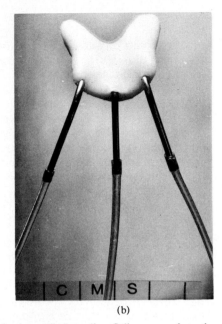

(a)   (b)

Figure 15.6 a, b. Suction cup for the collection of submandibular saliva. Saliva passes down the centre tube, whilst suction is applied from both lateral tubes.

SUBLINGUAL

Segregator appliance

This is the only method (Schneyer, 1955) which has been employed to collect sublingual saliva. It is the same appliance as described above for the submandibular. Hollow chambers are made in the lingual extension overlying the sublingual duct orifices.

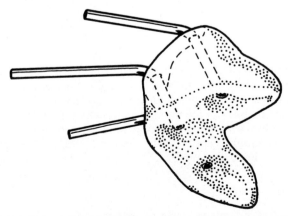

Figure 15.7. Diagram showing internal structure of appliance used to collect saliva from submandibular glands and illustrated in Figure 15.6.

MIXED SALIVA

There is no entirely satisfactory method of collecting 'resting' mixed saliva. In suction and to a lesser extent in spitting methods mechanical stimuli occur. The drainage method can be uncomfortable and inconvenient for some patients, especially those who are elderly or arthritic. Stimulated mixed saliva may be obtained by chewing on inert material such as rubber bands. Mixed saliva contains suspended matter, mostly bacteria, cells and mucoid. If this is not removed it may interfere with analytical techniques and for this reason mixed saliva is usually centrifuged after collection. An additional advantage of centrifugation is that air bubbles and foam are also spun down and the volume can therefore be measured more accurately.

Spitting

The subject is seated with his head inclined forward so that the saliva will collect in the floor of the mouth anteriorly, and he then spits the saliva produced into a collecting filter funnel once per minute for a certain period, depending on the purpose of the investigation (Zaus and Fosdick, 1934; Kerr, 1961). A bench clock with minute hand should be placed in front of the subject in order that he can regulate the spitting procedure himself.

Drainage

The subject again is seated with his head inclined forwards so that the saliva produced will collect anteriorly in the floor of the mouth from where, because of the head position, it will flow out over the lip. The saliva is again collected in a funnel connected to graduated measuring tubes (Becks and Wainwright, 1943; Kerr, 1961). Before starting the collection the subject should swallow all the saliva present in the mouth. At the end he should spit out all the saliva remaining in the mouth to ensure that the viscous minor gland secretion is also obtained.

Suction

The subject is placed with his head tilted slightly anteriorly and supported by a head rest posteriorly. This allows saliva to collect in the floor of the mouth when the mouth is held open and a saliva ejector placed in the anterior region behind the lower incisors. This method has been employed in several large surveys where saliva was being collected for measurement of flow rates or assessment of xerostomia (Faber, 1943; Ostlund, 1953; Schneyer and Levin, 1955; Kerr, 1961; Bertram, 1967).

Cotton wool rolls

A method of collecting mixed saliva for measurement of flow rate only has been described by Razran (1935). Pre-weighed dry cotton wool rolls are placed under the tongue for a two-minute period. The total volume is determined by reweighing and subtracting the dry weight. This method has been used extensively by Peck (1959) in studies of salivary flow in patients with depressive illness.

MINOR SALIVA

Capillary tubes

Saliva from the labial salivary glands may be collected using a technique which has been described by Kutscher et al (1967). The subject's lower lip is everted by an assistant, the mucosa dried with sterile gauze and a conventional dental aspirator placed in the floor of the mouth. A few drops of citric acid (5% solution) are applied to the dorsum of the tongue. Saliva may then be collected using 10 μl capillary tubes ("Microcaps", Drummond Scientific Company, U.S.A.) by capillary attraction (Figure 15.8). The saliva is expelled into weighed tubes which are then reweighed and the volume measured.

It is of interest that the minor salivary glands rapidly become depleted on continued stimulation so that measurable secretion is abolished after 8 to 10 minutes and a recovery phase is necessary before further secretions can be collected (Schneyer, 1956).

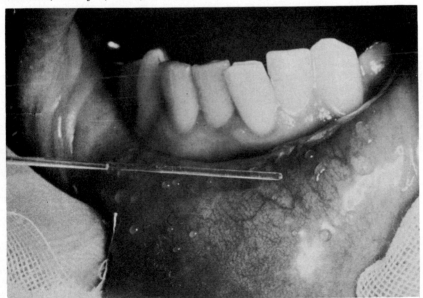

Figure 15.8. Technique employed to collect minor salivary secretion from the lower labial glands, using micro-capillary tubes.

REFERENCES

Becks, H. & Wainwright, W. W. (1943) Rate of flow of resting saliva of healthy individuals. *Journal of Dental Research,* **22,** 391.
Bertram, U. (1967) Xerostomia. *Acta Odontologica Scandinavica,* **25,** Supplement 49.

Block, P. L. & Brottman, S. (1962) À method of submaxillary saliva collection without cannulation. *New York State Dental Journal,* **28,** 116.
Carlson, A. J. & Crittenden, A. Z. (1910) The relation of ptyalin concentrations to the diet and rate of secretion. *American Journal of Physiology,* **26,** 169.
Curby, W. A. (1953) Device for collection of human parotid saliva. *Journal of Laboratory and Clinical Medicine,* **41,** 492.
Faber, M. (1943) The causes of xerostomia. *Acta Medica Scandinavica,* **113,** 69.
Finesinger, J. E. & Finesinger, G. L. (1937) Modification of Krasnogorski method for stimulating and measuring secretion from parotid glands in human beings. *Journal of Laboratory and Clinical Medicine,* **23,** 267.
Gore, J. T. (1938) Saliva and enamel decalcification. II. Saliva Separator. *Journal of Dental Research,* **17,** 69.
Kerr, A. C. (1955) Continuous recording of the rate of flow of parotid secretion in man (Abstract). *Journal of Dental Research,* **34,** 784.
Kerr, A. C. (1961) The physiological regulation of salivary secretion in man. In *International Series of Monographs on Oral Biology.* p. 9. Oxford: Pergamon Press.
Krasnogorski, N. I. (1931) Bedingte undebedingte Reflexe in Kindesalter und ihre Bedeutung für die Klinik. *Ergebnisse der inneren Medizin und Kinderheilkunde,* **39,** 613.
Kutschner, A. H., Mandel, I. D., Zegarelli, E. V., Denning, C., Eriv, A., Ruiz, L., Ellegood, K. & Phalen, J. (1967) A technique for collecting the secretion of minor salivary glands: I. Use of capillary tubes. *Journal of Oral Therapeutics and Pharmacology,* **3,** 391.
Lashley, K. S. (1916) Reflex secretion of the human parotid gland. *Journal of Experimental Psychology,* **1,** 461.
Miller, J. L. (1960) Method of pure parotid saliva collection without cannulisation. *Journal of Dental Research,* **39,** 1075.
Östlund, S. G. (1953) *Palatine Glands and Mucin.* Lund: Berlingska Boktryckeriet.
Peck, R. E. (1959) The S.H.P. Test—an aid in the detection and measurement of depression. *Archives of General Psychiatry* **1,** 35.
Razran, G. H. (1935) Conditioned responses: An experimental study and a theoretical analysis. *Archives of Psychology,* **28,** 1.
Richter, C. P. & Wada, T. (1924) Method of measuring salivary secretions in human beings. *Journal of Laboratory and Clinical Medicine,* **9,** 271.
Schneyer, L. H. (1955) Method for the collection of separate submaxillary and sublingual saliva in man. *Journal of Dental Research,* **34,** 257.
Schneyer, L. H. (1956) Source of resting total mixed saliva in man. *Journal of Applied Physiology,* **9,** 1.
Schneyer, L. H. & Levin, L. E. (1955) Rate of secretion by individual salivary gland pairs in man under two conditions of stimulation. *Journal of Dental Research,* **35,** 725.
Shannon, I. L., Prigmore, J. R. & Chauncey, H. H. (1962) Modified Carlston-Crittenden device for the collection of parotid fluid. *Journal of Dental Research,* **41,** 778.
Stephen, K. W. & Speirs, C. F. (1974) Methods for collection of mixed salivary constituents—the relevance in clinical pharmacology. *British Journal of Clinical Pharmacology.* In press.
Suhara, R. & Asakawa, H. (1959) On the composition of human parotid resting saliva and reflex saliva. *Journal of Nihon University School of Dentistry,* **1,** 153.
Terry, J. L. & Shannon, I. L. (1965) Modification of a self positioning device for the collection of parotid fluid. *Journal of Oral Therapeutics and Pharmacology,* **2,** 32.
Tiedemann, F. & Gmelin, L. (1826) *Récherches Expérimentale Physiologiques et Chimiques sur la Digestion* (trans. Jourdan). Paris: Baillière.
Truelove, E. L., Bixler, D. & Merritt, A. D. (1967) Simplified method for collection of pure submandibular saliva in large volumes. *Journal of Dental Research,* **46,** 1400.
Tsaturov, V. L. (1957) New modifications for the saliva collecting capsule. *Bulletin of Experimental Biology and Medicine U.S.S.R.,* **43,** 124.
Zaus, E. A. & Fosdick, L. S. (1934) Effects of saliva upon gastrin digestion. *Journal of Dental Research,* **14,** 3.

CHAPTER 16

Measurement of Salivary Flow Rate

SALIVARY FLOW RATE

The concentration of many salivary constituents varies with flow rate. Since the original work of Heidenhain (1883) many other workers have confirmed this observation. Some examples of changes in concentration with flow rate are shown in Figure 16.1. The changes which may occur with many salivary constituents are detailed in Tables 3.2 to 3.6 in Chapter 3. When saliva is being collected for analysis, it is therefore important to know whether it has been collected under 'resting' or stimulated conditions. There is probably no true 'resting' secretion of saliva. What most workers mean by this term is saliva collected under conditions of minimal stimulation. However, the term 'resting' is shorter, has a time-honoured usage and, with this reservation, has been used in this text.

Measurement of salivary volume

Before proceeding to discuss the measurement of salivary flow rate, the measurement of salivary volume should first be considered. The method adopted will depend upon the amount of saliva being collected. If small samples of 1 to 2 ml are required, this is accurately measured by weighing the collection bottle or tube before and after. The maximum error involved in assuming that the specific gravity of salivary sections is 1.000 is one per cent (Kerr, 1961). Where larger quantities are involved, graduated tubes or bottles may be used and the volume measured visually.

Measurement of salivary flow rate

In clinical practice, when saliva is collected for the analysis of a constituent, the rate of flow is usually obtained by dividing the volume of saliva secreted in unit time by the duration of the collection period.

Some research workers have devised methods of measuring salivary flow rate automatically. Earlier workers, Lashley (1916) and Krasnogorski (1931), measured the outflow of saliva using drop counters but these had the

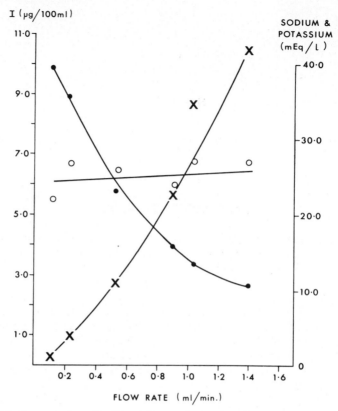

Figure 16.1. Concentration of iodide, sodium and potassium, in parotid saliva collected from one patient at different flow rates. O————O iodide; x————x sodium; ●————● potassium.

disadvantage that saliva coated the electrodes, causing corrosion. Richter and Wada (1924) and Kutscher et al (1964) have described methods whereby the volume of flow is measured along a calibrated tube, but the pattern of flow was not recorded. Kerr (1961) emphasised the desirability of a satisfactory automatic outflow recording method to measure sudden changes in secretion rate. He described two suitable methods, but each had the disadvantage that saliva could not be readily collected for subsequent analysis.

The pattern of salivary flow

If flow rate is measured by dividing the volume of saliva collected in unit time by the duration of the collection period, it cannot be assumed that the flow rate is constant throughout this period. It is well recognised that the flow rate varies with many factors—swallowing, chewing and the rate of application of the stimulus (Kerr, 1961). For example, if 5 ml of saliva are collected in 10 minutes, then the average flow rate is 0.5 ml/min. If 2 ml of this total volume are secreted in one minute and the remaining 3 ml in the other nine minutes, then the saliva collected is a mixture of saliva collected at 2 ml/min and 0.3 ml/min. Depending on the effect of flow rate, this could render inaccurate any comparative measurement of a constituent being carried out. One can only overcome these inaccuracies if the pattern of salivary flow is maintained constant throughout the collecting period.

A technique has been described (Mason et al, 1966), to monitor the pattern of salivary flow and is illustrated in Figures 16.2 and 16.3. The instrument is designed around three identical photo-electric detectors into which are inserted polyethylene catheters conveying saliva from the subject's salivary ducts. Each detector (Figure 16.2) consists of a glass drip chamber (A)

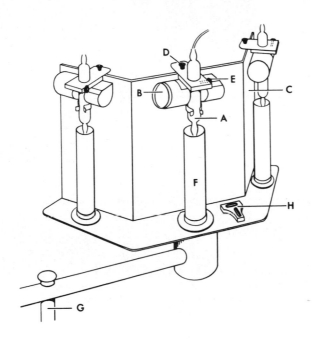

Figure 16.2. Diagram of apparatus for recording pattern of salivary flow. A. Glass drip chamber; B: Perspex housing containing photo-transistor; C: Angled metal plate; D: Perspex slide; E: Screw clamp; F: Collection bottle; G: Stand; H: Spirit level.

screwed to a perspex housing (B) which contains a photo-transistor and a 2.2-volt lens-ended lamp so arranged that the beam of light falling on the photo-transistor is interrupted by the falling drop. The detectors are mounted on an angled metal plate (C) so that each detector is equidistant from the patient's mouth. The stand (G) allows this plate to be positioned both vertically and horizontally to suit each patient. To ensure that the drip chamber is vertical, a spirit level (H) is incorporated in the side of the plate.

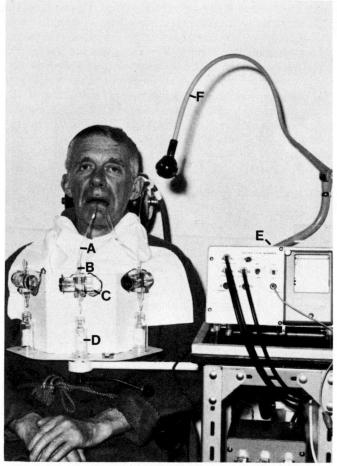

Figure 16.3. The 3-channel photo-electric salivary flowmeter in use. A: Catheter—saliva; B: Glass drip chamber; C: Photo-electric detector; D: Collecting bottle; E: Event recorder; F: Chairside lamp.

The drip chambers are easily interchangeable and can be accurately aligned by means of the perspex slide (D) and finally locked in position by a screw clamp (E). The saliva is collected for analysis in bottles or tubes (F) situated under each drip chamber.

A permanent record of salivary flow is made by the electronic 4-track recorder and examples of drop rate at different regular flow rates are shown in Figure 16.4. The effect of various factors influencing the flow rate is shown in Figure 16.5.

'Resting' and stimulated saliva

The type of saliva which should be collected for a particular investigation varies. 'Resting' saliva can be selected because it is more representative of the

264

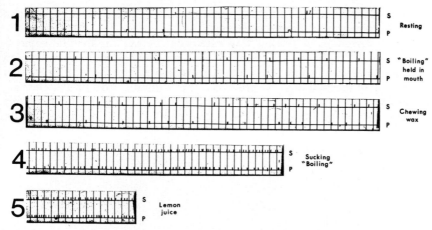

Figure 16.4. Records of parotid and submandibular salivary flow pattern. 1: 'Resting'; 2: Boiled sweet held in mouth; 3: Chewing paraffin wax; 4: Sucking boiled sweet; 5: Lemon juice. S = Submandibular saliva; P = Parotid saliva. Vertical lines on paper correspond to 5-second intervals.

secretion present throughout most of the day and night. Stimulated saliva is required when the functional reserve of a particular gland is being assessed. In order to study the metabolism of a salivary constituent fully, saliva should be collected, at least initially, at a range of flow rates. When the changes with flow rate are known, it may then be quite satisfactory, for comparative

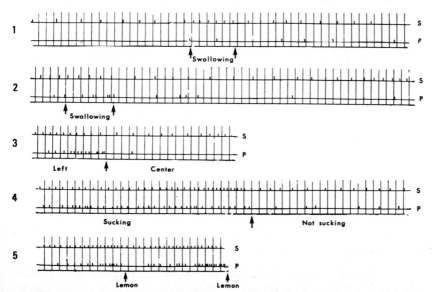

Figure 16.5. Records of parotid and submandibular salivary flow patterns showing irregularities. Tracings read from right to left. 1: Increased rate with swallowing; 2: Residual effect of lemon juice 1½ minutes after stimulus discontinued; 3: Effect of change in intra-oral position of boiled sweet on flow rate; 4: Effect of holding boiled sweet and sucking boiled sweet; 5: Effect of intermittent stimulation with lemon juice. S = Submandibular saliva; P = Parotid saliva.

265

analysis, to collect saliva using one stimulus only in different subjects, or in the same subject on different occasions.

Wide variations in 'resting' flow rate occur between individual subjects and to collect 1 ml of 'resting' parotid saliva may take 30 to 45 minutes. On the other hand, after stimulation, the salivary flow rate varies with the rate of application of the stimulus, the position of the stimulus intra-orally, chewing and swallowing. The remarkable difference in flow rate when chewing on one side and not on the other described by Kerr (1961) is illustrated in Figure 16.6.

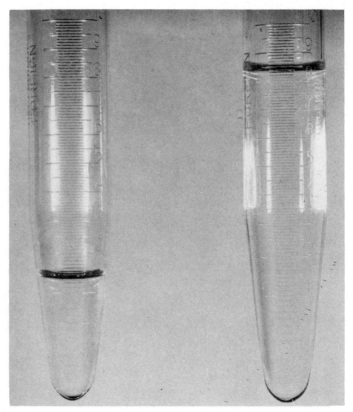

Figure 16.6. Salivary volumes collected from R parotid gland during two five-minute collection periods, chewing fruit gums as the stimulus. A: Chewing on L side only—volume = 1.5 cm³; B: Chewing on R side only—volume = 8.5 cm³.

Salivary stimuli

If stimulated saliva is to be collected, then either secretagogues or gustatory stimuli may be used. Pilocarpine, a parasympathomimetic drug has been given orally (Dawes, 1966), subcutaneously (Kullander and Sonesson, 1965) and intravenously by Curry and Patey (1964). Metacholine similarly has been used (Diamant, Diamant and Holmstedt, 1957; Thaysen, Thorn and Schwartz, 1954). However there are certain drawbacks associated with the use of parasympathomimetic drugs. Baxter (1933) has shown that pilocarpine in dogs is not a suitable physiological stimulus, as lowered concentrations of sodium and potassium occur. Dawes (1966) confirmed Baxter's observations in man and emphasised that pilocarpine stimulation does not reproduce the normal combined parasympathetic and sympathetic balance. Also para-sympathomimetic drugs in sufficient dosage to produce very high flow rates may produce undesirable side effects such as flushing, palpations, colicky abdominal pains and an urgent desire to micturate.

One problem associated with the collection of saliva for analysis is the possible occurrence of 'rest transients'. It has been observed that the concentration of potassium in saliva secreted at the start of a period of stimulation was greater than the concentration found after secretion had continued for a minute or two (Kestyüs and Martin, 1937). This phenomenon has been demonstrated for potassium and iodide in the dog submaxillary gland (Burgen and Seeman, 1958) and in the human parotid gland by Dawes (1967). It is important therefore to flush out stagnant secretions with a few drops of lemon juice and the saliva collected for a period of 15 minutes initially should be discarded, to avoid salivary rest transients. Also, it is necessary to apply stimuli for at least two minutes before the collection of an actual sample is started.

It is possible using different types of gustatory stimuli to produce a graded flow rate response as first described by Dawes and Jenkins (1964), and as demonstrated in Figure 16.7a and b. In this way, the concentration of a salivary constituent may be observed at different flow rates.

Clinical tests of gland function

Tests of gland function solely concerned with flow rate have been described using both parasympathomimetic drugs and gustatory stimuli.

Curry and Patey (1964) described a test of parotid function using intravenous pilocarpine. Its value in measurement of salivary function in 86 patients has been described by Sewards, Hamilton and Patey (1966). If analysis of salivary constituents as well as flow rate measurements are to be carried out, one has to realise the changes in salivary constituents which occur in pilocarpine-stimulated saliva referred to earlier in this chapter.

In some disease states, e.g. occult heart disease, pilocarpine would obviously be contra-indicated. For these reasons, the authors believe gustatory stimuli are to be preferred.

A suitable clinical test, using 5 per cent citric acid as a stimulus, is as follows:
1. The subject is seated comfortably in a dental chair and the procedure explained to him.
2. The collection device is applied. Five drops of 5 per cent citric acid solution are dropped on the tongue from a 10-ml disposable syringe to flush out stagnant secretions for 15 minutes to avoid rest transients.
3. Saliva is then collected under 'resting' conditions for 30 minutes, and after 5 per cent citric acid stimulation for two minutes. The citric acid is

267

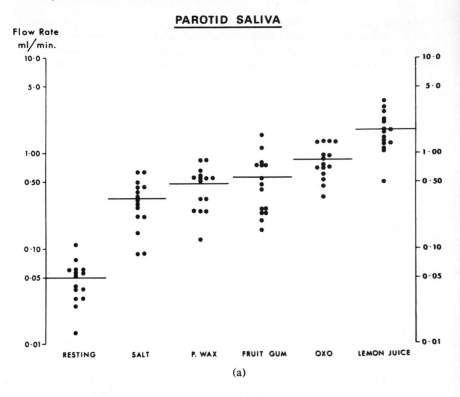

(a)

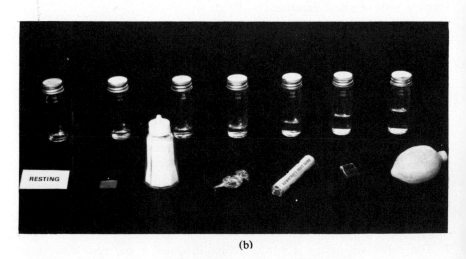

(b)

Figure 16.7. a. Salivary flow rate (log scale) under resting conditions and in response to various stimuli in 15 normal subjects. b. Stimuli used to produce different salivary flow rates: paraffin wax, salt, boiled sweet, fruit gums, Oxo, and lemon juice. The volumes of saliva collected in the same time period (5 minutes) in one subject are also shown.

268

Table 16.1. *Mean parotid salivary flow rates in normal subjects (ml/min).*

Age range (years)	Resting		Fruit gum		Lemon juice	
	Male	Female	Male	Female	Male	Female
<20 {18 M / 8 F	0.061±0.007 (0.02 —0.12)	0.083±0.02 (0.04 —0.16)	0.66±0.06 (0.36—1.07)	0.46±0.07 (0.27—0.80)	1.49±0.09 (0.60—2.10)	1.99±0.14 (1.25—2.50)
21-40 {20 M / 20 F	0.104±0.008 (0.06 —0.20)	0.09 ±0.01 (0.01 —0.19)	0.47±0.03 (0.32—0.85)	0.50±0.05 (0.09—1.04)	1.73±0.09 (0.85—2.99)	1.76±0.09 (1.03—2.70)
41-60 {27 M / 31 F	0.078±0.02 (0.01 —0.31)	0.064±0.01 (0.01 —0.34)	0.59±0.08 (0.15±1.76)	0.52±0.05 (0.13—1.15)	1.68±0.11 (0.85—3.20)	1.36±0.12 (0.50—3.02)
>61 {14 M / 31 F	0.084±0.02 (0.03 ±0.20)	0.06 ±0.02 (0.01 —0.5)	0.050±0.08 0.15—1.26)	0.43±0.03 (0.14—0.83)	1.58±0.16 (0.90—2.76)	1.15±0.08 (0.47—2.20)

Mean ± Standard error of the mean (S.E.M.).
Ranges indicated in parenthesis.

applied for at least one minute before the collection of the stimulated sample is commenced.

Using this method in over 170 subjects, normal values for resting and stimulated saliva have been defined (Table 16.1). The importance of age and sex on normal values is apparent and it is important that these parameters should be considered when interpreting salivary flow rates in disease states.

It is worthy of note, as Ericson (1969) has pointed out, that the results obtained from different sialometric methods are not comparable because individuals with a high secretory response to one stimulus do not necessarily have the same to another. Therefore, in clinical examinations of the salivary glands, standardisation of the stimuli to a limited number of internationally acceptable methods would be of great scientific value (Ericson, 1969).

REFERENCES

Baxter, H. (1933) Variations in the inorganic constituents of mixed and parotid saliva activated by reflex stimulation in the dog. *Journal of Biological Chemistry,* **102,** 203.

Burgen, A. S. V. & Seeman, P. (1958) The role of the salivary duct system in the formation of saliva. *Canadian Journal of Biochemistry and Physiology,* **36,** 119.

Chisholm, D. M. (1970) *The Salivary Glands in Connective Tissue Disease.* Ph.D. Thesis, University of Glasgow.

Curry, R. C. & Patey, D. H. (1964) A clinical test for parotid function. *British Journal of Surgery,* **51,** 891.

Dawes, C. (1966) The composition of human saliva secreted in response to a gustatory stimulus and to pilocarpine. *Journal of Physiology,* **183,** 360.

Dawes, C. (1967) The effect of flow rate and length of stimulation on the protein concentration in human parotid saliva. *Archives of Oral Biology,* **12,** 783.

Dawes, C. & Jenkins, G. N. (1964) The effects of different stimuli on the composition of saliva in man. *Journal of Physiology,* **170,** 86.

Diamant, B., Diamant, H. & Holmstedt, B. (1957) The salivary secretion in man under the influence of intravenously infused acetyl-beta-methylocholine iodide. *Archives Internationales de Pharmacodynamie et de Therapie,* **3,** 86.

Ericson, S. (1969) An investigation of human parotid saliva secretion rate in response to different types of stimulation. *Archives of Oral Biology,* **14,** 591.

Heidenhain, R. (1883) Physiologie der Absonderungsvorgange. In *Handbuch der Physiologie* (Ed.) Hermann, L. Vol. 5, Part I, 14. Leipzig: Vogel.

Kerr, A. C. (1961) The physiological regulation of salivary secretion in man. In *International Series of Monographs on Oral Biology.* Oxford: Pergamon Press.

Kestyüs, L. & Martin, J. (1937) Uber den Einfluss von Chorda und Sympathicusreizung aug die Zusammensetzung des Submaxillarspeichels. *Pflugers Archiv für diegesemte Physiologie des Menschen und der Tiere,* **239,** 408.

Krasnogorski, N. I. (1931) Bedingte undbedingte Reflexe in Kindesalter und ihre Bedeutung für die Klinik. *Ergebnisse der inneren Medizin und Kinderheilkunde,* **39,** 613.

Kullander, S. & Sonesson, B. (1965) Studies on saliva in menstruating, pregnant and post menopausal women. *Acta Endocrinologica,* **48,** 329.

Kutscher, A. H., Zegarelli, E. V., Wotman, S., Mandel, I. & Goldstein, J. (1964) A new saliva collection technique: for more accurate determination of salivary flow rate. *New York State Dental Journal,* **30,** 63.

Lashley, K. S. (1916) Reflex secretion of the human parotid gland. *Journal of Experimental Psychology,* **1,** 461.

Mason, D. K., Harden, R. McG., Rowan, D. & Alexander, W. D. (1966) Recording the pattern of salivary flow. *Journal of Dental Research,* **45,** 1458.

Richter, C. P. & Wada, T. (1924) Method of measuring salivary secretions in human beings. *Journal of Laboratory and Clinical Medicine,* **9,** 271.

Sewards, H. F. G., Hamilton, D. I. & Patey, D. H. (1966) An investigation of the value in clinical practice of the Curry test for parotid function. *British Journal of Surgery,* **53,** 190.

Thaysen, J. H., Thorn, N. A. & Schwartz, I. L. (1954) Excretion of sodium, potassium, chloride and carbon dioxide in human parotid saliva. *American Journal of Physiology,* **178,** 155.

CHAPTER 17

Radiology and Sialography

RADIOLOGY

Because of the superficial position of the glands, radiological examination is particularly suitable for the investigation of salivary gland disease. Plain films are helpful in the diagnosis of calculi in the submandibular and parotid glands and ducts. There are several views favoured by different radiologists, depending on the site of the calculus. These are demonstrated in Figures 17.1 to 17.4. Calculi may be wholly or partially radiolucent and sialography is helpful in these circumstances.

SIALOGRAPHY

Sialography is the term used to describe radiography of the salivary glands whose duct system has been filled with a radiopaque contrast medium. It was introduced as a diagnostic procedure by Bársony (1925) and Uslenghi (1925), each working independently, in 1925. Adequate demonstration of the duct system and, where possible, the acini, form the essential part of the examination. As in other radiographic methods, a high degree of diagnostic accuracy can only be obtained if clinical and radiological findings are considered together.

Some modifications to the original hand injection technique described by Bársony have been made. Fine rubber catheters were used instead of metal cannulae by Putney and Shapiro (1950) and tapered polyethylene tubing by Liverud (1959). Early workers used barium suspensions and potassium iodide which were replaced by fat soluble media (e.g. Lipiodol). Because of the relatively high viscosity, these media were expelled from the ducts slowly over a period of one to three days (Ollerenshaw and Rose, 1951). The vehicle of 'Lipiodol' poppy seed oil has irritant properties and foreign body reactions have been described in dogs (Epsteen and Bendix, 1954). Recently water soluble contrast media have been available but were not widely used initially because of their low viscosity and rapid emptying time from ducts. It was necessary, therefore, to use a 'closed system' of hand injection technique; the needle or catheter being maintained in position while the radiographs were

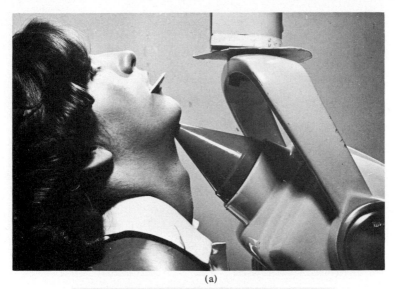

(a)

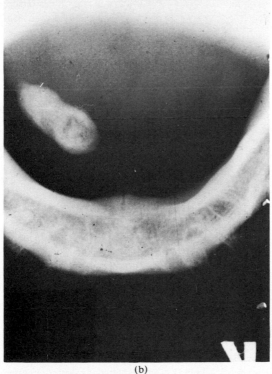

(b)

Figure 17.1. Radiographic localisation of submandibular calculus in the anterior part of the duct. a. Patient in position with occlusal plane 50° to the horizontal. Central ray—20° in midline under and behind chin. Occlusal film, centrally placed as far back as possible. b. Radiograph demonstrating calculus in anterior part of duct.

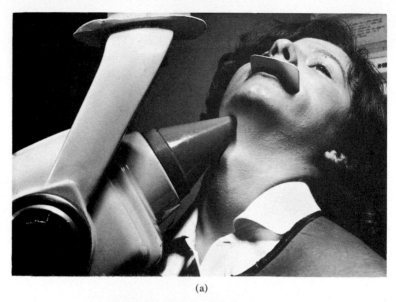

(a)

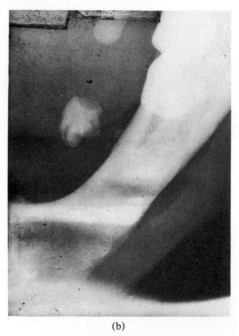

(b)

Figure 17.2. Radiographic localisation of submandibular calculus in posterior part of the duct.
a. Patient in position with occlusal plane 45° to horizontal and mid-sagittal plane 45° to
opposite (unaffected) side. The central ray—30°, directed under the 2nd premolar of the
affected side towards the opposite side. The film is placed centrally in the occlusal plane. b.
Radiograph demonstrating calculi in mid and posterior parts of the duct.

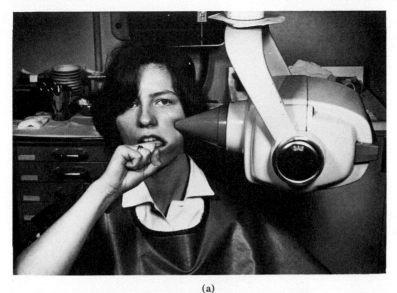

(a)

(b)

Figure 17.3. Radiographic localisation of calculus in parotid duct. a. Patient in position, occlusal plane horizontal and mid-sagittal plane vertical. Central ray horizontal (0°) directed through cheek to 1st molar area. A peri-apical film is held in position by the patient against the cheek intra-orally, centred to the parotid duct orifice. b. Radiograph demonstrating parotid duct calculus.

275

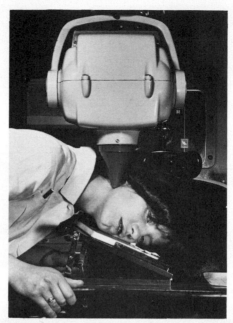

(a)

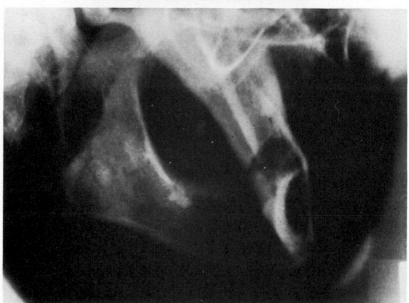

(b)

Figure 17.4. Radiographic localisation of calculus in parotid duct. a. Patient in position with head placed on the film with chin extended forward, and the lower border of the mandible on the affected side parallel to the edge of the cassette. A 5 inch $\times$ 7 inch film is placed in the 25° angle board. The central ray is directed vertically (90°), 1 inch below the angle of the mandible of the opposite side towards the molar region of the affected side. b. Radiograph demonstrating parotid duct calculus.

276

exposed (Rubin and Holt, 1957). Gullmo and Böök-Hederstrom (1957) described a hydrostatic technique in which the contrast medium was allowed to flow into the gland using only the force of gravity. Modifications of this method have been described by Drevattne and Stiris (1964) and Park and Mason (1966).

Sialography has been used by the authors as one of the screening tests in patients suspected of having Sjögren's syndrome. It was clear early in these investigations that the conventional method of performing sialography, i.e. by hand injection technique, was unsatisfactory. In diseased glands where destructive changes have occurred the salivary ducts may be more friable and the pain sensation normally felt when the ducts are distended may be absent in some patients. Thus, overdistension and extravasation of radiopaque medium into the surrounding tissues is a not infrequent occurrence with hand injection techniques. Figure 17.5 demonstrates the retention of contrast medium in the adjacent tissues in a patient with Sjögren's syndrome who presented with a history of sialography six months previously (Figure 17.5).

Ideally for sialography, the radiopaque contrast medium should have similar physical characteristics to saliva and the water soluble contrast media are therefore more suitable than the preparations previously used. It should be introduced into the duct at a constant pressure just greater than the secreting pressure of the salivary gland. Hand injection techniques, except perhaps in the most experienced hands, allow only crude control of the pressure which makes any standardisation difficult and may cause artefacts. The secreting pressure in a group of 18 subjects has been measured by Mason (1966), as shown in Table 17.1. As a result of these findings Park and Mason (1966) suggested 70 to 90 cm of H_2O as a suitable pressure for the contrast medium to be introduced.

Table 17.1. *Secreting pressures (cm of H_2O) of parotid and submandibular glands under 'resting' and stimulated conditions in 18 adult subjects.*

	Parotid		Submandibular	
	'Resting	Stimulated	'Resting'	Stimulated
Range	0-40	54-72	12-25	58-74
Mean	16.4	63.5	17.1	69.6
S.E.M.	2.48	1.41	0.97	1.26

In summary, while recognising that some radiologists have through their experience obtained excellent results with hand injection techniques, we would advocate the hydrostatic method for the following reasons:
1. Constant pressure is obtained during the introduction of the radiopaque medium and overfilling is a rare occurrence as compared with the hand injection technique.
2. As films are exposed during the filling phase, no reflux of contrast medium occurs.
3. A water-soluble contrast medium can be used which is rapidly expelled from the duct system. One gland examination including the emptying

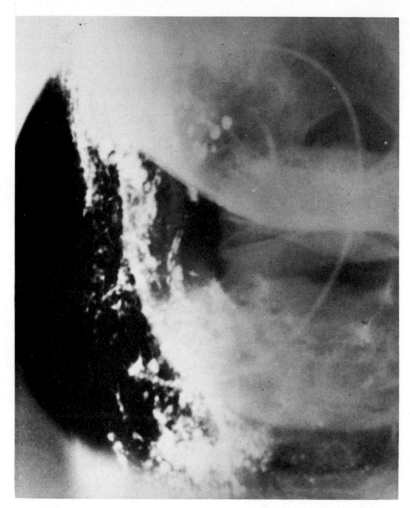

Figure 17.5. Retention of contrast medium in tissues around parotid and submandibular glands. Patient with Sjögren's syndrome reported having had sialographic examination six months previously by hand injection technique.

phase takes 15 to 20 minutes and several glands may be examined at the one visit. In comparison, contrast media containing iodised oils are retained for one to three days (Schultz and Weisberger, 1947; Ollerenshaw and Rose, 1951).

INDICATIONS AND CONTRA-INDICATIONS FOR SIALOGRAPHY

Sialography is a useful technique in the diagnosis of calculi (especially radio-lucent stones), duct strictures, chronic inflammatory conditions, fistulae and neoplastic disease of the salivary glands.

278

Contra-indications are few but important. Sialography is contra-indicated in any acute sialadenitis of whatever cause; also, although uncommonly, when there is a history of allergy to iodine, as this is a main constituent of the radiopaque contrast medium.

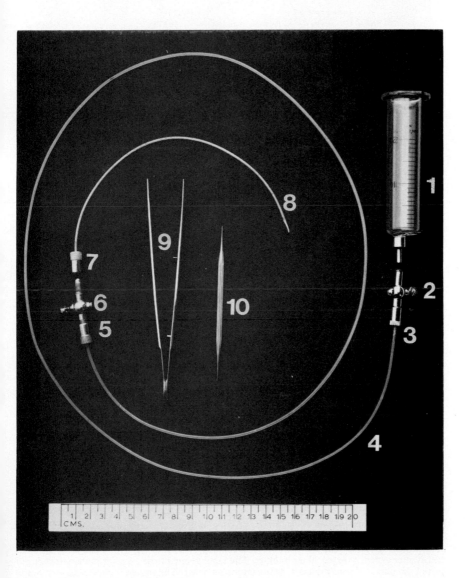

Figure 17.6. Instrumentation for hydrostatic sialography. 1: 20 cm³ glass syringe barrel; 2: Adapter; 3: Cap; 4: Portex polythene tubing P.E. 205; 5: Cap; 6: Adapter; 7: Cap; 8: Portex polythene tubing P.E. 160, tapered at one end; 9: Tissue forceps, non-toothed; 10: Lacrimal probe dilator.

279

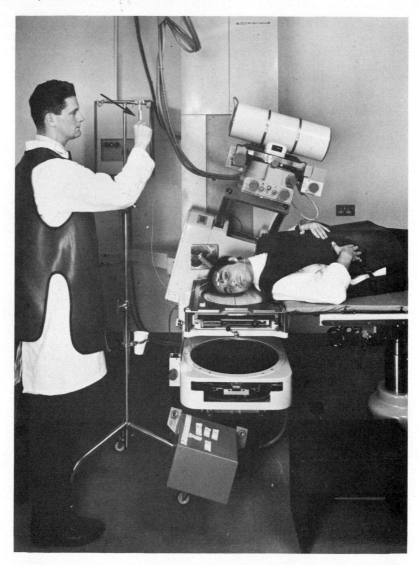

Figure 17.7. Apparatus assembled prior to sialography. a. Passive filling phase: With the apparatus assembled and the patient lying horizontally on an Elema-Schonander Skull Table, the syringe barrel (arrowed) is filled with contrast. The contrast is allowed to run freely through the catheter system to expel all air bubbles. The tapered end of the catheter is then introduced 0.5 to 1 cm into the salivary duct. b. Active emptying phase: The patient is given a slice of lemon to suck immediately after the passive phase exposures have been completed and the catheter removed from the duct. After a 5-minute period a further two exposures are made—postero-anterior and lateral oblique of the parotid gland region and a lateral view of the submandibular gland. If the gland is functioning normally no contrast medium should be demonstrated.

METHOD

Descriptions of hand injection techniques are available in standard textbooks and we have no recent direct experience of them. During the past five years we have used a hydrostatic method and this will now be described in detail.

EQUIPMENT (Figure 17.6)

A 20 cm³ glass syringe barrel.
Two catheters: (1) Portex polythene tubing P.E. 205 100 cm in length.
                  (2) Portex polythene tubing P.E. 160, finely tapered at one end, 25 cm in length.
Two metal connectors.
Adaptors and tap for polythene tubing, size P.E. 205 with Luer-Lock fitting.
Adaptor and tap especially designed with a screw cap to fit tubing P.E. 205 at one end and to take tubing P.E. 160 at the other end.
Lacrimal probe dilator.
Elema-Schonander skull table.
No. 13 cone with slit diaphragm.
8 × 6 Ilford Blue brand film with fast tungstate screen.
Conroy 280 or other similar water soluble contrast medium (May and Baker, Ltd., Dagenham, Essex, England).
Slices of fresh lemon.

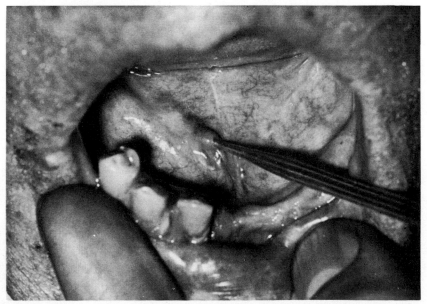

Figure 17.8. Dilation of the submandibular duct orifice using a lacrimal probe dilator, prior to catheterisation.

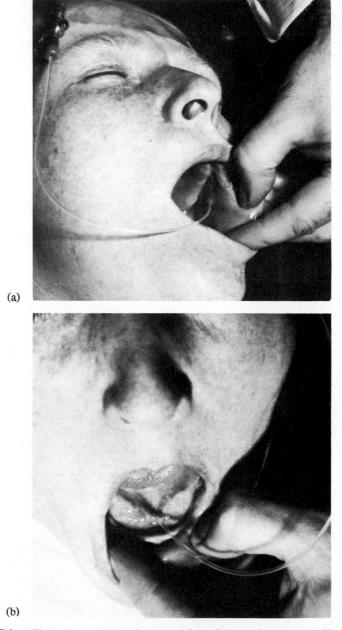

(a)

(b)

Figure 17.9. a. The catheter has been introduced for a distance of about 1 cm. The elasticity of the soft tissues around the orifice holds the catheter in position and prevents leakage. The catheter is looped round the face and taped to the forehead to avoid superimposition over the parotid gland. b. The submandibular duct orifice has been dilated, and the catheter lies about 0.5 cm within the duct. This patient is edentulous and in these cases the cannulation of the duct is easier.

SIALOGRAPHIC METHOD

1. Passive filling phase. With the apparatus assembled, the syringe barrel is filled with contrast material and set at a height of 70 to 90 cm above the level of the patient's mouth (Figure 17.7). The medium is allowed to run through the catheter system freely to expel all air bubbles. The duct orifice is located with a lacrimal probe and, where necessary, gently dilated (Figure 17.8). The tapered end of the catheter is then introduced 0.5 to 1 cm into the duct (Figure 17.9) and the patient asked to grip the catheter gently with the lips (Figure 17.10). Before commencing the examination, it is briefly explained to the patient, who is asked to indicate when discomfort or pain is felt, by raising the right hand. At this point, the exposure is made at once while the contrast agent is flowing. The tap is then closed to prevent unnecessary distention of the gland. The same procedure is repeated for each view. The short catheter may then be replaced by a fresh one and contrast material run through it. The apparatus is then ready for the next examination.

2. Active emptying phase. The patient is given a slice of lemon to suck immediately after the passive filling phase is completed, and the catheter is removed from the mouth. After a five-minute interval, further exposures are obtained. A normal secretory phase film shows no evidence of residual contrast medium.

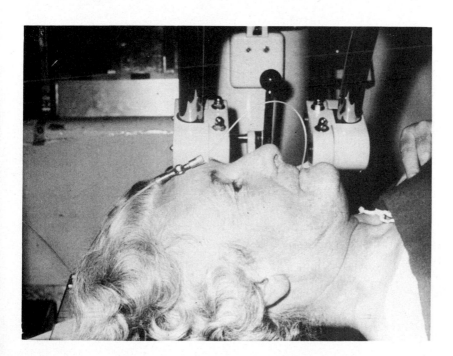

Figure 17.10. Patient in supine position, prior to sialography. Valve and catheter are strapped to patient's forehead, whilst extension of catheter is held by lip pressure.

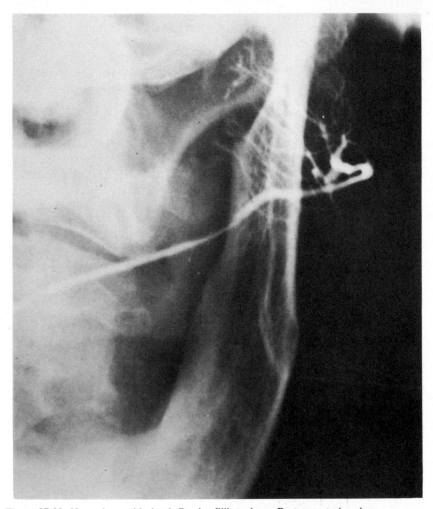

Figure 17.11. Normal parotid gland. Passive filling phase. Postero-anterior view.

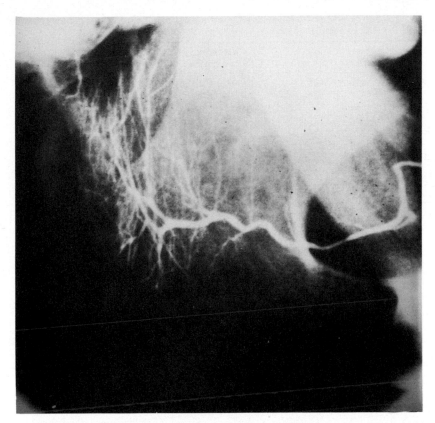

Figure 17.12. Normal parotid gland. Passive filling phase. Lateral view.

Examples of the results obtained in normal and pathological glands are shown in Figures 17.11 to 17.18. The results obtained by this method in large groups of patients in Glasgow have been described by Blair (1973) and are summarised in Tables 17.2, 17.3 and 17.4.

PROBLEMS ENCOUNTERED USING THE HYDROSTATIC TECHNIQUE

These were encountered in a large series of over 700 patients (Blair, 1973). They included the occasional patient who was unable to control his tongue movements sufficiently and dislodged the polyethylene catheter from the duct orifice. Underfilling in the apprehensive patient and overfilling in the stoic or less sensitive occurred in a few patients. In only eight of 746 patients in Blair's series was sialography unsuccessful; in five patients this was due to duct orifice obstruction and in the remaining three it was because of involuntary tongue movements causing catheter displacement (Blair, 1973).

285

Table 17.2. *The parotid gland: the ages and sex of the patients examined, the glands examined, and the volumes of contrast medium needed to outline them* (Blair, 1973).

	Total	M	F	Age (years) Range	Mean	R	L	Volume (ml) Range	Mean
All cases	657	187	470	8-94	(51)	282	375	0.1-3.0	(0.8)
Normal	439	127	312	8.94	(52)	181	257	0.2-3.0	(0.8)
Abnormal	218	60	158	8-82	(49)	101	118	0.1-3.0	(0.8)
Normal local	93	30	63	16-74	(49)	43	50	0.2-2.0	(0.8)
Normal general	346	97	249	8-94	(53)	138	208	0.2-3.0	(0.7)
Abnormal local	96	46	50	8-74	(46)	51	45	0.1-3.0	(0.9)
Abnormal general	122	14	108	15-82	(51)	50	72	0.2-2.0	(0.7)

Table 17.3. *The submandibular gland: the ages and sex of the patients examined, the glands examined, and the volumes of contrast medium needed to outline them* (Blair, 1973).

	Total	M	F	Age (years) Range	Mean	R	L	Volume (ml) Range	Mean
All cases	81	26	55	16-73	(45)	38	43	0.2-2.5	(0.9)
Normal	32	11	21	16-72	(42)	15	17	0.2-2.0	(0.9)
Abnormal	49	15	34	18-73	(23)	23	26	0.2-2.5	(0.8)

Table 17.4. *Analysis of sialographic findings in patients referred with pain and/or swelling in the region of a major salivary gland* (Blair, 1973).

	Normal	Inflam- matory	Fistulas	Space occupying lesions	Obstructive Radio- lucent calculi	Radio- paque calculi	Stricture or stenosis
All cases	125	75	5	11	15	18	21
Parotid	93	57	5	10	11	6	7
Submandibular	32	18	—	1	4	12	14

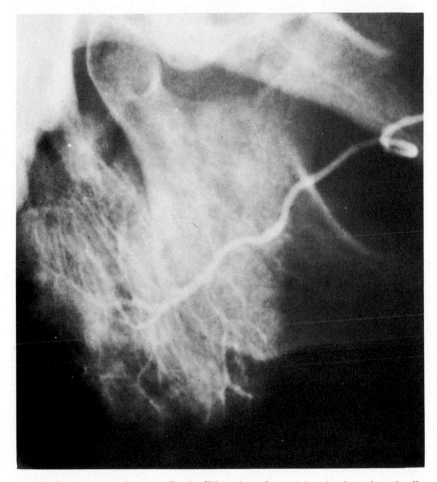

Figure 17.13. Normal parotid gland. Passive filling phase. Lateral view showing acinar clouding.

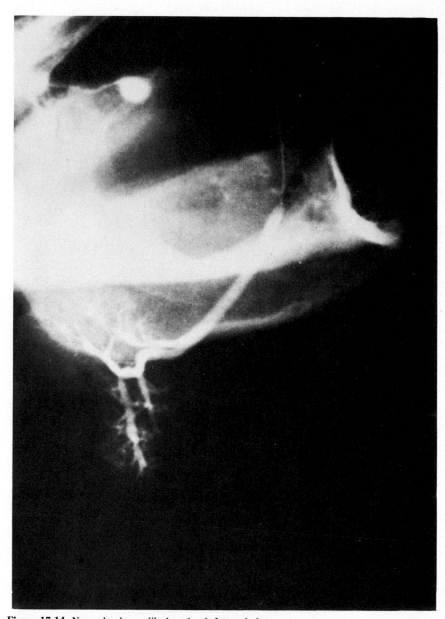

Figure 17.14. Normal submandibular gland. Lateral view.

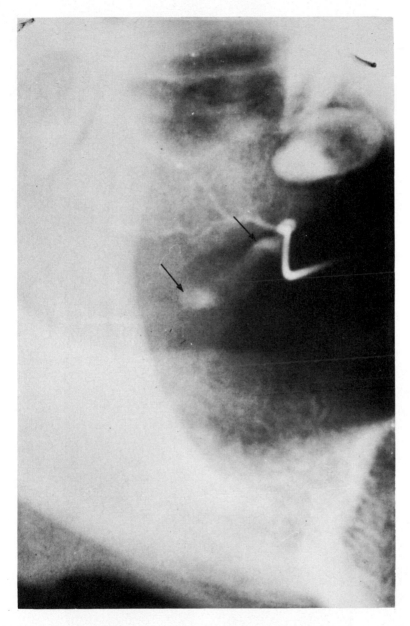

Figure 17.15. Parotid sialogram. This is an example of where sialography was unnecessary. Plain film would have revealed this calculus. Lateral oblique view.

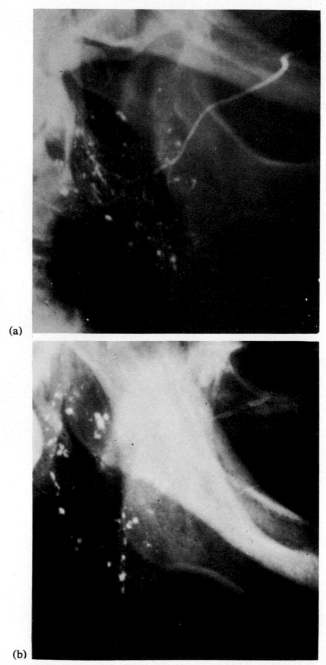

(a)

(b)

Figure 17.16. Sjögren's syndrome. a. Lateral view of the filling phase reveals poor peripheral duct filling and punctate contrast collections of 'mulberry bush' type, indicating moderate changes of the disease. b. Lateral view in the secretory phase, showing characteristic retention of contrast agent in the punctate areas after the main ducts have emptied.

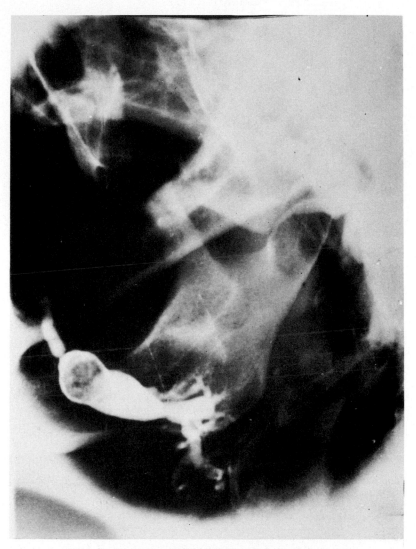

Figure 17.17. Large submandibular calculus. The water soluble radiopaque contrast medium outlines the calculus, the dilated duct system posteriorly extending into the submandibular gland itself.

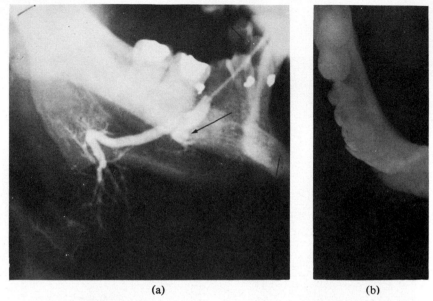

(a)   (b)

Figure 17.18. Small submandibular calculus. a. The submandibular duct is dilated, and a calculus (arrowed) is lodged at the junction with the sublingual duct. b. Occlusal view showing the calculus in the floor of the mouth.

REFERENCES

Bársony, T. (1925) Idiopathische stenongang—dilation. *Klinische Wochenschrift,* **52,** 2500.

Blair, G. S. (1973) Hydrostatic sialography. *Oral Surgery, Oral Medicine and Oral Pathology,* **36,** 116.

Drevattne, T. & Stiris, G. (1964) Sialography by means of a polyethylene catheter and water soluble contrast medium. *British Journal of Radiology,* **37,** 317.

Epsteen, C. M. & Bendix, R. (1954) Effect of non volatile substances on salivary glands in sialography. *Journal of Plastic and Reconstructive Surgery,* **13,** 299.

Gullmo, A. & Böök Hederstrom, G. (1957) A method of sialography. *Acta Radiologica (Stockholm),* **49,** 17.

Liverud, K. (1959) Sialographic technique with a polythene catheter. *British Journal of Radiology,* **32,** 627.

Mason, D. K. (1966) *Studies in Salivary Glands and their Secretions in Health and Disease.* M.D. Thesis, University of Glasgow.

Ollerenshaw, R. G. W. & Rose, S. S. (1951) Radiological diagnosis of salivary gland disease. *British Journal of Radiology,* **24,** 538.

Park, W. M. & Mason, D. K. (1966) Hydrostatic sialography. *Radiology,* **86,** 116.

Putney, F. J. & Shapiro, M. J. (1950) Sialography. *Archives of Otolaryngology,* **51,** 526.

Rubin, P. & Holt, J. F. (1957) Secretory sialography in diseases of the major salivary glands. *American Journal of Roentgenology,* **77,** 575.

Schultz, M. D. & Weisberger, D. (1947) Sialograms in the diagnosis of swelling about the salivary glands. *Surgical Clinics in North America,* **27,** 1156.

Uslenghi, J. P. (1925) Nueva technica para la investigacion radiologica de las glandulas salivaires. *Revista de la Sociedad Argentina de Radiologica Electrologia,* **1,** 4.

CHAPTER 18

Radio-isotopes and Salivary Gland Function

It is probably a fair analogy to compare the use of radio-active materials or radio-isotopes at the present time to the situation with regard to the introduction of x-rays into clinical medicine and dentistry earlier in this century. Since radio-isotopes were first used in clinical tests in 1937 they have been more and more widely applied to the investigation of disease and the subsequent development of the subject has resulted in the creation of the specialty of Nuclear Medicine. Although the equipment and facilities required for radio-isotopic tests are expensive, they are becoming available in many countries. The reason why radio-active materials are of use in diagnostic work is simply because of two basic properties. Firstly, they emit radiations which can be detected and are measurable; secondly radio-isotopes have the same chemical properties as their stable chemical counterparts.

As far as salivary glands are concerned, investigative tests have been of two types:
1. Those in which isotopes have been detected and measured in saliva;
2. Those in which uptake of the isotopes by the salivary glands has been detected within the glands themselves.

RADIO-ISOTOPES IN SALIVA

Measurement of the concentration of salivary radio iodine has been used in investigation of patients with defects in iodide trapping (Chapter 10). In patients with Sjögren's syndrome low saliva/plasma ratios have been demonstrated by Mason, Harden and Alexander (1967). The most common use of salivary radio iodine in investigation has been in the routine measurement of the plasma inorganic iodine in patients with thyroid disease. The basis of this test is as follows. The inorganic iodine in the plasma is too small a concentration to measure directly. After a tracer dose of ^{132}I is given orally, the specific activity of iodine is the same in plasma and saliva. That is:

$$\frac{^{132}I \text{ plasma}}{I \text{ plasma}} = \frac{^{132}I \text{ saliva}}{I \text{ saliva}}$$

Inorganic iodide is concentrated in the saliva to many times the plasma level; it therefore is large enough to be measured directly. It is thus possible to determine from the above equation the iodide in the plasma, that is:

$$I \text{ plasma} = \frac{^{132}I \text{ plasma} \times I \text{ saliva}}{^{132}I \text{ saliva}}$$

Clinical studies using this technique have been reported by Harden, Mason and Buchanan (1965a, b), Wayne (1967) and Mason, Harden and Alexander (1967).

Other isotopes, which have similar biological properties to iodine and also members of the 7th Periodic Group, such as $^{99m}TcO_4$, ^{82}Br, have been used in studies of thyroid and salivary concentrating mechanisms (Harden et al, 1968; Stephen et al, 1973; Lazarus et al, 1973).

Other radio-isotopes which have been measured in saliva in various investigations are as follows: ^{42}K, ^{86}Rb, ^{131}Cs, which have been used in ionic exchange experiments in animals and humans; and ^{18}F, used in studies of fluoride distribution and excretion and deposition in teeth.

The radio-activity of the salivary sample is counted in an automatic scintillation counter. A standard containing an aliquot of the initial dose is also counted. Sample counts are corrected for background and for radio-active decay between counting of sample and standard. Activities of plasma and saliva may be expressed as percentage of dose per ml of sample.

RADIO-ISOTOPES IN SALIVARY GLANDS AND SALIVA

There has been a great deal of interest recently in the use of gamma radio-isotopic visualisation of salivary glands as a test of function (Gates and Work, 1967; Harden et al, 1967, 1968; Stephen et al, 1971). The basis of these methods is that according to their physiological and metabolic function organs and tissues may contain different concentrations of a suitable isotope after it has been administered as a clinical tracer. This difference in radio-activity between an organ and surrounding tissues can be recorded and charted using a rectilinear scintiscanner or gamma camera.

Using this principle various isotopes have been used to visualise many different organs including brain, liver, kidney, spleen, pancreas, stomach, bone, lymph nodes, lungs and placenta (Mallard, 1966). Scanning can thus be used as an additional diagnostic aid in the detection of disease or of a tumour mass within an organ. It may also be of value in the location of tumour metastases. Because of its iodide concentrating ability the thyroid gland is particularly suitable and scanning is now a standard technique in the diagnosis of thyroid disease. Until recently, the measurement of the uptake of radio-isotopes in the salivary glands was not possible because of the high background radio-activity in the neck region. However, with the development of isotope scanning techniques, one can now quantitate the amount of isotope in the glands, and also observe its distribution within them. [99m]Tc pertechnetate is used in preference to radio-isotopes of iodine because of its shorter biological half-life and very low radiation dosage to the tissues.

More recently an alternative to the scintiscanner, the gamma camera, has been used by some workers (Sorsdahl, Williams and Bruno, 1969; Schall et al, 1971). The technique is essentially the same but instead of the scanner head moving backwards and forwards across the head and neck area the gamma camera records the whole field at once.

Clinical studies using these tests have been reported by Harden et al (1967), Veronesi, Cascinelli and Damascelli (1967), Grove and Di Chiro (1968), Stebner et al (1968), Abramson et al (1969), Stephen et al (1971), Szabo and Laudenbach (1971), Schall et al (1971) and Fourestier et al (1973).

The main uses for radio-isotope visualisation using either the scanner or the gamma camera have been in the assessment of:
1. Physiological function, e.g. comparing the function of the parotid and submandibular glands.
2. Pathological function, e.g. observing local or generalised decrease or increase in function as in tumours or Sjögren's syndrome.
3. The localisation of ectopic tissue, e.g. determining whether a lump in the neck is of thyroid or salivary origin.

A full description of the two current methods in use, scintigraphy and the gamma camera, will now be given.

Method

The patient to be studied is placed comfortably in position on the scanner table, or in front of the gamma camera. In order to avoid head and neck movement a head rest is used. For both scanner or gamma camera (scintigraphy), a 1 mCi sample of ^{99m}Tc labelled sodium pertechnetate is injected intravenously in an arm vein, though doses up to 10 mCi may be used.

Scanning

A Selo DS4/4 superscanner or other rectilinear scanner is used to scan the subject in the antero-posterior position over an area between the bridge of the nose and cricoid cartilage which includes all the salivary glands; scans commence at 1 min, 6 min and 11 min after the tracer dose, each scan taking approximately 4 min. A line spacing of 4 mm and a scan speed of 20 mm/sec is used. A sample of the dose solution is scanned under identical conditions. Slow scans more suitable for visualisation are obtained by adjusting the speed to 10 mm/sec and the line spacing to 2 mm. Such scans take approximately 20 min. The technique is demonstrated in Figure 18.1 and

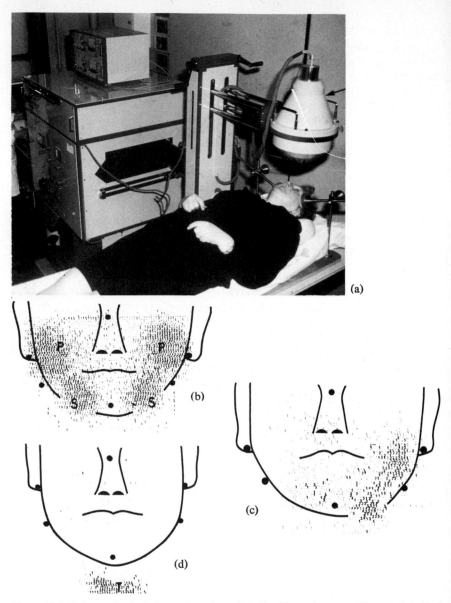

Figure 18.1. Salivary gland scintiscanning using a Selo Rectilinear Scanner. All scans described are 20 to 40 mins post ^{99m}Tc injection i.v. Solid circles represent anatomical landmarks used in aligning the detector head.

a. Patient in position for antero-posterior scan. Detector head of scintiscanner is indicated.

b. Normal scan. Gland areas (P = parotid; S = submandibular) are defined and located in relation to superimposed outline of face. Dot markers indicate anatomical features used to align the scanner head prior to commencement of scanning.

c. Scan obtained in patient with an adenoid cystic carcinoma affecting right parotid and submandibular areas.

d. Scan obtained in patient with advanced Sjögren's syndrome. No detectable uptake of ^{99m}Tc is obvious in salivary glands. However, downward extension of the scanning field to include the thyroid region (T) exhibits normal isotope uptake by the thyroid gland.

296

some normal and abnormal scans are shown. The uptake of isotope over the salivary gland can be quantified as described by Harden et al (1967) and Shimmins et al (1969) and expressed as a percentage of the injected dose at the mid-time of the scan.

Scintigraphy

Salivary scintigraphy is a visual recording with a gamma camera of the uptake concentration and excretion of an isotope by the salivary glands. The isotope is detected by sequential scintigraphs taken at 2, 6, 10, 20, 40 and 60 minutes after the injection of the isotope intravenously (Schall et al, 1971). Simultaneously the data can be recorded on video tape for quantification. Sequential scintigraphs of normal and abnormal are shown in Figures 18.2 and 18.3.

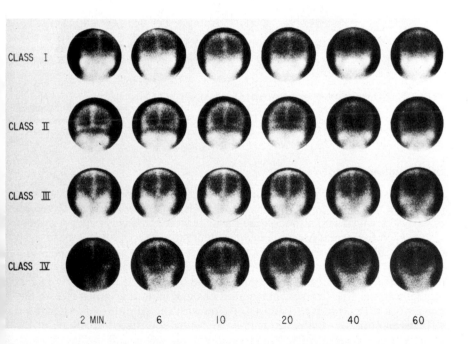

Figure 18.2. Scintigrams in patients with Sjögren's syndrome (after Schall et al, 1971). Class I: Uptake of isotope occurs immediately after injection and concentration increases progressively. Mouth activity appears at 8 to 10 min. Class II: Active concentration begins at 6 min and increases with time, but absolute level of uptake is less than normal. Mouth activity appears at 60 min. Class III: Active concentration begins at 10 min in submandibular glands and 40 min in parotid glands. No mouth activity. Class IV: No active concentration.
Class I: Normal; Class II: Mild to moderate gland involvement; Class III: Severe involvement; Class IV: Very severe involvement.

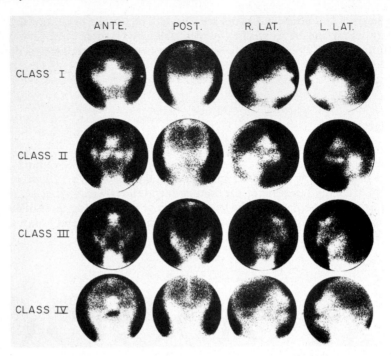

Figure 18.3. Comparison of four-view static studies, one hour after injection of isotope, in patients with Sjögren's syndrome (after Schall et al, 1971). Class I: Mouth activity surpasses gland activity. Class II: Mouth and gland activity approximately equal. Class III: Shows reduced uptake. Class IV: Displays only background activity. For definition of classes see Figure 18.2.

Evaluation of these tests

At the present time scintiscanning or sequential scintigraphy of the salivary glands can only be regarded as promising investigative techniques. These are relatively new tests and although the basic parameters have been worked out with regard to normal ranges and reproducibility, they have not been used enough in disease states for us to assess their potential in diagnosis. Their main attraction is that there is little inconvenience to the patient and all four major salivary glands can be examined at the one time. Scintigraphy in this respect is better than the scanner in that one can look at a larger area at one moment in time. However, good resolution with the gamma camera is more difficult to obtain at the present time. With the equipment available at the present time detection of tumours smaller than 1.5 to 2.0 cm is impracticable. It is likely, therefore that any tumours which can be detected by scintigraphy will be apparent clinically. Tumours are usually detectable by an area of decreased radio-activity except for one type, the adenolymphoma or Warthin's tumour (Veronesi, Cascinelli and Damascelli, 1967; Stebner et al, 1968; Grove and Di Chiro, 1968; Abramson et al, 1969). It is of interest therefore, that these techniques can contribute to tumour recognition, e.g. adenolymphoma, and in this way can aid the surgeon in his management and operative procedure (Schall, personal communication, 1974). Other tests of salivary gland function, e.g. biopsy, flow rate determination and sialography, give more localised information about salivary gland disease. Radio-isotopes which are concentrated in disease tissues, e.g. gallium or seleno-methionine, which are more specific for lymphosarcoma and Hodgkin's disease, can be used when these conditions are suspected. There is much work in this field at the present time and new developments can be anticipated.

REFERENCES

Abramson, A. L., Levy, L. M., Goodman, M. & Attie, J. N. (1969) Salivary gland scintiscanning with technetium 99m pertechnetate. *Laryngoscope (St. Louis)*, **79**, 1105.

Fourestier, J., Gacon, J., Esvan, J., Le Stir, A. & Morcelet, J. -L. (1973) Scintigraphie salivaire: Intérêt dans le traitement des bouches sèches provoquées par les médicaments psychotropes. *La Nouvelle Presse Medicale,* **2**, No. 13, 839.

Gates, G. A. & Work, W. P. (1967) Radioisotope scanning of the salivary glands. *Laryngoscope (St. Louis)*, **77**, 861.

Grove, A. S. jr. & Di Chiro, G. (1968) Salivary gland scanning with technetium 99mpertechnetate. *American Journal of Roentgenology, Radium Therapy, and Nuclear Medicine,* **102**, 109.

Harden, R.McG., Mason, D. K. & Buchanan, W. W. (1965a) Estimation of the plasma inorganic iodine in man: A comparison of methods. *Journal of Laboratory and Clinical Medicine,* **65**, 500.

Harden, R. McG., Mason, D. K. & Buchanan, W. W. (1965b) Quantitative studies of iodide excretion in saliva in euthyroid, hypothyroid and thyrotoxic patients. *Journal of Clinical Endocrinology and Metabolism,* **25**, 957.

Harden, R. McG., Hilditch, T. E., Kennedy, I., Mason, D. K., Papadopoulos, S. & Alexander, W. D. (1967) Uptake and scanning of the salivary glands in man using pertechnetate 99mTc. *Clinical Science,* **32**, 49.

Harden, R. McG., Alexander, W. D., Shimmins, J. & Russell, R. I. (1968) Quantitative uptake measurements of 99mTc in salivary glands and stomach and concentration of 99mTc, 132I and 82Br in gastric juice and saliva. In *Radioaktive Isotope in Klinik und Forschung,* **8**, 76. (Eds.) Fellinger, K. & Hofer, R. Munich: Urban und Schwarzenberg.

Lazarus, J. H., Stephen, K. W., Harden, R. McG., Robertson, J. W. K. & Lister, G. (1973) Simultaneous quantitative measurement of 131I-Iodine and 99mTc-Pertechnetate uptake by human salivary glands using scintiscanning with validation by direct estimation in biopsy samples. *European Journal of Clinical Investigation,* **3**, 156.

Mallard, J. R. (1966) Medical radioisotope visualisation. *International Journal of Applied Radiation,* **17**, 205.

Mason, D. K., Harden, R. McG. & Alexander, W. D. (1967) Salivary and thyroid glands—a comparison. *British Dental Journal,* **122**, 485.

Schall, G. L. (1974) Personal communication.

Schall, G. L., Anderson, L. G., Wolf, R. O., Herdt, J. R., Tarpley, T. M., Cummings, N. A., Zeiger, L. S. & Talal, N. (1971) Xerostomia in Sjögren's syndrome. *Journal of the American Medical Association,* **216**, 2109.

Shimmins, J., Hilditch, T. E., Harden, R. McG. & Alexander, W. D. (1969) Neck extra-thyroidal activity of 99mTc pertechnetate. *Journal of Nuclear Medicine,* **10**, 483.

Sorsdahl, O. A., Williams, C. M. & Bruno, F. P. (1969) Scintillation camera scanning of the salivary glands. *Radiology,* **92**, 1477.

Stebner, F. C., Eyler, W. R., Du Salt, L. A., Black, M. A., Kelly, A. P. & Nichols, R. (1968) 99mTc pertechnetate scanning of the salivary glands. *Radiology,* **90**, 583.

Stephen, K. W., Chisholm, D. M., Harden, R. McG., Robertson, J. W. K., Whaley, K. & Stuart, A. (1971) Diagnostic value of quantitative scintiscanning of the salivary glands in Sjögren's syndrome and rheumatoid arthritis. *Clinical Science,* **41**, 555.

Stephen, K. W., Robertson, J. W. K., Harden, R. McG. & Chisholm, D. M. (1973) Concentration of iodide, pertechnetate thiocyanate, and bromide in saliva from parotid, submandibular, and minor salivary glands in man. *Journal of Laboratory and Clinical Medicine,* **81,** 219.

Szabo, G. & Laudenbach, P. (1973) Quantitative isotope diagnostic method of the salivary glands in Sjögren's syndrome. *Journal of the International Association of Maxillofacial Radiology,* **2,** 29.

Veronesi, U., Cascinelli, N. & Damascelli, B. (1967) [131]I accumulation in a cystadenoma lymphomatosum of the parotid gland. *British Journal of Radiology,* **40,** 862.

Wayne, E. J. (1967) The value of inorganic iodine studies in the clinical assessment of thyroid disease. *Journal of Clinical Pathology (Supplement),* **20,** 253.

CHAPTER 19

Biopsy

MAJOR SALIVARY GLANDS

Biopsy of the salivary glands has obvious advantages to the clinician for it is the one investigative test which gives an indication of the nature of the disease process. This diagnostic information allows better assessment of the further treatment and management of an individual case. However, incisional biopsy of the major salivary glands is not without risk. Damage to important neuro-vascular structures, the creation of salivary fistulas and the contamination of tissue planes by altered cells are factors to be seriously considered when biopsy is contemplated. Furthermore, repair tissue at the site of biopsy can make later surgery more difficult. For these reasons biopsy of the major salivary glands is rarely undertaken unless the lesion is fairly superficial and a malignant neoplasm is suspected. It is clear that the clinical appearance and history of a salivary gland swelling are of the utmost importance when consideration is given to the differential diagnosis. The use of frozen sections made during operation overcomes some of these disadvantages outlined above. However, the histopathology of salivary gland neoplasia is a complex field and interpretation, especially of frozen sections, can be difficult.

Recently much interest has been shown in aspiration or needle biopsy to obtain neoplastic salivary or other tumour tissue for cytological diagnosis (Berge and Söderström, 1963; Söderström, 1966; Eneroth and Zajicek, 1965, 1966, 1969). Here again the procedure is not without the attendant risks outlined above for incisional biopsy. The small amounts of tissue obtained by this method make interpretation difficult.

These two techniques of major salivary gland biopsy are now described.

Incisional biopsy

The salivary gland lesion should be carefully palpated and a readily accessible portion located. To approach the mass a short incision is to be preferred. A lateral wound opening should be avoided and the wound closed carefully when the specimen has been taken. Whenever possible the biopsy site should be chosen so that when subsequent surgical excision is performed it may readily be included in the excised mass.

Imprint cytology may be a valuable adjuct to incisional biopsy. Imprints are made by touching a freshly cut surface of the biopsy on to clean glass slides. These are then fixed in methyl alcohol and stained by the Papanicoleou technique. This procedure may be of great practical importance, since an imprint can be stained and examined in less than an hour, while other rapid methods for microscopic examination are often not available to the clinician performing the biopsy (Medak et al, 1970).

Aspiration biopsy

The apparatus consists of an ordinary 22-gauge needle attached to a 10 ml syringe. A special handle of the syringe has been developed (Franzén, Giertz and Zajicek, 1960) which permits a one-hand grip while the biopsy is being performed. Although a fine needle minimises the risk of contamination by blood constituents a thicker needle may be required for lesions in which a connective tissue element predominates.

No anaesthesia is required and using an antiseptic technique the needle is inserted into the tumour area. The plunger of the syringe is withdrawn in order to create a vacuum in the system. As the needle advances through the lesion material is thus aspirated into the needle. When aspiration is complete the pressure in the syringe is allowed to equalise before the needle is withdrawn. This prevents aspiration of tumour cells into the needle track. The contents are then expressed on to a glass slide and allowed to dry at room temperature before being stained. Using this technique Eneroth, Franzén and Zajicek (1967) were able to provide positive tumour diagnosis in 92 per cent of 1000 cases with histologically verified tumours. In addition information concerning the histological type of tumour was obtained in 70 per cent of their material.

MINOR SALIVARY GLANDS

Where a neoplasm of the minor salivary glands is suspected an excision biopsy is generally undertaken. However, in non-neoplastic disease of a systemic nature such as Sjögren's syndrome, cystic fibrosis and sarcoidosis where the salivary glands may be generally involved, then an incisional biopsy of minor salivary gland tissue may be of great value. Not only may the technique provide diagnostic information, but it also permits the relatively safe and easy collection of tissue which may be submitted for specialised laboratory studies. It is plain that biopsy of the minor salivary glands overcomes the operational complications which are inherent in biopsy of their major gland counterparts. The two techniques for biopsy of the minor salivary glands—incisional and punch biopsy—are now described.

Incisional biopsy

Although biopsy of the buccal and palatal glands have been described we prefer to biopsy the minor salivary glands of the lower lip. This is a readily accessible site and the procedure is more convenient for the patient.

The glands lie above the muscle layer of the lip and are located close to the surface epithelium (Figure 19.1). A small incision approximately 2 cm in length is generally sufficient to expose several lobules of salivary tissue and these should be carefully removed. In our unit, the practice is to submit tissue not only for routine histopathological examination but also for electronmicroscopy and immunofluorescent studies. An elliptical incision is used when both epithelial and supporting connective tissue changes may be considered of diagnostic importance (Figures 19.2 and 19.3).

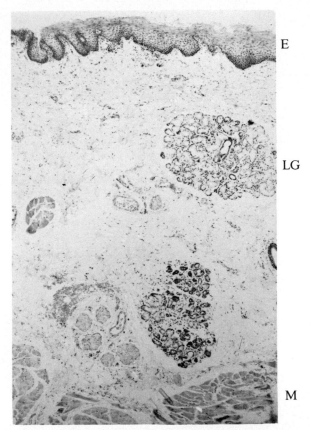

E

LG

M

Figure 19.1. Labial salivary glands (LG) lying in connective tissue stroma above the muscle layer (M) and in close proximity to overlying oral epithelium (E). (× 25.)

Punch biopsy

A 3 mm skin biopsy punch may be usefully employed to biopsy minor salivary gland tissue. The area to be biopsied is injected with local anaesthetic. The biopsy site is stretched and the skin biopsy punch is placed perpendicular to the surface. It is then rotated to cut through the mucous membranes and underlying connective tissue. Several sites may be biopsied in this way. The

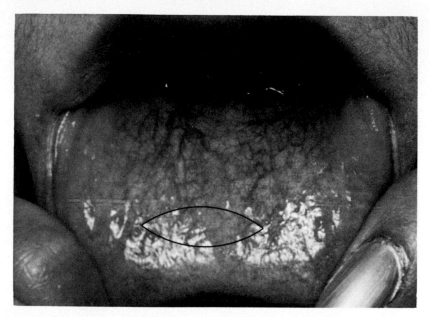

Figure 19.2. Eversion of lower lip prior to labial salivary gland biopsy. Site of biopsy is indicated.

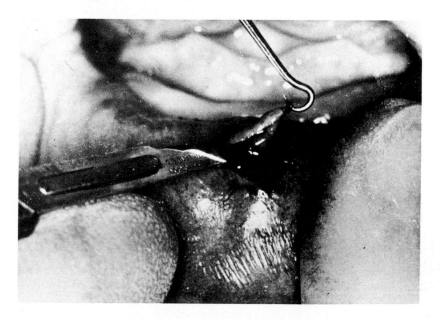

Figure 19.3. Removal of labial salivary gland tissue.

punch biopsy technique has been used to diagnose sarcoidosis (Cahn et al, 1964), cystic fibrosis (Meskin, Bernard and Warwick, 1964) and Sjögren's syndrome (Bertram, 1967).

Of these two methods of biopsy we prefer the incisional biopsy technique. In our experience, this technique is well tolerated by the patient. The biopsy wound is closed with fine black silk sutures and heals with little evidence of fibrous contraction. The incisional technique is more reliable in locating salivary tissue, especially where the glands may be atrophic. Thus, the relatively less traumatised material may be submitted not only for routine laboratory investigation but also for the more specialised and exacting techniques of electronmicroscopy and immunohistopathology.

REFERENCES

Berge, T. & Söderström, N. (1963) Fine-needle cytologic biopsy in diseases of the salivary glands. *Acta Pathologica,* **58,** 1.
Bertram, U. (1967) Xerostomia. *Acta Odontologica Scandinavica,* **25,** Suppl. 49, 1.
Cahn, L. R., Eisenbud, L., Blake, M. N. & Stern, D. (1964) Biopsies of normal appearing palates of patients with known sarcoidosis. *Oral Surgery, Oral Medicine and Oral Pathology,* **18,** 342.
Eneroth, C. M. & Zajicek, J. (1965) Aspiration biopsy of salivary gland tumours. II. Morphologic studies on smears and histologic sections from oncocytic tumours. *Acta Cytologica,* **9,** 355.
Eneroth, C. M. & Zajicek, J. (1966) Aspiration biopsy of salivary gland tumours. III. Morphologic studies on smears and histologic sections from 368 mixed tumours. *Acta Cytologica,* **10,** 440.
Eneroth, C. M. & Zajicek, J. (1969) Aspiration biopsy of salivary gland tumours. IV. Morphologic studies on smears and histologic sections from 45 cases of adenoid cystic carcinoma. *Acta Cytologica,* **13,** 59.
Eneroth, C. M., Franzen, S. & Zajicek, J. (1967) Cytologic diagnosis on aspirate from 1000 salivary gland tumours. *Acta Otolaryngologica,* Suppl. 224, 168.
Franzén, S., Giertz, G. & Zajicek, J. (1960) Cytological diagnosis of prostatic tumours by transrectal aspiration biopsy: A preliminary report. *British Journal of Urology,* **32,** 193.
Medak, H., McGrew, E. A., Burlakow, P. & Tiecke, R. W. (1970) *Atlas of Oral Cytology.* Washington, D.C.: U.S. Government Printing Office.
Meskin, L. H., Bernard, B. & Warwick, W. J. (1964) Biopsy of the labial mucous salivary glands in cystic fibrosis. *Journal of the American Medical Association,* **188,** 82.
Söderström, N. (1966) *Fine-needle Aspiration Biopsy.* Stockholm, Göteborg, Uppsala: Almquist & Wiksell.

CHAPTER 20

Microbiology and Immunology

This chapter is concerned with microbiological and immunological approaches to the investigation, diagnosis and treatment of salivary gland disease.

MICROBIOLOGY

Microbiological examinations in salivary gland disease can be of value in the diagnosis and treatment of non-specific bacterial parotitis, and in specific infections such as tuberculosis, syphilis, mumps, cytomegalic inclusion disease, infectious mononucleosis and various other viral infections which exhibit sialadenotrophism. The close association between Sjögren's syndrome and oral candidosis also warrants routine microbiological investigation.

Acute and Chronic Septic Parotitis

Acute non-specific parotitis is commonly associated with post-operative abdominal surgery, prolonged fever and generally disorders which disturb water balance. Chronic non-specific parotitis of the submandibular gland is often associated with salivary calculi, but in the parotid gland an abnormally low salivary flow rate is often involved in the pathogenesis of the infection.

As soon as the possibility of acute septic parotitis is suspected a specimen of pus should be obtained from the parotid duct orifice. The specimen should be taken by the dentist or doctor and not by a junior nurse or ward orderly who is unlikely to know the site of the parotid duct orifice. The area around the duct orifice should be wiped dry by using a sterile cotton wool swab. Exudate should be 'milked' from the gland and collected with a second sterile swab. If no exudate can be milked out, the duct can be cannulated with a fine polythene catheter and irrigated with sterile physiological saline to obtain a specimen for culture. Blood cultures should be taken if septicaemia is suspected as this condition is associated with acute parotitis.

Smears are made from the pus swab or irrigation fluid from the infected gland, and stained by Gram's method. The specimens are also cultured and antibiotic sensitivity tests are carried out on blood agar plates. The bacteria isolated from the infection are identified by routine bacteriological tests. The most common causal organisms are *Staphylococcus aureus,* followed by *Streptococcus viridans,* non-haemolytic streptococci and β-haemolytic streptococci (Speirs and Mason, 1972).

Specific Parotitis

Tuberculosis

The parotid gland is affected more commonly than the submandibular, with the sublingual and mixed salivary glands more rarely affected. The gland alone may be affected without evidence of tuberculosis elsewhere or it may be involved in the course of haematogenous spread. In the former localised variety a salivary tumour is usually suspected clinically and the diagnosis made after excision and histopathological examination including Ziehl Neelsen staining. In the more diffuse form the diagnosis is made by general clinical, radiological and haematological findings.

Syphilis

The major salivary glands may be involved during the secondary or tertiary stages of the disease. Diagnosis is usually made by serological examination. 10 ml of clotted blood are required and most laboratories perform the VD RL slide test, the Wasserman and Reiter protein complement fixation test routinely, with the Fluorescent Treponemal antibody test and the *Treponema pallidum* immobilisation test for doubtful results. A gumma may have been excised as a suspected tumour and histopathological examination will then be helpful.

Oral Candidosis

Sjögren's syndrome

In up to 70 per cent of patients with Sjögren's syndrome, in which xerostomia is a main complaint, oral candidosis may occur and can be diagnosed by investigating smears and swabs from the affected areas (MacFarlane and Mason, 1974).

The smear is made directly from the lesion by firmly scraping the area with the edge of a metal plastic instrument. The smears are then fixed by passing above the flame of a bunsen burner, or by spraying with a cytology fixative. Finally the smears are stained by Gram or Periodic acid Schiff (PAS). Microscopic examination, if positive, reveals Candida in the mycelial or hyphal phase (Figure 20.1). Smears of dentures are also taken when present. Swabs are cultured on Sabouraud's medium, for 24 hours at 37°C. This medium does not support the growth of most oral bacteria due to its low pH and high content of glucose. The plates are then examined and the number of colonies assessed. A heavy or moderate growth of a yeast together with a positive smear is usually taken as evidence of infection. The yeast is then identified by Germ tube production, chlamydospore formation and sugar fermentation reactions. If the diagnosis is in doubt a biopsy or the

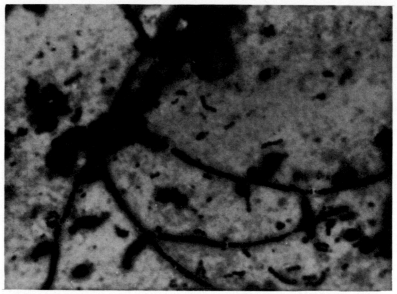

Figure 20.1. Smear demonstrating *Candida albicans* in the hyphal phase. Gram stain.

quantitative indirect fluorescent antibody technique described by Lehner (1965 and 1966) can be applied to serum and saliva for further evidence of candidosis.

Viral Sialadenitis

Collection of specimens

The usual requirements for a virology investigation are a cotton wool swab of saliva from the affected gland and a sample of venous blood (Figure 20.2). The swab is immediately immersed in virus transport medium (VTM), and sent as quickly as possible to the virus laboratory. If delay is unavoidable, the VTM can be stored at 4°C until transport can be arranged. The viability of virus under these conditions varies considerably and as a general rule three days storage is the absolute maximum. 10 ml of venous blood is taken from the patient at the first visit (acute serum) and a second sample taken 10 to 14 days later (convalescent serum). By means of a complement fixation test the antibody titre of each of these samples to various viral antigens is compared, and, where there is a fourfold or greater than fourfold difference between the two samples, a diagnosis of a recent infection with the virus tested can be made. Details of the isolation and identification of viruses are outside the scope of this book and are described in standard textbooks of virology.

Mumps

Mumps or epidemic parotitis is caused by a paramyxo virus. The saliva of patients with the infection is highly infectious. When saliva swabs arrive in

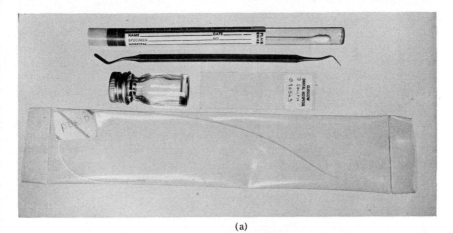

(a)

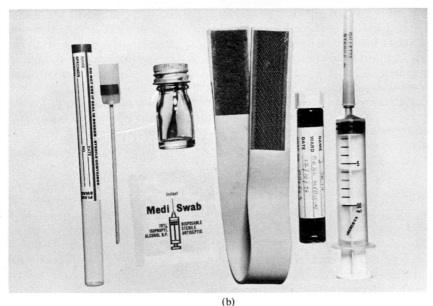

(b)

Figure 20.2. a. Bacteriological investigation. Saliva may be collected aseptically in a sterile container via a plastic catheter. If pus is flowing from the duct a conventional cotton wool swab can be used. Smears of lesions involving the oral mucosa can be prepared by using the edge of a dental plastic instrument. b. Virological investigation. The lesion is sampled by means of a cotton wool swab, which is then broken into a bottle of virus transport medium. Venous blood is collected using the instruments and materials shown above.

the virus laboratory they are inoculated in Rhesus monkey kidney tissue cultures, and incubated at 37°C for two to three weeks. Mumps virus produces a mild cytopathic effect in tissue culture, and since it agglutinates fowl red blood cells its presence can be detected by the phenomenon of haemadsorption. However, since isolation and identification of this virus is

309

difficult and time consuming, mumps is usually diagnosed by serological means. The blood samples are collected as mentioned earlier. Mumps virus possesses two complement-fixing antigens. The 'S' or soluble antigen is the nucleoprotein core of the virus particle and the 'V' or viral antigen is contained in the protein coat or capsid of intact particles. Tests for complement fixation are carried out using both these antigens. Antibody to the 'S' antigen appears early in infections and wanes rapidly. Antibody to the 'V' antigen appears more slowly but persists for several years. By testing for antibodies against the two antigens it can readily be determined if the patient has recently had infection with mumps or whether the infection occurred many months or years ago.

Cytomegalo virus

Cytomegalo virus probably produces an unapparent and probably common infection of salivary glands during early childhood, since about 80 per cent of healthy adults have antibody to the virus. Infections in older children and adults are not well defined in clinical terms, although cytomegalo virus has been implicated in the aetiology of heterophile antibody-negative cases of infectious mononucleosis. CMV is an extremely labile virus and optimal isolation rates are achieved when clinical specimens are inoculated into human embryo fibroblast cultures with the minimum of delay. Virus growth is recognised by the appearance of a cytopathic effect (CPE) which may take four to six weeks to develop. For this reason the complement fixation test is usually used for diagnosis.

Infectious mononucleosis or glandular fever

This is a mild febrile illness, often prolonged, and is associated with lymphadenopathy, hepatitis, mononucleosis and occasionally salivary gland involvement and swelling. There seems little doubt that the causative agent is the Epstein-Barr virus. The diagnosis is usually made by carrying out the Paul-Bunnell test. Agglutinins to sheep erythrocytes (heterophile antibodies) appear in the serum of most patients with the disease and the Paul-Bunnell test measures the titre of these antibodies. 10 ml of clotted blood are required for the test.

Other viral causes of sialadenitis

Coxsackie Group A and B, influenza and para-influenza viruses and Echo type 9 have been isolated from cases of sialadenitis. With the exception of Coxsackie A, all these viruses can be isolated in rhesus monkey kidney. Since Coxsackie A virus does not readily grow in tissue culture, part of the sample is injected by the combined subcutaneous and intra-cerebral route into new-born mice. A positive test results in flaccid paralysis of one or more limbs or back muscles.

Viruses and Saliva

There are probably five main ways in which viruses enter saliva, and it is important to understand these since infected saliva is commonly involved in the transmission of many viral infections. However, little detailed work has been carried out to investigate the source of viruses found in the mouth, and much of the information available is based on impression rather than on fact. For example, polio virus has been isolated from the pharynx, and it is believed to proliferate in this area, but whether it gains access to this site by the spread of intestinal contents, or via the salivary secretions, or via the gingival exudate, is not known. The five sources are as follows.

1. The virus may primarily infect the oral or tonsillar mucosa and thus find its way into saliva. Examples of these viruses are *Herpes simplex* virus, and the viruses associated with hand foot and mouth disease, herpangina, and infectious mononucleosis.

2. The virus may primarily infect the upper or lower respiratory tract and gain access to the mouth in sputum, e.g. influenza and para-influenza viruses, adenovirus and rhinoviruses.

3. The virus may infect the salivary gland tissue and enter the mouth in the salivary secretions, e.g. mumps virus, cytomegalo virus and rabies virus.

4. Viruses which have a latent period during their life cycle can be reactivated many years after the primary infection, and cause lesions in the oral mucosa, which rupture and release viruses into saliva, e.g. *Herpes simplex* virus, *Varicella zoster*.

5. The virus may produce a generalised infection, but during the viraemic stage of the disease, settle out, proliferate and cause a lesion on the oral mucosa, e.g. measles, chickenpox and smallpox. In addition, during the viraemic stage of the infection the virus may enter the mouth in the gingival exudate, e.g. serum hepatitis.

It is of interest to examine serum hepatitis in more detail due to the current problems in the transmission of the virus, especially in relation to dentistry. Two types of viral hepatitis have been clearly differentiated; infectious hepatitis caused by virus A and serum hepatitis caused by virus B. Serum hepatitis is usually transmitted by parenteral inoculation of infected blood or blood products, by means of blood transfusion or inadequately sterilised instruments, especially syringes. The virus-like particles which have been found in the blood of patients with virus B hepatitis are believed to be closely associated with Australia antigen and this antigen can be detected by a number of laboratory tests (Almeida, Ruberstein and Stott, 1971). In recent years Australia antigen has been isolated from the saliva of some patients with serum hepatitis and a few carriers of the disease (Ward et al, 1972; Heathcote, Cameron and Dane, 1974). The presence of occult blood in saliva does not appear to account for these findings, and it is possible that the antigen enters saliva in the gingival exudate. However, the presence of Australia antigen in pure parotid or submandibular saliva has not been investigated to date, and the possibility that the antigen enters saliva via the salivary glands cannot be ruled out.

IMMUNOLOGY

The oral cavity as a part of the body is subject to all the variations of host environment reactions. Many of the oral inflammatory reactions are mediated by systemic immunological defence mechanisms. However, there is also a local immune system derived from salivary secretory antibodies which may be of importance in defence against bacterial and viral infection. The salivary immunoglobulins have been reviewed in Chapter 3. The main salivary immunoglobulin is IgA which is secreted along with its component transport piece. Much smaller amounts of IgG are also contained in saliva.

The role of these secretory immunoglobulins in saliva is still controversial. It has been suggested that salivary secretory IgG may prevent adhesion of bacteria to tissue surfaces and contribute to bacterial opsonisation and bactericidal activities with or without lysozyme or complement derived from gingival fluid. It has been suggested that it may provide protection in various bacterial diseases such as cholera, dental caries and periodontal disease. In some immunological deficiency diseases salivary as well as humoral immuno-globulins may be decreased or absent and oral Candida infections may be an early manifestation in a severe case. Quantitative measurements of these secretory salivary immunoglobulins may be required in the investigation of patients with immunological deficiencies or in other clinical research projects. This can be done by a radial immunodiffusion technique.

Radial immunodiffusion or Mancini technique for measurement of salivary immunoglobulins

This method depends upon the halo of precipitation that occurs when a small volume of saliva fluid is introduced into a circular wall cut in an agar plate into which specific antiserum has been incorporated. As diffusion occurs from the well the precipitation halo increases in diameter until all the antigenic protein has been expended. A linear relation exists between the antigen concentration and the area of the precipitate or halo at the end of the diffusion. A series of dilutions of standard antigens is set up as a reference on the same agar plate and by comparison of the halo diameters of the unknown sera with these controls an estimate of antigen concentration can be made.

Salivary Gland 'Auto-immune' Disease

Recently, certain diseases have been described as 'auto-immune'; in these humoral antibodies are present which react against host tissue. It has been suggested that Sjögren's syndrome is an 'auto-immune' disease although proof of this is still lacking. What cannot be disputed is that in the sera of patients with Sjögren's syndrome there are certain antibodies, most of which are non-organ specific such as rheumatoid factor and antinuclear factor, and others which are organ specific such as salivary duct and thyroid antibodies which react with certain body tissues or cells.

In a patient suspected of having Sjögren's syndrome a serological examination is an essential part of the examination. The percentage of patients having different types of antibodies in two large series (Bloch et al, 1965; Whaley et al, 1973) is shown in Table 10.7. While elevated gastric parietal cell, thyroid microsomal and thyroglobulin antibodies have been demonstrated, the most consistently elevated auto-antibodies were rheumatoid factor, antinuclear factor and salivary duct antibody (see Chapter 10). Not all of these antibodies are therefore found in each patient.

Serological Tests for Auto-antibodies in a Patient Suspected of Having Sjögren's Syndrome

20 ml of venous blood is obtained by venepuncture and serum prepared. The following specific serological tests are carried out using an indirect immuno-fluorescent technique for detection of auto-antibodies in the patient's serum.

Indirect immunofluorescent technique

For routine purposes a 'sandwich' technique is used in which the serum being tested is placed in contact with a section of appropriate tissue. The section is then washed to remove unbound serum proteins and is then treated with a fluorochrome-labelled antibody to human gamma globulins, washed again and examined using a fluorescent microscope.

Reagents

Veronal buffer

pH 7.2
Sodium barbitone   20.6 g
Sodium chloride   85 g
$2N$ hydrochloric acid   40.3 cm³ (approximately)

Dissolve salts in 2 l ion-exchange water. Make quantity up to 5 l. Adjust pH with $2N$ hydrochloric acid, ensuring adequate mixing. Dilute 1:2 (i.e. with an equal volume of distilled water) for use.

Mounting medium
Sodium barbitone   0.10309 g
Sodium chloride   0.85 g
Glycerol AR   90 ml

Add $2N$ HCl to adjust pH to 7.2 (i.e. approx. 0.23 ml). Dissolve salts in 10 ml distilled H_2O. Adjust pH to 7.2 with $2N$ HCl (i.e. approx. 0.23 ml). Add glycerol. Shake well and allow to settle.

Conjugates

These are fluorescein isothyocyanate conjugated anti-human γ-globulins and are obtained commercially. Prior to use they are absorbed with rat liver powder and/or washed human muscle in order to reduce non-specific staining.

Rat liver powder

1. Homogenise rat liver tissue in an equal volume of normal saline.
2. Add 4 vol. acetone AR with stirring, and allow to stand for 10 min.
3. Centrifuge, discard supernatant.
4. Wash several times with saline until supernatant is free of Hb, i.e. clear.
5. Resuspend residue in equal vol. saline.
6. Add approx. 4 vol acetone with stirring.
7. Centrifuge, discard supernatant and add further 4 vol. acetone.
8. Dry on Buchner funnel and wash with 2 aliquots acetone.
9. Leave to dry.
10. Store in sealed containers at room temperature.

Washed human muscle

1. Homogenise muscle and wash about 4 times in saline.
2. Wash twice in diluted veronal buffer.
3. Store at —20°C.

Method for absorption of conjugates

Place enough rat liver powder to cover base of 3 inch by $\frac{3}{8}$ inch rimless test tube (approx. 100 mg/ml conjugate). Add veronal buffer and mix. Centrifuge and discard supernatant. Add 2 ml of conjugate, stopper and incubate for one hour at 37° in water bath, with occasional shaking. Centrifuge and transfer supernatant into another tube similarly prepared. Incubate for another hour. Centrifuge. Transfer supernatant into tube containing washed human muscle. Incubate ½ hr. Centrifuge and store supernatant conjugate at —20°C.

Preparation of frozen sections

Suitable fresh unfixed tissues are used:

Tissues

1. Fresh post-mortem salivary gland tissue can be used, not more than 10 h after death.
2. Toxic thyroid from fresh thyroidectomy specimens.
3. Gastric fundal mucosa from fresh post-operative partial gastrectomy specimens.
4. Rat liver from freshly killed young adult rat.
   Blocks of tissue may be stored at —70°, with the exception of rat liver for which a fresh block must be made each week and sections cut for use in that week only.

A small block of tissue is snap-frozen on to a metal microtome chuck by applying Dri-kold. Cut sections of approx. 4μ and thaw each section onto a microscope slide. Allow to dry at room temperature; store at $-20°$C. Allow to dry completely before use.

General technique

1. Apply appropriate dilution of patient's serum to section in moist chamber for ½ hour at room temperature.
2. Wash off excess serum in veronal buffer with shaking for 15 min.
3. Apply conjugate at suitable dilution for ½ hour.
4. Wash off excess conjugate in veronal buffer with shaking for 15 min.
5. Mount in buffered glycerol.
6. Examine in fluorescent microscope.

Specific tests

Anti-nuclear factor. Rat liver as substrate. Positive and negative controls included. The positive control is used at dilutions of 1/64 and 1/1000, ensuring that its end-point of staining is approx. 1/1000. Patient's serum is screened at 1/16, and if positive at 1/16, is then titrated at 1/16, 1/64, 1/256, 1/1000, using sterile saline as diluent. Positive result is indicated by fluorescent staining of nuclei; (1) speckled; (2) nucleolar; (3) homogeneous; (4) membranous.

Salivary duct antibody. Human salivary gland as substrate. Positive and negative controls included. Patient's serum is used undiluted. Positive result indicated by fluorescence of salivary duct epithelium.

Gastric parietal cell antibody. Human gastric fundal mucosa as substrate. Positive and negative controls included. Patient's serum is used undiluted. Positive result is indicated by fluorescent staining of the cytoplasm of parietal cells.

Thyroid microsomal antibody. Human toxic thyroid tissue as substrate. Positive and negative controls included. Patient's serum diluted ¼ with saline. Positive result is indicated by fluorescence of thyroid epithelium.

Test for detection of rheumatoid factor in serum

Rheumatoid factor is an antibody directed against normal protein of the serum globulin class, and is demonstrated by a method similar to the tanned red cell agglutination method, different in that latex particles are used instead of red cells as the carrier of the antigen.

315

RA latex test

The latex-coated reagent is commercially obtained (Hyland Laboratories). One drop of serum, diluted 1/20 with saline, is placed on a slide. One drop of reagent is added, and the slide rocked to and fro for approximately 45 sec.

Positive result shows visible flocculation with large aggregates and complete clumping.

Weakly positive result shows visible flocculation with only partial clumping.

Negative result shows a smooth suspension, with no visible flocculation.

REFERENCES

Almeida, J. D., Ruberstein, D. & Stott, E. J. (1971) A new antigen-antibody system in Australia-antigen-positive hepatitis. *Lancet,* **ii,** 1225.

Bloch, K. J., Buchanan, W. W., Wohl, M. J. & Bunim, J. J., (1965) Sjögren's syndrome. *Medicine (Baltimore),* **44,** 187.

Heathcote, J., Cameron, C. H. & Dane, D. S. (1974) Hepatitis B antigen in saliva and semen. *Lancet,* **i,** 71.

Lehner, T. (1965) Immunofluorescent investigation of Candida albicans antibodies in human saliva. *Archives of Oral Biology,* **10,** 975.

Lehner, T. (1966) Immunofluorescent study of Candida albicans in candidiasis, carriers and controls. *Journal of Pathology and Bacteriology,* **91,** 97.

MacFarlane, T. W. & Mason, D. K. (1974) Changes in the oral flora in Sjögren's syndrome. *Journal of Clinical Pathology,* **27,** 416.

Speirs, C. F. & Mason, D. K. (1972) Acute septic parotitis: Incidence, aetiology and management. *Scottish Medical Journal,* **17,** 62.

Ward, R., Borchert, P., Wright, A. & Kline, E. (1972) Hepatitis B antigen in saliva and mouth washings. *Lancet,* **ii,** 726.

Whaley, K., Webb, J., McAvoy, B. A., Hughes, G. R. V., Lee, P., MacSween, R. N. M. & Buchanan, W. W. (1973) Sjögren's syndrome. 2. Clinical associations and immunological phenomena. *Quarterly Journal of Medicine,* **42,** 513.

Index

317

Index

Sialadenitis—*Continued*
  in Sjögren's syndrome, 174, 176, 194-200
  and syphilis, 95-99
  and tuberculosis, 95-99
  viral, 99-101, 308
    inclusion disease, 101
    mumps, 99-101, 308-310
    other, 101
Sialography
  in disease, 286
  general, 272, 277, 278
  indications, 278, 279
  method, 280-285
  normal range, 286
  problems, 285
  in Sjögren's syndrome, 185
Sialolithiasis
  major gland, 106-108
  minor gland, 117
Sialorrhoea, *see* Excessive saliva
Sialosis, 129, 213-221
  drug-induced, 218
  dysenzymatic, 216
  experimental, 219-221
  hormonal, 214-215
  malnutritional, 216
  neurohumoral, 216
  ultrastructure, 219
Sjögren's syndrome, 167-202
  auto-antibodies, 313-315
  clinical features, 168-170
  diagnosis, 187
  diagnostic techniques, 176-190
  evaluation of tests of gland function, 185, 187
  flow rate estimation, 178
  general features, 167-168
  histopathology, 194-200
  immunological abnormalities, 190-194
  labial gland biopsy, 178-184
  laboratory investigations, 190-194
  and lymphoepithelial lesions, 207-211
  and lymphoreticular neoplasia, 194-200
  oral manifestations, 170-176
  pathogenesis, 194-200
  salivary duct antibody, 193
  salivary gland enlargement, 174, 176
  scintiscanning, 185
  sialography, 185
  treatment, 200-202
  xerostomia, 170-174
Stomatitis nicotina, 103
Sublingual duct, 11
Sublingual gland
  anatomy, 11
  blood supply, 12
  embryology, 3
  innervation, 14, 15
  lymph drainage, 12

Sublingual gland—*Continued*
  surgery, 244
Submandibular duct, 10
Submandibular gland
  anatomy, 10
  blood supply, 11
  embryology, 3
  innervation, 14, 15
  lymph drainage, 11
  surgery, 232-245
Suction cup, 252, 255
Surgical treatment, 232-245
  biopsy, 233, 234
  complications, 237, 240, 241
  indications, 232-233
  minor gland lesions, 244, 245
  parotid gland excision, 243
  sublingual gland excision, 244
  submandibular gland excision, 243
Swelling, 73, 74, 92-104, 174, 176
Syphilis, 95, 307

Taste abnormality
  as clinical symptom, 74
Thiocyanate
  concentration in duct, 39
  dependent factors, 57
Thyroid disease
  congenital iodide trapping disease, 129
  and saliva composition, 129
Tuberculosis, 95, 307

Unclassified tumours, 161
Undifferentiated carcinoma, 159, 160

Viruses
  cytomegalo, 310
  in disease, 99-101
  infectious mononucleosis, 310
  mumps, 308-310
  and saliva, 311
  in Sjögren's syndrome, 200
Volume of saliva
  measurement of, 261

Xerostomia
  causes, 52, 120-124
  and drugs, 120-124
  sign, 74
  in Sjögren's syndrome, 170-174
  symptom, 74
  treatment, 124